A Complete System of Land-surveying, Both in Theory and Practice, Containing the Best, the Most Accurate, and Commodious Methods of Surveying and Planning of Ground by all the Instruments now in use
The Second Edition

A
COMPLETE SYSTEM
OF
LAND-SURVEYING,
Both in THEORY and PRACTICE,

Containing the Best, the most Accurate, and Commodious
METHODS of SURVEYING and PLANNING of GROUND
by all the INSTRUMENTS now in Use, with regular Forms
of keeping a FIELD BOOK or JOURNAL

The METHOD of
DIVIDING of COMMONS, &c. according to QUAN-
TITY and QUALITY.

To which is added,
The NEW ART of SURVEYING
By the PLAIN TABLE.

Containing a NEW METHOD of
SURVEYING and PLANNING by that INSTRUMENT.

To this WORK is annexed
A True and Correct TABLE of the LOGARITHMS of all
Numbers, from 1 to 10000, as also a TABLE of the LOGARITHMIC
SINES and TANGENTS to every Degree and Minute of the QUADRANT,
together with a TABLE of LOGISTICAL LOGARITHMS

By THOMAS BREAKS.

The SECOND EDITION.

Οὐδεὶς ἀγεωμέτρητος εἴτω.

LONDON
PRINTED for J MURRAY, No 32, FLEET-STREET;
FACING St DUNSTAN'S CHURCH.
M,DCC,LXXVIII.

PREFACE.

AMong the Multiplicity of Books relative to that useful and entertaining Branch of Mathematical Learning, called *Geodesia*, or *Land-Surveying*, I could not perceive in any one of them, the Subject handled after such a Method as is necessary, or might be expected from Treatises of this Nature.

The many Irregularities and Obscurities with which Works of this Sort abound, have induced me to undertake a Performance of this Kind, in order to remove Difficulties, clear Obscurities, and render that which has hitherto been deemed dark and mysterious, plain and intelligent to the meanest Capacity.

I have all along been anxious and solicitous not to omit or neglect any thing which might be of Use or Benefit therein, so as to render the Work of perfect Utility to every one who has any Delight or Pleasure in the Pursuit of Mathematical Knowledge.

In Pursuance of this my Design, I have in the first Book given you the most useful Geometrical Problems and Theorems.

The second Book contains the Use of the Table of Logarithms, as also the Table of artificial Signs and Tangents; together with a complete Course of Mensuration both of Superficies and Solids.

In the third Book you have Plain Trigonometry, both right and oblique angled, with the Solution of the several Cases thereof.

The fourth Book contains the Projection of the Sphere orthographically and stereographically, on the Planes of the Meridian, Solstitial Colure, and the Horizon.

In the fifth Book is given Spheric Trigonometry, containing the Resolution of all the Cases of right and oblique angled Spherical Triangles.

The sixth Book contains a few Astronomical Problems relating to the Variation of the Magnetical Needle, necessary in finding a true Meridian Line to any Plan; I have also given Tables of the Sun's mean Motion, by which the Sun's true Ecliptic Place may be readily found for any Time, past, present, or to come.

a

In

(ii)

In the seventh Book I have given the Description and Use of the several Instruments used in Surveying.

The eighth Book contains a clear, comprehensive, and practical Method of Surveying and Planning all Sorts of Ground, by the Chain, Plain Table, and Theodolite.

In the ninth Book I have given Altimetry and Longimetry, (or the Method of measuring accessible and inaccessible Heights and Distances), together with the Method of finding the Horizontal Lines of Hills and Valleys, as also the Form of reducing Plans, with County-Surveying, and an easy, practical, and expeditious Method of taking the Perspective of any Gentleman's Seat or Building with the Theodolite.

The tenth Book contains the whole Art of dividing of Ground, according to Quantity and Quality, with the Theory and Practice of Levelling, as also the Manner of finding the Variation of the Compass, with the Method of Washing or Colouring Maps or Plans.

Lastly, I have given a new Method of Surveying and Planning all Sorts of Ground by the Plain Table only, by which the Angles (or rather Bearings) are taken and protracted at one and the same Instant in the Field, and that too upon one Sheet of Paper, by means of which the Trouble and Inconvenience of shifting the Paper is entirely removed.

I have also given a correct Table of the Logarithms of all Numbers from 1 to 10000; together with a Table of Logarithmic Sines and Tangents, to every Degree and Minute of the Quadrant. I have also given a Table of Logistical Logarithms in Street's Form. The Table for converting Time into Motion, or Motion into Time, I have omitted, as it is of little or no Use in practical Surveying.

Having thus given a brief Recital of the Substance of what is herein contained, and being perfectly satisfied, that every Endeavour has been used to omit nothing essentially necessary, nor at the same Time to add any Thing superfluous, I hope I may, without Vanity, stile it, *A Complete System of Land-Surveying, both in Theory and Practice.*

THE

A COMPLETE SYSTEM OF LAND-SURVEYING.

BOOK I.
PRACTICAL GEOMETRY.

DEFINITIONS.

1. A POINT has undergone various Definitions, according to the different Sentiments of different Geometricians, who all seem to correspond at last, in allowing it to be a very small imaginary something, and incapable of being divided, for as several Authors have allowed it to be a Matter of Substance, it might thence be argued, that every Substance or Magnitude is capable of being parted or divided, but then at the same Time it is considered to be the smallest Thing possible to be conceived, and thence incapable of any further Division.

FIG. 1.

2. A Line is generated by the Motion of a Point, for if the Point A be conceived to move from A to B, it will generate the right Line AB, and is the neareſt Diſtance between any two given Things in a ſtraight Courſe. But a curve Line is not the neareſt diſtance between two points, being generated by the crooked Motion of the Point A, which deſcribes the Arch or Curve ACB. And hence a Line is accounted the firſt Magnitude in Geometry, having Length without Breadth or Thickneſs.

2. A Superficies is the ſecond Magnitude in Geometry, being generated by the Motion of a Line, for if the Line AC be conceived to move in a parallel Direction to itſelf along the Lines AB, CD, it will produce the Superficies $ABCD$.

4. The third Geometrical Magnitude is a Solid, whoſe Dimenſions are Length, Breadth, and Thickneſs, but it is no Ways concerned in the Practice of Surveying, although it be a Part of Menſuration.

5. An Angle is the Inclination of two Lines meeting in a Point called the Angle Point, and is moſt commonly expreſſed by three Letters, the Middlemoſt of which denotes the Angle, as ABD ſignifieth the Angle B in the Triangle ABD, and BDC expreſſes the Angle D in the Triangle BDC, &c.

3.

6. A right Angle containeth juſt 90 Degrees of the Arch of a Circle, or it is the Meeting

of two Lines perpendicular to each other, as Fig. *ABC*. 3.

7. An acute Angle is less than a right Angle or 90 Degrees, as the Angle *A* or *C* in the Triangle *ABC*.

8. An obtuse Angle is greater than a right Angle, and therefore any Angle which containeth more than 90 Degrees of the Arch of a Circle (as the Angle *C* in the obtuse Triangle *BCD*) is an obtuse Angle, and contains as many 3. degrees above 90, as the Sum of the other two Angles *B* and *D* fall short of 90.

9. A Perpendicular is a Line drawn down upon another Line, making a right Angle (or an Angle of 90 Degrees) as the Line *CD* is ⊥ 4. to the Line *AB*; making the Angles *ADC*, *BDC* each equal to 90 Degrees, or a right Angle.

10. Of superficial Figures, some are regular, and some irregular.

11. Regular Superficies are either three-sided, four-sided, five-sided, many-sided or circular.

12. A Figure consisting of three sides, is called a Triangle, of which there are two Sorts, viz. right-angled and oblique-angled.

13. Right-angled Triangles are such, as have one right Angle, and two acute Angles, as in the Triangle *ABC*, the Angle *B* is a right 5. Angle, and containeth just 90 Degrees, and the other two Angles *A* and *C* are acute, each containing less than 90 Degrees (or a right Angle,)

of

Fig. of the three sides, the longest Side AC is called the Hypothenuse, and the other two are named Legs.

6. 14. Oblique Triangles are such as have no right Angle, but all the Angles oblique, as ABC. Of these there be three Kinds, viz. an equilateral Triangle, an isosceles Triangle, and a scalenous Triangle.

7. 15. An equilateral Triangle hath all its Sides (and consequently all its Angles) equal, as BCD.

16. An isosceles Triangle hath two of its Sides equal, and consequently their opposite Angles

8. equal, as in the Triangle ABC, the Sides AC, BC are equal to each other, and therefore the Angle B is $=$ the Angle A.

17. A scalenous Triangle hath all its Sides
6 (and consequently all its Angles) unequal, as ABC.

These and all other Sorts of oblique-angled Triangles whatsoever, are under the Denomination of acute-angled and obtuse-angled Triangles.

18. An obtuse-angled Triangle hath one of its Angles obtuse, and more than 90 Degrees, as
6 in the Triangle ABC, the Angle C is obtuse, and more than 90 Degrees.

19. Acute-angled Triangles have all their Angles acute, as BCD. And therefore all equi-
7 lateral Triangles have every Angle acute; but
8 of isosceles Triangles, some are acute-angled, as
9. ABC, and some are obtuse-angled, as EFG.

20. A

DEFINITIONS.

20. A Geometrical Square hath all its Sides equal, and Angles right, as $ABCD$.   FIG. 10.

21. A Parallelogram or long Square hath four right Angles, but the opposite Sides are only equal, as $ABCD$.   2.

22. A Rhombus hath four equal Sides, but not four right Angles, as $BCDE$, two of the Angles B and D are acute, and the other two C and E obtuse.   11.

23. A Rhomboides hath four Sides, the Opposites only are equal; as in the Rhomboides $ABCD$, the Side AB is $=$ to the Side CD, and the Side $AC =$ to the Side BD, it hath also four Angles, viz. two acute and two obtuse.   12.

24. All four-sided Figures, except those above-mentioned, are called Trapezia or Trapeziums, as $ABCD$.   13.

25. A Diagonal is a Line BD drawn from one Corner to another in any four-sided Figure $ABCD$.   13.

26. Figures consisting of more than four Sides, are called Polygons, some of which are regular, and some irregular.

27. A regular Polygon consisteth of equal Sides and equal Angles, and taketh its Name from the Number of its Sides, as the five-sided Figure $ABCDE$ is called a Pentagon, and the eight-sided Figure $FGHIKLMN$ is called an Octagon, &c. As   14. 15.

A re-

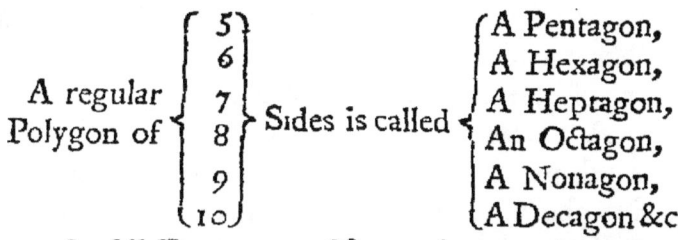

A regular Polygon of { 5, 6, 7, 8, 9, 10 } Sides is called { A Pentagon, A Hexagon, A Heptagon, An Octagon, A Nonagon, A Decagon &c.

28. All Figures consisting of more than four Sides, and having unequal Sides, are called irregular Polygons, and are distinguished by the Number of their Sides; as *ABCDE* is an irregular Polygon, &c. and may consist of fifteen, twenty, thirty, &c Sides.

29. A Circle is a Figure formed by the Motion of a Point round its Center, till the Motion end where it first begun. Every Circle contains 360 Degrees or four right Angles. A Circle comprehends a greater Space than any other superficial Figure, for a Line equal in Length to the Periphery or Circumference thereof, will comprehend a greater Area than any other Figure whatsoever.

30. The Periphery or Circumference of a Circle, is the Out-line or Bound thereof, as *DXZE*, every Part of which is equally distant from its Center *A*.

31. The Diameter of a Circle is a right Line drawn through its Center, as *DAZ*, and is the longest Line that can possibly be drawn therein, dividing the whole Circle into two equal Parts. Half the said Line (*AD*) is called the Semi-diameter or Radius of the Circle.

32. An

32. An Arch of a Circle is a Part of the Periphery or Circumference, as ZY is an Arch, or Part of the Periphery $DXZE$. Fig. 17.

33. A Sector of a Circle, is a Part cut out by two Lines drawn from the Center through the Periphery, and bounded by these and the Arch contained between the two Semi-diameters; as the Part AXY is bounded by the Lines AX, AY, and the Arch XY, and is termed the Sector of a Circle. 17.

34. A Segment of a Circle is a Part cut off by a right Line drawn across the Circle, as the Part CEB cut off by the Line CB, is called the Segment of a Circle. 17.

35 An Ellipsis is a curve-lined Figure of unequal Diameters, being longer one Way than the other, the longer Diameter AC is called the transverse Diameter, and the shorter BD is named the conjugate Diameter. 18.

Axioms *drawn from the first Book of* Euclid's Elements *of* Geometry.

1. THINGS that are equal to one and the same Thing, are equal to one another.
2. If equal Quantities be added to equal Quantities, the Sum of those Quantities will be equal.
3. If from equal Quantities be deducted equal Quantities, the Remainder will be equal.
4. If equal Quantities be added to unequal Quantities, the Sum will be unequal.
5. If from equal Quantities be taken unequal Quantities, the Remainder will be unequal.
6. Things that are double to one and the same Thing, are equal between themselves.
7. Those Things that are half one and the same Thing, are equal among themselves.
8. Things mutually agreeing together, are equal to one another.
9. The Whole of any Thing is greater than its Parts.
10. Two right Lines cannot contain a Space.
11. All right Angles are between themselves equal.
12. If a right Line fall upon two other right Lines, and make the inward Angles on the same both together, less than the right Angles, then those two right Lines infinitely produced, will meet each other on that Side where the Angles are less than right ones.

SIGNS *and* CHARACTERS; *their Names and Significations in Geometry and Surveying.*

= EQUAL to, as 8 = 8, i.e 8 is equal to 8.

+ Plus or more; as $a + e = z$. i.e. a more or added to e is equal to z.

− Minus or less, as $a - e = z$. i.e e taken or subtracted from a leaves z

× Multiplied, as $a \times e$, or ae, either of which shews the Product of a and e.

− Divided by; as $a - e$, or $\frac{a}{e}$, either of these denotes the Quotient of a divided by e.

√ Square Root, $\sqrt{16} = 4$, the Square Root of 16 is equal to 4.

□ Square; as □ 12, the Square of 12 is to be taken.

:, ·, : Proportional, as 2 : 4 ∷ 8 · 16; that is, as 2 is to 4, so is 8 to 16.

∠ An Angle less than 180°; ⟩ An Angle greater than 180₀. ⊙ A Station.

△ A Triangle; ▭ A Parallelogram; ∥ Parallel to.

∠s Angles; △s Triangles; ∠r Corner, □s Squares.

▭s Parallelograms, ⊥s Perpendiculars.

C   SEC-

SECT. I.

GEOMETRICAL PROBLEMS.

FIG

PROP. I. PROB.

19. *To divide a given Line* AB *into two equal Parts.*

RULE.

With any Diſtance greater than Half *AB*, and one Foot on *A* and *B*, deſcribe two Arches cutting each other in *C* and *D*; through the interſecting Points *C*, *D*, draw a Line *CD* which will divide *AB* into two equal Parts in *I*.

PROP. II. PROB.

20. *To draw a Line parallel to a given Line* CD, *to paſs through any aſſigned Point* A.

RULE.

From the given Point *A* take the neareſt Diſtance to the given Line *CD*; with that Diſtance, and one Foot any where towards *C*, deſcribe an Arch *O*; through *A* draw a Line *AB* juſt to touch the Arch *O* in *O*, ſo ſhall the Line *AB* be the Parallel required.

Or

Or thus;

Chuse any Point O in the given Line CD, on which as a Center describe a Semi-circle $CABD$; make $DB = CA$, and through the Points A, B, draw the Line AB which will be ∥ CD as was required.

PROP. III. PROB.

To raise a Perpendicular from a given Point P in a given Line AB.

RULE.

Make $PA = PB =$ any Distance; and from A and B describe two Arches to cut each other in D, from P draw a Line PD to pass through the intersecting Point D, which will be ⊥ to AB.

Or thus

On the given Point P describe the Arch FD; take PF and set from F to C and from C to D; with any convenient Distance, on C and D describe the Arches O, and through their Point of Intersection, from the given Point P draw the Line PO the Perpendicular required.

PROP. IV. PROB.

To raise a Perpendicular from a given Point A, at the End of a given Line AB.

12   Geometrical Problems.   Book I.

Fig.

Rule.

24. Set one Foot in *A*, and extend the other to any Point *C* above the Line *AB*, on the Center *C* defcribe the femi-circle *FAP*, to cut *AB* in *F*, draw *FC* cutting the femi-circle in *P*. Then draw *AP*, which will be ⊥ to *AB*.

PROP. V. Prob.

25. *From a given Point* P *to let fall a Perpendicular upon a given Line* AB.

Rule.

On the given Point *P* as a Center, defcribe the Arch *EF* to cut *AB* in *E* and *F*. With any convenient Diftance, and one Foot on *E* and *F*, defcribe two Arches to cut each other in *I*, through *P* and *I*, draw *PI*, which is perpendicular to *AB*.

PROP. VI. Prob.

26. *To make an Angle* ABC *equal to a given Angle* CDE.

Rule.

With any convenient Extent of the Compaffes, and one Foot on *D*, draw the Arch *FG* = the Meafure of the given ∠*D*. Draw a Line *BC*, and with the Diftance *DF* defcribe the Arch *HI*; then make the Arch *HI* = to the Arch *FG*,

Sect. I.   Geometrical Problems.   13

FG, and through I draw the Line BA bounding the Angle; so is the Angle ABC = the Angle CDE.

PROP. VII. Prob.

To lay down an Angle FDG = *to any determinate Number of Degrees,* &c. (suppose 35°.)   27.

Rule.

Draw the Line DF at Pleasure, and with 60° off the Scale of Chords describe the Arch EH on the Center D. From the same Chords take 35° (the Quantity of the Angle) and lay upon the Arch from E to H, through which from D draw the Line DG, and it is done, for the Angle FDG will contain just 35°, as was required.

PROP. VIII. Prob.

To make a Triangle of three given Lines A, B, C, *any two of which being longer than the third.*   28.

Rule.

Make DE = to the Line A; take B and C in your Compasses, and with one Foot on E and D, describe two Arches to cross each other in F; then draw DF and EF, which will form the $\triangle DEF$.

PROP.

PROP. IX. PROB.

Upon a given Line A *to make a Square.*

RULE.

Draw BC and CD perpendicular to each other, and make each $=$ to A, with the Distance A, and one Foot on B and D, describe two Arches to cut each other in I. Then draw BI and DI, which will complete the Square BD.

PROP. X. PROB.

To make a Parallelogram on two given Lines A *and* B.

RULE.

Take $CD =$ to B, also make $DE \perp$ to CD, (by Prob 4) and $DE = A$; then with the Distances CD and DE, from E and C describe two Arches to cross each other in F; draw EF, CF; so is DF the parallelogram required

PROP. XI. PROB

To draw a Circle through any three Points A, B, C, *not in a right Line.*

RULE.

With any Extent greater than Half AB, and with one Foot on A and B severally, describe two Arches cutting each other in D and E;

also,

Sect. I.   GEOMETRICAL PROBLEMS.   15

also with any Extent greater than Half *BC*, de- Fig. scribe as before, on the Points *B*, *C*, two Arches 31. intersecting each other in *F* and *G*. Through the intersecting Points *D*, *E*, draw the indefinite Line *DI*, also through the intersecting Points *F*, *G*, draw an indefinite Line *FI* to cut *DI* in *I* the Center of the Circle. With the Radius *IA* (= *IB* = *IC*) sweep the Circle *ABC* as required.

PROP. XII. PROB.

To divide a given right Line AB *into any proposed Number of equal Parts (suppose six).*   32.

RULE.

At each End *A* and *B* of the given Line *AB*, set off an equal acute Angle *BAD*, *CBA*, that is, make the ∠*A* = the ∠*B*, and draw the Lines *AD*, *BC* of any sufficient Length, which (by Theor. 3) will be parallel. Take any little Distance in your Compasses and lay it six Times upon the Lines *BC*, *AD*, each Way from *B* and *A* towards *C* and *D*, and note each with the Figures 1, 2, 3, &c. Then draw the Lines 15, 24, 33, 42, 51, which will divide *AB* into six equal Parts.

PROP. XIII. PROB.

Given two Lines S *and* T, *to find a third* 33. *in geometrical Proportion.*

RULE

16   GEOMETRICAL PROBLEMS.   Book I.
FIG.
                    R U L E.

33.   Draw LM to make any acute Angle with LN; make $LO =$ to S, and LQ and LP each $= T$, draw OQ, and from P draw PR parallel to OQ, to cut LN in R. Then it will be, as $LO (= S) \ LQ (= T) :: LP (= LQ) \cdot LR$, the third Proportional required, and therefore $S . T .. T : LR$.

                PROP. XIV. PROB.

To divide a Line AB *into two Parts, in Pro-*
34. *portion to each other as the Line* S *is to the Line* T.

                    R U L E.

From either End A or B of the given Line AB, draw a Line AD to make an acute Angle (BAD) at Pleasure, make $AE = S$, and $ED = T$. Join BD, and from E draw EF ‖ to BD, to cut AB in F. therefore, as $S : T .: AF . FB$.

                PROP. XV. PROB.

35.   *Given three Lines* A, B *and* C; *to find a fourth in Proportion to them.*

                    R U L E.

Draw DH and DG, to make any acute Angle HDG, make $DH =$ the Line A, $DG =$ the Line B, and $DI =$ the Line C, join the
                                Points

Points H, G, and from I draw IF ‖ to HG, which will cut DF in F, so is DF the fourth Proportional required; for $DH:DG::DI:DF$.

FIG. 35.

PROP. XVI. PROB.

To divide any Circle KLMN *into any Number of equal Parts not exceeding ten.*

36.

RULE.

Quarter the Circle by drawing the Diameters KM, LN perpendicular to each other; make KO and KP each $=$ to LQ, and draw $PO =$ One-third of the Circle. Join KL which will be one-fourth Part thereof. On R, with the Distance RL, describe the Arch LS, and draw the Line $LS =$ one-fifth Part of the Circle. KQ ($= LQ$) is one-sixth Part. Also RP ($= RO$) is one-seventh Part. KA is one-eighth Part. Divide the Arch OKP into three equal Parts, so will OZ be one-ninth Part, and QS one-tenth Part thereof.

After this Manner you may make a Pentagon, Hexagon, Heptagon, Octagon, Nonagon, &c.

PROP. XVII. PROB.

Given the Transverse Diameter AB, *and the Conjugate* CD *of an Oval, to describe the same.*

37.

RULE

18   GEOMETRICAL PROBLEMS.   Book I.

FIG.

RULE.

37. Bisect AB by drawing CD through the middle a. Make $A\odot = CD$, and divide $\odot B$ into three equal Parts; set two of those Parts from a to b and I; with the Distance Ib make two equilateral Triangles Idb, Ieb, whose Angles are the Centers. Then with one Foot of the Compasses on b and I severally, describe the Arches fBh, iAg with the Radius bB $(= IA:)$ Then with the Distance eC $(= dD)$ and with one Foot on the Centers e, d, severally describe the Arches iCf, hDg, completing the Ellipsis or Oval $ACBD$. But the true Method of delineating an Ellipsis, is by the Line of Sines on the Sector, as performed in the following Proposition.

PROP. XVIII. PROB.

To lay down an Ellipsis by the Line of Sines
38 *on the Sector, having the Diameters AC and BD both given.*

RULE.

Draw the Diameter AC, and make $AE = EC$; through E draw $BD \perp AC$, and make $BE = ED$. Make EA $(= EC)$ a parallel Radius of 90 · 90 on the Line of Sines; then take the parallel Sines of 10, 20, 30, &c. and set respectively from E towards A and C, both Ways,

Ways, which will give the Points 10, 20, 30, 40, &c. through every one of these Points draw Lines ‖ *BD*, as 80 80, 70 70, 60 60, &c then make *EB* (= *ED*) a parallel Radius of 90 : 90 on the Sines, and take parallelwise the Sines of 80, 70, 60, &c. and set all Ways from 10, 20, 30, &c. to 80, 70, 60, &c. then through these Points, with an even Hand draw a Curve which will give the Ellipsis required, and is every Way true and perfectly mathematical.

If an Ellipsis thus drawn be cut out on Pasteboard or very stiff Paper, it may afterwards be neatly taken off upon Paper, by following the Edges thereof with a drawing Pen.

PROP. XIX. PROB.

To delineate a Parabola, having the Ordinate AB *and its Axis* CD *both given.*

RULE.

Draw a Circle through the three Points *ACB*, (by Prob. 11) Also through *C* draw as many Circles as may seem convenient, each of which must cut the Axis *CD* somewhere between *C* and *D*, as in *a*, *b*, and *c*. Make *ad*, *be*, and *cf* each equal to *DE*, and through *d*, *e*, and *f*, draw *gh*, *ik*, *lm*, all parallel to *AB*, to cut their respective Circles in *g*, *h*, *i*, *k*, *l*, *m*, through which from *C*, with an even Hand draw the parabolic Curves *CiA*, *CkB*. This is *Fletcher*'s Method, as also is the following Problem.

PROP. XX. PROB.

40. *To draw an Hyperbola* ABC, *having its Transverse Axis* BD, *and* BE (= DF) *the Distance of the Focus from the Ends* B *and* D *of the Axis given.*

RULE.

Continue BE any convenient Length, as to G; also divide BG into any Number of Parts equal or unequal, in a, b, c. With the Distances Da, Db, and Dc, and one Foot on F, describe the Arches dd, dd, dd, &c. Also with the Distances Ba, Bb, bc, &c and one Foot in E cross the Arches first drawn, with other Arches ee, ee, ee, &c. Through the Points of Intersection draw the Curve ABC.

PROP. XXI. PROB.

41. *To reduce any Quadrilateral (or four-sided Figure)* ABCD, *to a Triangle.*

RULE.

Draw AC, also from B draw BE ‖ to AC, which will cut DC extended, in E; then draw AE, so is DAE the Triangle.

For the Triangles ACB, ACE, standing upon the same Base AC, and between the same Parallels AC and BE, are equal (by Theor. 13.) and by adding the Triangle ADC (which is common to both Triangles), we have the Triangle ADE equal to the Quadrilateral $ABCD$.

PROP.

Sect. I. GEOMETRICAL PROBLEMS. 21

PROP. XXII. PROB.

To reduce the Pentagonal Figure ABCDE to a Triangle whose vertical Angle shall be at C.

FIG. 42.

RULE.

Extend the Side AE (opposite to the vertical Angle C) both Ways to G and H, and draw the Diagonals EC, AC; then, through D draw DG ∥ to CE, to cut AE extended in G; and through B draw BH ∥ to CA, which will cut AE extended in H; then draw GC and HC, which will make the Triangle HCG equal to the Pentagon $ABCDE$.

PROP. XXIII. PROB.

To reduce the Octagonal Figure ABCDEFGH to a Triangle.

FIG. 43.

RULE.

Continue its Sides AB, BC, CD, DE, EF; then beginning at H, draw GI ∥ HF, to cut EF extended in I; also draw IK ∥ HE, which will cut DE extended in K, also draw KL ∥ HD, to cut CD extended in L; also draw LM ∥ HC, to cut BC extended in M, and lastly, draw MN ∥ HB, which will cut AB extended in N. Then draw HN, so is AHN the Triangle.

Note, The Work of this and the following Problem will become perfectly easy, if you use a parallel Ruler.

PROP.

PROP. XXIV. PROB.

To reduce an irregular Figure ABC *&c. as a Field whose Hedges contain many Bendings, Angles, &c to a Trapezium.*

Rule.

First reduce the Sides AB, BC to one Side AM, by the last Prob then beginning at M, lay the Edge of a parallel Ruler on M and E, and extend the other Edge to D, which will cut AM in a, then lay the Ruler on a and the the next Corner F, and its Edge extended to E will cut AM in c; then apply the Ruler to c and the next Corner G, and its Edge being extended to F will intersect AM in b; again, lay the Edge of the Ruler on b and the next Corner H, and its Edge being extended to G will cut AM in P. Draw HP, which has reduced the crooked Side CDE, &c. to a straight one. Thus reduce the other Sides, and you will have a Trapezium equal to the Figure ABC &c This Trapezium may be further reduced to a Triangle (by Prob 21.) if required.

Sect. II.   Geometrical Theorems.   23

SECT II.

Geometrical Theorems.

PROP. I. Theor.   Fig. 17.

IF any right Line A Y *stand upon the Middle of another right Line* D Z, *it will make therewith two right Angles, or two Angles whose Sum is equal to two right Angles*   Euc. 1. 13.

Draw the Diameter DZ, which will divide the Circle $DXZE$ into two equal Parts DXZ and DEZ, each containing a Semi-circle (or 180°,) if therefore a Line XA be drawn from the Point X to the Center A, it will divide the Semi-circle DXZ into two equal Parts, making two right Angles DAX, ZAX; or if a Line AY be drawn down from another Part (Y) of the Circumference to A, it will divide the Semi-circle into two unequal Parts, making the Angles DAY, ZAY unequal, but $DAY + ZAY$ are equal to a Semi-circle or two right Angles.   Q. E. D.

PROP.

PROP. II. THEOR.

If two right Lines IL, KM *intersect each other, the opposite Angles* A *and* C, *as also* B *and* D *are equal, that is, the Angle* A = *the Angle* C, *and the Angle* B = *the Angle* D. Euc. I. 15.

The Sum of the Angles $A + B$ (by Theor. 1.) is = to a Semi-circle, also the Sum of the Angles $A + D$ (by the same Theor.) is = to a Semi-circle; then $A + B = A + D$ (by Axiom 1.) Throw away A from both Sides of the Equation, and there will remain the $\angle B = \angle D$ (by Axiom 3.) Q. E. D.

PROP. III. THEOR.

If a right Line OR *cut two parallel right Lines* NP, SQ, *the alternate Angles* NaR, QbO *are equal, and consequently the Lines parallel.* Euc. I. 29.

The Angles NaR, and PaO (by Theor. 2) are equal; and because the Lines are parallel, the $\angle NaR$ is $= \angle QbO = \angle PaO$, which (by Theor. 2.) $= \angle QbO$. Q. E. D.

PROP. IV. THEOR.

If any Side of a right-lined Triangle be continued, the external Angle is equal to the Sum of the two opposite internal ones. Euc. I. 32.

Let

Sect. II.   GEOMETRICAL THEOREMS.   25

Let UST be the given Triangle; continue the Side UT to Z, and from T draw TY parallel to the Side US (by Prob. 2.). Then will the external $\angle STZ$ be equal to the Sum of the internal $\angle$s SUT, UST; for the Lines SU, TY being parallel, the $\angle STY$ is $= \angle UST$ (by Theor. 3); also the $\angle ZTY$ is $= \angle SUT$, and consequently the $\angle STZ$ $(= STY + ZTY) = \angle SUT + \angle UST =$ Sum of the opposite internal Angles. Q.E.D

FIG. 47.

PROP. V. THEOR.

The three Angles of any rectilinear Triangle are together equal to two right Angles, or 180 Degrees. Euc. 1. 32.

The Line ST falling on the Line UZ, makes the Angles STU and STZ together equal to two right Angles (by Theor. 1.). Also the Sum of the Angles S and U is equal to the $\angle STZ$ (Theor. 4.). Therefore the Angles S, U and STU are $=$ 180 Degrees. Q.E.D

47.

Or the same may be demonstrated thus.

Let the Triangle be ABC; through A draw DE parallel to the Side CB, so is the $\angle DAC$ $=$ the $\angle ACB$ (by Theor. 3); as also the $\angle EAB =$ the $\angle CBA$; but the $\angle DAC$ $+ \angle CAB + \angle EAB = 180°$, or two right

48.

E   Angles

Fig. 48. Angles (by Theor. 1); and confequently the three Angles $ACB + CAB + CBA$ are equal to a Semi-circle, or 180 Degrees. Q.E.D.

PROP. VI THEOR.

The Sides of fimilar Triangles are proportional, and the Angles fubtended by proportional or equal Sides, are equal.

47. 48. In the Triangles STU and ABC, the Sides ST and AB are proportional, as are alfo the other Sides, then it will be as $SU : AC :: TU : BC$; and as $ST : AB :: SU : AC$, alfo the $\angle T$ will be equal the $\angle B$, the $\angle U =$ the $\angle C$, and the $\angle S =$ the $\angle A$, and therefore Triangles whofe Angles are equal, have the Sides fubtending thofe Angles, equal or proportional. 6 *Euc* 4. 5. Q.E.D.

PROP VII. THEOR.

In any four-fided right-lined Figure, commonly called a Trapezium, the Sum of the four Angles is equal to four right Angles, or 360 Degrees

49. Let $FGHI$ be the Figure given, through which draw the Diagonal IG, dividing the Trapezium into two △s IFG, IHG, each of which is equal to two right Angles (by Theor. 5.). Therefore the four Angles of the Quadrangle are equal to four right Angles. Q.E.D.

PROP.

Sect. II.   GEOMETRICAL THEOREMS.   27

PROP. VIII. THEOR.   FIG

The Sum of all the Angles of any right-lined Figure (though it contain never so many Sides,) is equal to double the Number of right Angles (abating four) that there are Sides in the Figure

In the irregular Polygon $KLMNOP$ con- 50
sisting of six unequal Sides, assume a Point Q, from which draw Lines $QK, QL, QM, QN, QO, QP,$ to the Corners K, L, M, N, O, P, reducing the Polygon into as many Triangles (viz 6) as it hath Sides. Each of these Triangles contains two right Angles (by Theor 5.), and therefore the Number of right Angles contained in all the six Triangles is $= 12$ ($=$ double the Number of the Polygon's Sides), but from these take four right Angles ($=$ the Sum of all the Angles at Q,) and the Remainder 8 is the Number of right Angles equal to the Sum of the Angles $K, L, M, N, O, P.$ $Q.E.D.$

PROP. IX. THEOR.

In right-lined Triangles, equal Sides subtend equal Angles (Euc. 1. 5) *The greatest Side subtends the greatest Angle* (Euc. 1. 19) *and the least Side subtends the least Angle.*

PROP. X. THEOR.

An Angle in a Semi-circle is a right Angle; 51.
or if two Lines, as TR *and* SR, *be drawn from*
                                        T *and*

Fig. T and S (*the Ends of the Diameter*) *to* R *in the Circumference, they will form a right Angle* TRS, *being perpendicular to each other.*

51. Through the Center U draw the Diameter TS; let R be a Point assumed in the Circumference, to which draw SR, UR, TR, and you will have two Triangles UTR, URS. Then because UT is $= UR = US$, therefore the $\angle UTR = \angle TRU$, and $\angle URS = \angle USR$, by Theor. 9. And because the three Angles of the Triangle TRS are equal to two right Angles, (Theor. 5.) and the $\angle T = \angle URT$, and the $\angle S = \angle URS$, therefore the Sum of the Angles URT and URS is equal the Sum of the Angles T and S, which is equal to Half the Sum of two right Angles, which is one right Angle. Q.E.D.

Or thus;

51   The $\angle SUR + \angle TUR =$ to two right Angles (Theor. 1). Also the $\angle UTR + \angle URT = \angle SUR$, and the Angles USR and URS are together equal to the Angle TUR (Theor. 4); therefore the $\angle URS (= \angle USR) + \angle URT (= \angle UTR) =$ to one right Angle. Q.E.D.

PROP. XI. Theor.

52. *Parallelograms standing upon the same or equal Bases, and between the same or equal Parallels, are equal. That is,* ▱YZCB *is* $=$ ▱VXCB.

It

Sect. II.   GEOMETRICAL THEOREMS.   29

It is evident that VX is $= CB = YZ$; alſo XY being common to both, VY is $= XZ$, (Ax. 2.); alſo VC is $= XB$ (Def 21.). Therefore the Triangles VCY, XBZ are equal. If therefore DXY (which is a Part of both Triangles) be taken away, there will remain $VXDC$ and $DYZB$, which (by Ax. 3) are equal. Alſo CDB being common to both Parallelograms, makes $VXCB =$ to $YZCB$. Q. E. D.

FIG. 52.

PROP. XII. THEOR.

If a Triangle have the ſame Baſe that a Parallelogram hath, and be between the ſame Parallels, the Triangle is equal to Half the Parallelogram.

In the Parallelogram $FGIK$ draw the Diagonal KG, which divides it into two equal Triangles KFG, GIK, for the Side FG is equal to the Side KI, and the Side FK is equal to the Side GI, and KG is common to both Triangles, and conſequently the Triangles are equal, and each equal to Half the Parallelogram. Q. E. D.

53.

PROP. XIII. THEOR.

All Triangles having the ſame or equal Baſes, and being between the ſame or equal Parallels, are equal.

It is evident from Theor. 11. that Parallelograms ſtanding upon the ſame Baſe, and between the

FIG. the fame or equal Parallels, are equal to one another, and that fuch Triangles (Theor. 12) are the Half of thefe Parallelograms, therefore all fuch Triangles ftanding upon the fame or equal Bafes, are (Ax. 7.) equal. Q E D.

PROP. XIV. Theor.

Such Parallelograms and Triangles as ftand upon and between the fame Parallels, are proportional to their Bafes.

53. Let EK and FI be two Parallelograms lying between the Parallels EG, LH, then $LK : KI \square EK \cdot \square FI$: Alfo in the Triangles KGI, IGH, it is, as $KI \quad IH \quad \triangle KGI \cdot \triangle IGH$. Euc. 6. 1.

PROP. XV. Theor.

If a Line be drawn parallel to any Side of a Triangle, it will cut the other two Sides proportionally.

47. Draw WX parallel to UT, to cut the Sides SU and ST in W, X, then $SW \quad SU : SX : ST$, draw WT and UX, making the Triangles WUT and XTU, which (by Theor. 13) are equal, as alfo are the Triangles UWX and TXW, therefore it will be, as $SWX : WUX :: SW . WU$; and, as $SWX : WUX$ (the Triangles

Sect. II.   GEOMETRICAL THEOREMS.   51

angles UWX and TXW being equal) SX : FIG. XT, then throw away the two firſt Terms 47. SWX, WUX, and it will be, as $SW:WU::SX$ XT. Q.E.D.

PROP XVI THEOR.

If in any right-angled Triangle a Perpendicular be let fall from the right Angle, upon its oppoſite or longeſt Side, it will divide the given Triangle into two right-angled ones, ſimilar and proportional to the firſt, and alſo to each other.

In the right-angled Triangle PMN, let fall 54. the Perpendicular MO, which will divide it into two right-angled Triangles PMO, OMN, which are alike (by Theor. 6). Alſo the Angle P is common to both Triangles, *i.e.* it is common to the Triangles PMN and PMO, alſo, by the ſame Theorem, PMN and PMO are alike, as are alſo PMN and NOM, becauſe the Angles POM and NOM are right, and ſo the Triangles POM and NOM are alike (by Ax. 1.); and therefore in the Triangles PMN, POM, it will always be, as PO PM PM PN That is, the Square of PM is $= PO \times PN$. Alſo in the Triangles NOM and PMN, as $ON:MN:MN\cdot PN$; and therefore the Square of MN is $= ON \times PN$. Q.E.D.

PROP.

PROP XVII. THEOR.

In any right-angled Triangle, the Square of the Hypothenuse (or longest Side) is equal to the Sum of the Squares of the other two Sides or Legs.

Let SQR be the given Triangle. On the Hypothenuse SR construct a Square, each Side of which shall be $= SR$, (as the Square SY), and from the right Angle Q let fall the Perpendicular QB upon the Hypothenuse, and continue it to Z, which will divide the $\square SY$ into two $\square$s BY and SZ. It is evident that SR is $= RY = SA$, and therefore $RY \times BR$ $= \square$ of the $\square BY$, which (by the last Theor.) is $= \square QR$, also $SA \times BS = \square$ of the $\square SZ$, which (by the same Theor.) is $= \square SQ$. But if the $\square BY$ be $= \square QR$, and the $\square SZ$ be $= \square SQ$, as hath been demonstrated, then the Sum of these two $\square$s $(= \square SR)$ will be $= \square QR + \square SQ =$ the Sum of the Squares of the two Sides or Legs. Q.E.D.

BOOK. II.

MENSURATION *of* SUPERFICIES *and* SOLIDS.

SECT. I.

The Use of the Tables *of* LOGARITHMS, *as also of the* Tables *of* ARTIFICIAL SINES *and* TANGENTS.

DEFINITIONS.

1. LOGARITHMS are a Series of Numbers which differ among themselves in arithmetical Proportion, as the Numbers they represent differ in geometrical Proportion.

2. The Index, or Characteristic of the Logarithm of any integral Number, is always less by 1 than the Number of Figures the said Integer consists of, as the Characteristic of 1 is 0, of 10 is 1, of 100 is 2, of 1000 is 3, &c. And therefore the Characteristic being known, will always shew the Number of Places of Figures the absolute correspondent Number must possess, which will be a Place more than the Characteristic contains Units. The Characteristic is separated from the Figures of the Logarithm by a Point (·) much after the Form of a Decimal, as 2·361728 is the Logarithm of the Number 230.

3. The

3. The Characteriſtic of a Decimal, is commonly called negative, and ſhews the Place the firſt ſignificant Figure of its correſpondent Decimal muſt poſſeſs below Units; as ſuppoſe the Characteriſtic be 1, the firſt ſignificant Figure muſt poſſeſs the firſt Place of Decimals; if 2, the ſecond Place, 3, the third, &c. Theſe Characteriſtics have a Point before and after them, to diſtinguiſh them from affirmative Characteriſtics, and to ſhew them to be negative; as ·1·740363 is the Logarithm of ·55, and 2·740363 is the Logarithm of ·055, &c.

4. If the Characteriſtic of 1 be accounted 10 or 100, then the Characteriſtic of ·1 will be ·9 or ·99, of ·01 will be ·8 or ·98, of ·001 will be ·7 or 97, &c. So that by thus doing, we obtain affirmative Characteriſtics to negative numbers, though it is neceſſary to prefix a Point, to ſignify their being negative. Theſe are a ſecond Sort of negative Indices, and are managed after a different Manner from the former, to which I give the Preference, and which I ſhall make Uſe of in the Sequel of this Work. Thoſe who are deſirous of ſeeing the Forms of working by theſe laſt-mentioned Characteriſtics, may conſult *Martin's Logarithms*.

5. The Tables of Logarithms, are the Logarithms of all Numbers from 1 to 10000, carefully ſelected from the moſt accurate Tables of the ingenious Mr *H. Sherwin*, and abbreviated, and reduced to a compendious Form, without their Indices.

6. The Canon of the logarithmic Sines and Tangents, is a Table of the Logarithms of the natural

Sines

Sines and Tangents to every Degree and Minute of the Quadrant, classed in a plain and obvious Manner, so as to render their Use easy.

P R O B. I.

To find the Logarithm of any Number not exceeding three Places of Figures.

R U L E.

Find the given Number in some one of the Columns of the Table, marked at Top (N°) and opposite to it, in the adjoining Column is the required Logarithm, to which prefix its proper Chrracteristic.

E X A M P L E I.

Given the Number 48, to find its Logarithm.

The Logarithm of 48 — — = 1·681241

E X A M P L E II.

Given the Number 436; required its Logarithm.

The Logarithm of 436 — — = 2·639486

Note, If Part of the given Number be a Decimal, find the Logarithm for the Whole, to which annex the Index belonging to the integral Part.

Prob. II.

To find the Logarithm of a Number confisting of four Figures.

Rule.

Seek out the firſt three Figures in ſome of the Columns mark'd at Top (N°) and take out the permanent Part of the Logarithm, then oppoſite to the Number laſt found (and in the Column ſigned by the laſt Figure thereof) take out the laſt Figures, which annexed to the Figures in the parmanent Part (firſt taken out) makes up the Logarithm ſought, to which annex its proper Index

Example.

Let it be required to find the Logarithm for the Number 643 6.

The Logarithm of 643 6 — — = 2·808616

Prob. III.

To find the Logarithm of a Number, of five Figures.

Rule.

Find the Logarithm of the firſt four Figures by Prob 2. Multiply the Difference between this and the next greater Logarithm, by the remaining Figure of the given Number, and from the Product cut off one

Sect. I. *of* Numbers. 37

one Figure to the right Hand; the remaining Figures of the Product added to the Logarithm firſt found, is the Logarithm sought.

Example.

Given the Number 68543, to find its Logarithm.

The Log of the firſt 4 Figures 68540 = 4.835944
The Log. next following is of 68550 = 4.836007

The Diff. of Numb. and Log.   10   63
                                          3
                                        ———
                                        18|9
Add the firſt Logarithm   —   —   4.835944

Sum is the Log. of 68543   —   = 4.835963

Prob. IV.

To find the Logarithm of any Number not exceeding seven Places of Figures.

Rule.

Find the Logarithm of the firſt four Figures (by Prob 2.) Then multiply the Difference between this and the next greater Logarithm, by the remaining Figure or Figures of the given Number, and from the Product cut off as many Figures on the right Side, as you multiplied by; to the remaining Figures of the Product add the Logarithm firſt found, the Sum ſhall be the Log. of the Number.

Ex-

Example I.

Required the Logarithm of the Number 436587.

The Log. of 436500 = 5·639984, the Log. of 436600 = 5·640084.

Then $\frac{5 \cdot 640084 - 5 \cdot 639984 \times 87}{100} + 5 \cdot 639984 = 5 \cdot 640071$ = Log. of 436587, as required.

Example II.

Given the Number 5436·875, to find its Log.

The Log. of 5436000 = 3·735279, the Log. of 5437000 = 3·735359.

Then $\frac{\text{Log. } 3 \cdot 735359 - \text{Log. } 3 \cdot 735279 \times 875}{1000} + 3 \cdot 735279$ = 3·735349 = Log of 5436 875.

Prob V

To find the Number belonging to a Logarithm.

Rule.

This is just the Reverse of the foregoing Rules for finding the Logarithm for any Number: And therefore seek in the Table for a Logarithm equal to, or the nearest less than the given Logarithm, and if you find a Logarithm exactly the same, then the Number corresponding thereto is the Number required. But if you cannot find exactly the Logarithm, take the Difference between the given Logarithm and the next less, and to the Remainder annex as many Cyphers

Sect. I.   *of* NUMBERS.   39

phers as you seek Figures for, which divide by the Difference between the Logarithm next greater and next less than the given Logarithm, and the Quotient annexed to the four first Figures will give the compleat Number.

EXAMPLE I.

Given the Logarithm 4·835963; to find the Number corresponding thereto.

The Log. next less is of 6854 — = 4·835944
The given Logarithm — — = 4·835963

Difference — — — — 19

The Log. next greater is of 6855   = 4·836007

Diff. between greatest and least Logs.   63

Then $\frac{19 \times 10}{63}$ = 3; which annexed to 6854, make 68543, the Number required.

EXAMPLE II.

Given the Logarithm 5·640071; the absolute Number thereto is required.

The Log next less is of 4365 — = 5·639984
The given Logarithm — — = 5·640071

Difference of these two Logs. — 87

The next greater Log. is of 4366   = 5·640084

Diff. between greatest and least Logs.   100

Then $\frac{87 \times 100}{100}$ = 87; which annexed to 4365 is = 436587 = the Number required.   PROB.

Prob VI.

To find the Sine, Co-sine, Tangent, Co-tangent, Secant, and Co-secant of any Arc to 90°.

Rule I.

To find the logarithmic Sine or Tangent of any Arc. If the given Arc consists of Degrees, or of Degrees and Minutes, the logarithmic Sine or Tangent thereof is had by Inspection in the Tables, which are too plain to need Explanation. But if the Arc consists of Degrees, Minutes, Seconds, Thirds, &c take the logarithmic Sine of the Degrees and Minutes given, and of the next greater by 1 Min. then multiply that Difference by the Decimal of the intermediate Part of a Minute, and add the Product to the Sine or Tangent of the given Degrees and Minutes, the Sum will be the logarithmic Sine and Tangent of the given Degrees, Minutes, &c. required.

Example I

Required the Log. Sine of 5° 36′ 48″.

The Log. Sine of 5° 36′ = 8·989374, the Log. Sine of 5° 37 = 8·990660, 48″ = 0′·8.

Then $\overline{8·990660 - 8·989374} \times 0·8 + 8·989374 =$ 8·990403 = Log. Sine of 5° 36′ 48″.

Sect. I.   *of* NUMBERS.   41

EXAMPLE II.

Required the Log. Tangent of $5°-36'-48''$.

The Log. Tangent of $5°-36' = 8.991451$, the Log. Tangent of $5°-37' = 8.992750$, $48'' = 0'.8$.

Then $8.992750 - \overline{8.991451 \times 0.8} + 8.991451 = 8.992490 =$ Log Tangent of $5°-36'-48''$.

Note, If great Exactness is required, (especially in small Arcs) it is better to find the natural Sine or Tangent of the Arc, and it is no more than finding the absolute Number to the Logarithm given in the Tables, by Prob. 5, and then work for the natural Sine or Tangent as you did before for the Logarithmic; after which find its Logarithm by Prob 4. See the last Example performed by this Method.

The natural Tangent of $5°-36'$ is 980507, the natural Tangent of $5°-37'$ is 983445.

Then $\frac{983445 - 980507 \times 8}{10} = 982857 =$ natural Tangent of $5°-36'-48''$; whose Log (by Prob. 4) is 992490, and is exactly the same with that found by the first Method, though in very small Arcs there will be some little Variation; to which annex its proper Index, and the complete Logarithm will be $8.992490 =$ the Log. Tang. of $5°-36'-48''$.

RULE. II.

To find the logarithmic Co-sine and Co-tangent of any Arc. Find the log. Sine and log. Tangent of that Arc's Complement, (by Rule 1) which will be the

G   logarithmic

logarithmic Co-fine and Co-tangent. Note, the Complement of an Arc is what that Arc wants of 90° or a Quadrant. This is so plain it needs no Example.

Rule III

From the double Radius subtract the Co-fine of any Arc, the Remainder is the log. Secant; also the log. Secant of any Arc's Complement is the Co-secant, or logarithmic Co-secant.

Example I.

Required the log. Secant of 43° — 38'.

90° — 43° 38' = 46° 22' = Complement of 43° — 38'.
From the double Radius — 20·000000
Subtract the Sine 46° — 22' (= Co-fine 43° — 38') } 9·859601

The Remainder is the log. Sec. 43° — 38' 10·140399

Example II.

Required the log. Co-secant of 24° — 14' — 35".
From the double Radius — — 20·000000
Subtract Sine 24° — 14' — 35" (= Co-fine 65° — 45' — 25") } 9·613428

Remains the log Co-sec. of 24° — 14' — 35" 10·386572

Prob. VII.

To find the Complement Arithmetical of a Logarithm.
Note, The Complement Arithmetical of a Logarithm

Sect. I. *of* NUMBERS. 43

is the Difference between that Logarithm and the Log of Radius, which is ever 10·000000.

RULE.

Take the Difference between the given Logarithm and the log. Radius, the Remainder is the Complement Arithmetical of that Logarithm. Or it may be found mentally, by taking each Figure's Complement to 9, except the first, which you must take to 10.

EXAMPLE I.

Required the Complement Arithmetical of the Logarithm 6 843783.

From the Log of Radius	—	10·000000
Take the given Log.	— —	6 843783
Remainder is the Comp Arithmet.		3 156217

EXAMPLE II.

Required the Comp. Arithmet. Log. Tang. 10·816940.

From — — — —	20 000000
Subtract the Log. Tangent —	10·816940
Remainder is the Comp. Arithmet.	9 183060

Note, The Comp. Arithmet. of a Tang. Log. is the Co-tangent, or of a Co-tangent the Tangent. Also, if 10 be added to the Index of the Arithmetical Complement of the Logarithm of a Sine or Tangent, it will be the Co-secant.

G 2 SECT

SECT. II
Logarithmetical Arithmetic.

Prob. VIII.
To multiply Numbers together

Rule I.

WHEN the Indices of the Logarithms of the Factors are both affirmative, then the Sum of these Logarithms is the Logarithm of the Product.

Note, If you carry 10 to the Indices, it is affirmative.

Example I.

		Logarithms.
Multiply — — —	34 =	1·531479
By — — —	26 =	1·414973
Product,	884 =	2·946452

Example II.

Multiply — —	20·8 =	1·318063
By — —	7·6 =	0·880814
Product,	158 =	2·198877

Example III.

Multiply — —	464·36 =	2·666854
By — —	88·4 =	1·946452
Product,	41049·424 =	4·613306

Rule II.

When the Indices of the Logarithms of the Factors are both negative, then the Sum of their Logarithms is the Logarithm of the Product, and the Sum of the Indices is also negative.

Note, If you carry 10 to the Indices, it is affirmative, and must be subtracted from their Sum.

Example I.

		Logarithms.
Multiply		·025 = ·2 397940
By		·41 = 1 623249
Product,		·0105 = ·2 021189

Example II.

Multiply		·418 = ·1 621176
By		·18 = ·1 255272
Product,		·07524 = 2·876448

Example III.

Multiply		·0076 = ·3 880814
By		·09 = 2·954242
Product,		·000684 = 4 835056

Rule III.

When the Indices are the one affirmative and the other negative, add the Logarithms together, to which Sum annex the Difference of the Indices, which shall be the Index of the Product, making it either affirmative

mative or negative, according to the Affection of the greater.

Note, If you carry any Thing to the Indices, it is affirmative, and muſt be added to the Index affirmative.

EXAMPLE I.

		Logarithms.
Multiply	348 =	2·541579
By	·64 =	·1 806180
Product,	222 72 =	2·347759

EXAMPLE II.

Multiply	64 8 =	1·811575
By	·007 =	·3·845098
Product,	·4536 =	1 656673

EXAMPLE III.

Multiply	·237 =	·1·374748
By	1·81 =	0 257679
Product,	·42897 =	·1·632427

PROB. IX

To divide one Number by another.

RULE I.

When the Indices of the Logarithms of the Dividend and Divifor are both affirmative, ſubtract the Logarithm of the Divifor from the Logarithm of the Dividend,

Sect. II.   ARITHMETIC.   47

Dividend, the Remainder is the Log. of the Quotient; and if you borrow 10 from the Indices, it is affirmative.

EXAMPLE I.

		Logarithms.
Divide	468 =	2.670246
By	12 =	1.079181
Quotient,	39 =	1.591065

EXAMPLE II.

Divide	144 =	2.158362
By	16 =	1.204120
Quotient,	9 =	0.954242

RULE II.

If the Indices of the Logarithms of the Dividend and Divisor be both negative, subtract the Logarithm of the Divisor from the Logarithm of the Dividend, the Remainder is the Logarithm of the Quotient; if you borrow 10, pay it again to the Index of the Divisor affirmatively.

EXAMPLE I.

Divide	48 =	·1·681241
By	·12 =	·1·079181
Quotient,	4 =	0.602060

Ex-

Example II.

			Logarithms.
Divide	—	—	·0096 = 3̄·982271
By	—	—	·038 = ·2̄579784
		Quotient,	·2526 = ·1̄402487

Rule III

When the Indices of the Logarithms of the Dividend and Divisor are homogenial, and the Index of the Divisor is greater than the Index of the Dividend, then subtract the Index of the Dividend from the Index of the Divisor, and the Remainder shall be the Index of the Quotient, changing its Sign, viz. if it be affirmative make it negative, and if it be negative make it affirmative. If you borrow any Thing from the Indices, work according to the last Rule.

Example I.

Divide	—	—	64 = 0·806180
By	—	—	80 = 1·903090
		Quotient,	·08 = ·2̄903090

Example II.

Divide	—	—	·75 = ·1̄875061
By	—	—	·0015 = ·3̄176091
		Quotient,	500 = 2·698970

Sect. II.   ARITHMETIC.   49

Rule IV.

When the Indices are the one affirmative and the other negative, subtract the Log. of the Divisor out of the Log. of the Dividend; and changing the Sign of the Index of the Divisor, add them together; so shall the Sum be the Index of the Quotient, which must be of the same Kind with the Index of the Dividend.

Note, If you borrow, pay it again to the Index of the Divisor affirmatively.

Example I.

		Logarithms.
Divide	·144 =	·1·158362
By	12 =	1·079181
Quotient,	·012 =	·2·079181

Example II.

Divide	64 =	1·806180
By	·08 =	·2·903090
Quotient,	800 =	2·903090

Example III.

Divide	·64 =	·1·806180
By	800 =	2·903090
Quotient,	·0008 =	·4·903090

H   Prob.

Prob. X.

To work Examples in the Rule of Three.

Rule.

Subtract the Log of the first Term in the Analogy from the Sum of the Logs of the other two, or add the Complement Arithmet of the Log of the first Term to the Sum of the Logs. of the second and third, the Remainder in the first Case, or the Sum in the latter, (one in the ten's Place of the Index of the Sum being abated for each Comp) is the Log. of the fourth Term or Answer.

Example

If eight Yards of Cloth cost 1*l* 4*s*. what will 96 Yards cost?—Answ 14*l*. 8*s*.

Log of 8 is	0 903090	Or thus
Log of 1 2	0 079181	Comp Log 8 is 9·096910
Log of 96	1 982271	The Log. 1 2 0 079181
Log of 115·2	2 061452	The Log 96 1·982271
Log of 14·4	1·158362	The Log. 144 1 158362

After the same Method may all Questions belonging the Rule of Three be solv'd.

Prob XI

To find mean Proportionals between any two Numbers

Rule.

Divide the Difference of the Logs. of the greatest and

Sect. II.   ARITHMETIC.   51

and least Terms by a Number more by one than the Number of Means required; then to the Log. of the least Term, or from the Log of the greatest, add or subtract the Quotient continually, the Sums or Remainders will be the Logs of the Proportionals required.

EXAMPLE I.

Let four mean Proportionals be sought between 108 and 80.

Log. of 108 ——— 2.033424
Log. of 80 ——— 1.903090

Divide by 5) 0.130334 (0.0260668

Log of the least Term	80	1.903090
Log of the first Mean	84.948	1.9291568
Log. of the second	90.203	1.9552236
Log. of the third	95.783	1.9812904
Log. of the fourth	101.70	2.0073572
Log of the greatest Term	108	2.033424

Wherefore the Proportionals found, are as 80 . 84.948 . 90.203 : 95.783 :: 101.7 . 108.

EXAMPLE II.

Required eight mean Proportionals between 16 and 84.

Log. of 84 ——— ——— 1.924279
Log. of 16 ——— ——— 1.204120

Divide by 9) 0.720159

0.0800176

Log. of the greateſt Term	84	1·924279
Log of the eighth Mean	69·865	1·844261·4
Log of the ſeventh	58 109	1 764243 8
Log of the ſixth	48·331	1·684226·2
Log. of the fifth	40 198	1 604208·6
Log of the fourth	33 434	1 524191·0
Log. of the third	27 808	1·444173·4
Log of the ſecond	23·128	1 364155 8
Log. of the firſt	19 237	1·284138·2
Log. of the leaſt Term	16	1 204120

The Series therefore is this:

16. 19·237. 23 128 27·808 33 434 40 198. 48 331. 58·109. 69·865 84.

Prob. XII.

To find the Logarithm of a Vulgar Fraction.

Rule I.

From the Logarithm of the Numerator take the Logarithm of the Denominator; the Remainder is the Log of the Fraction.

Or thus:

Add the Log of the Numerator to the Complement Arithmetical of the Log of the Denominator; the Sum is the Log. of the Fraction.

Sect. II.   ARITHMETIC.   53

EXAMPLE I.

What is the Log. of the Fraction $\frac{3}{4}$?

From the Log Numerator	3 =	0.477121
Subtract the Log. Denominator	4 =	0.602060
There remains the Log. of $\frac{3}{4}$ = .75	=	ˉ1.875061

Or thus:

To the Comp. Arith. Log Denom.	4 =	9.397940
Add the Log of the Numerator	3 =	0.477121
The Sum is the Log. of the Fract $\frac{3}{4}$	=	ˉ1.875061

EXAMPLE II.

What is the Log. of the Fraction $\frac{36}{15}$?

From the Log. of the Numerator	36 =	1.556302
Subtract the Log of the Denom	15 =	1.176091
Remainder is the Log. of $\frac{36}{15}$ = $2\frac{2}{5}$	=	0.380211

Or thus:

To the Log. Numerator	36 =	1.556302
Add the Comp. Arith Log. Denom.	15 =	8.823909
Sum is the Log of $\frac{36}{15}$ = $2\frac{2}{5}$	=	0.380211

By this it appears, that the Index of the Log. of an improper Fraction is affirmative, as that of a proper one negative.

RULE II.

Reduce mix'd Fractions to improper ones, and then proceed as before.

Ex-

EXAMPLE

What is the Log of $12\frac{5}{8}$ $(=\frac{101}{8})$?

From the Log Numerator $101 = 2.004321$
Subtract the Log Denominator $8 = 0.929419$

Differ. is the Log. of $12\frac{5}{8}$ $= 1.074902$

Note, If the mix'd Fraction consists of large Numbers, it may most easily be reduced by the Logarithms, by the following

RULE.

To the Log of the Integral Part add the Log of the Denominator of the Fractional Part, to the Number belonging the Sum of the Logs add the Numerator of the Fractional Part, and the Sum is the Numerator of the Fraction.

EXAMPLE.

Reduce $4345\frac{43}{684}$ to a Fraction

To the Log. of the Integral Part $4345 = 3.637990$
Add the Log of the Denom. $684 = 2.835056$

Sum is the Log of 2971980 $= 6.473046$
Numerator add 43

Sum $2972023 =$ the new Numerator; therefore $4345\frac{43}{684} = \frac{2972023}{684}$ In like Manner may any other mix'd Number be reduced to an equivalent Fraction.

PROB

Prob XIII.

To multiply Vulgar Fractions

Rule I.

Add the Logs of the Numerators together, for the Log of a new Numerator, and the Logs. of the Denominators for the Log of a new Denominator.

Example.

What is the Product of $\frac{365}{436}$ by $\frac{5}{8}$?

The Logs of the Numerators $\begin{cases} 365 = 2.562293 \\ 5 = 0.698970 \end{cases}$

Sum is the Log new Numerator $1825 = 3.261263$

The Logs of the Denominators $\begin{cases} 436 = 2.639487 \\ 8 = 0.903090 \end{cases}$

Sum is the Log new Denomin $3488 = 4.542577$

Therefore $\frac{365}{436} \times \frac{5}{8} = \frac{1825}{3488}$ as required.

Rule II

If the Product of several Fractions be required, add the Logs of the several Numerators and the Arithmetical Complements of the Logs. of the several Denominators together; the Sum is the Log. of the Product.

Example.

What is the Product of $\frac{68}{84} \times \frac{34}{63} \times \frac{3}{4}$?

The Logs. of the Numerators $\begin{cases} 68 = 1{\cdot}832509 \\ 34 = 1{\cdot}531479 \\ 3 = 0{\cdot}477121 \end{cases}$

The Arith. Compl. Logs. Denom. $\begin{cases} 84 = 8{\cdot}075721 \\ 63 = 8{\cdot}200660 \\ 4 = 9{\cdot}397940 \end{cases}$

Product of $\frac{68}{84} \times \frac{34}{63} \times \frac{3}{4} = \frac{6936}{21168} = {\cdot}32766 = 1{\cdot}515430.$

Prob XIV.

To divide one Vulgar Fraction by another.

Rule

Add the Logarithm of the Denominator of the Divisor to the Logarithm of the Numerator of the Dividend; the Sum is the Logarithm of a new Numerator: Also the Sum of the Logarithms of the Numerator of the Divisor and Denominator of the Dividend, is the Logarithm of the new Denominator.

Example.

What is the Quotient $\frac{352}{4382}$ by $\frac{7}{8}$?

Add the Logarithms $\begin{cases} 7 = 0{\cdot}845098 \\ 4382 = 3{\cdot}641672 \end{cases}$

The Sum is the Log new Denom. $30674 = 4{\cdot}486770$

Add

Sect II. ARITHMETIC. 57

Add the Logarithms $\begin{cases} 8 = 0{\cdot}903090 \\ 352 = 2{\cdot}546543 \end{cases}$

The Sum is the Log. new Numer $2816 = 3{\cdot}449633$

Therefore $\frac{352}{4382} - \frac{7}{8} = \frac{2816}{30674} = \frac{1408}{15337}$.

Or thus, by Rule 2, Prob. 12.

The Logarithms $\begin{cases} 8 = 0{\cdot}903090 \\ 352 = 2{\cdot}546543 \end{cases}$

The Comp. Arith Logs. $\begin{cases} 7 = 9{\cdot}154902 \\ 4382 = 6{\cdot}358328 \end{cases}$

The Sum is the Log. $\frac{352}{4382} - \frac{7}{8} = {\cdot}091804 = 2{\cdot}962863$

PROB. XV

To involve Numbers, integral or fractional, to any Power.

RULE.

Multiply the Logarithm of the Number by the Index of the Power required, the Product is the Logarithm of the Power

EXAMPLE I.

What is the Square of 48?

Multiply the Logarithm of $48 = 1{\cdot}681241$
By the Index of the Power 2

The Prod. is the Log. of the Square $2304 = 3{\cdot}362482$

I   Ex-

Example II.

What is the Square of 4·8?

Multiply the Log of   4·8 = 0·681241
By the Index of the Power   2

The Prod. is the Log of the Square 23 04 = 1·362482

Example III.

What is the Square of 48?

Multiply the Log of   48 = 1·681241
By the Index of the Power   2

The Prod. is the Log of the Square 2304 = ·1 362482

Example IV.

Required the several Powers of 4 to the sixth?

1. Multiply the Log. of   4 = 0 602060
By   2

The Prod is the Log of the Square 16 = 1 204120

2. Multiply the Log. of   4 = 0 602060
By   3

The Prod. is the Log of the Cube 64 = 1 806180

3. Multiply the Log. of   4 = 0 602060
By   4

The Prod is the Log Biquadrate 256 = 2 408240

4. Multiply the Log of   4 = 0·602060
By   5

The Prod. is the Surfolid   1024 = 3 010300

5. Multiply

Sect. II.   ARITHMETIC.   59

   5. Multiply the Log. of   4 = 0·602060
   By   6
   ―――――――――――――――――
   The Prod. is the Cubo-cube   4096 = 3·612360

EXAMPLE V.

Required the $\frac{1}{4}$ Power of 12?
The Log of   12 = 1·079181
Multiplied by $\frac{1}{4}$
―――――――――――――――――
The Prod. is the Log of $\frac{1}{4}$ Power 1·8612 = 0·269795

EXAMPLE VI.

Required the $\frac{5}{12}$ Power of 16?
The Logarithm of   16 = 1·204120
Multiplied by $\frac{5}{12}$
―――――――――――――――――
The Prod. is the Log $\frac{5}{12}$ Power 3·1748 = 0·501716

EXAMPLE VII.

Required the $6\frac{2}{3}$ Power of 3?
The Logarithm of   3 = 0·477121
Multiplied by $6\frac{2}{3}$
―――――――――――――――――
The Prod. is the Log. of $6\frac{2}{3}$ Power 1516·3 = 3·180807

EXAMPLE VIII.

What is the $\frac{1}{4}$ Power of ·0436?
The Logarithm of   ·0436 = ¯2·639487
Multiplied by $\frac{1}{4}$
―――――――――――――――――
The Prod. is the Log. of the $\frac{1}{4}$ Power ·45695 = ¯1·659871

I 2   *Note*

Note, When the Index of the Logarithm is negative, and cannot be divided by a given Number without a Remainder, a new Index must be assumed, equal to the former, which will admit of an equal Division without any Remainder. As in the last Example, the Index 2 (being negative) cannot be divided by 4 without a Remainder, therefore it is changed to ·4 + 2 = 2, and so the Log. will be (with its new Index annexed to it) ·4 + 2 639487, which divided by 4, quotes the Log. ·1 659871.

Prob XVI

To extract the Root of any Power.

Rule.

Divide the Logarithm of the Power by the Index of the Root, the Quotient shall be the Log. of the Root required.

Example I.

What is the Square Root of 2304?

| Divide the Logarithm of | 2304 = 3·362482 |
| By the Index of the Root | 2 |

The Quotient is the Log of the Root 48 = 1 681241

Example II.

What is the Cube Root of 64?

| Divide the Log of | 64 = 1·806180 |
| By the Index of the Root | 3 |

The Quot. is the Log. Root 4 = 0·602060

Sect. II.   ARITHMETIC.   61

EXAMPLE III.

What is the $\frac{1}{4}$ Root of the Power 1·8612, &c ?

The Log of ——— 18612 = 0·269795
Which divided by the Index of Root $\frac{1}{4}$

The Quot is the Log. of the $\frac{1}{4}$ Root 12 = 1·079181

EXAMPLE IV.

What is the $6\frac{2}{3}$ Root of 1516·3, &c ?

The Log. of ——— 1516·3, &c. = 3·180807
Which divided by the Index $6\frac{2}{3}$

The Quot is the Log of the $6\frac{2}{3}$ Root 3 = 0·477121

EXAMPLE V.

What is the $\frac{1}{4}$ Root of 45695, &c. ?

The Log. of ——— 45695, &c. = ·1·659871
Which divided by the Index $\frac{1}{4}$

The Quot is the Log of the $\frac{1}{4}$ Root 0436 = 2·639487

SECT. III

The CONSTRUCTION *and* USE *of the* LOGISTICAL LOGARITHMS.

THE Logistical Logarithms were first of all invented by Mr *Jeremiah Shakerly*, as may be seen in his *Tabulæ Britannicæ;* and afterwards improved

proved by Mr *Thomas Street*, who in his *Astronomia Carolina* hath compiled a much more convenient Form of Logistical Logarithms than those of *Shakerly*.

These Sort of Logarithms are principally used in Astronomical Calculations, in working Proportions of Degrees, Minutes, and Seconds, but more especially of Minutes and Seconds. They may be also applied to finding the Proportional Parts of the Logarithms of Artificial Sines, Tangents, and Secants.

PROB XVII

To find the Logistical Logarithm for any Number of Degrees, Minutes and Seconds, in Shakerly's *Form*

RULE.

From the Logarithm of the given Degrees, Minutes, and Seconds, (reduced to Seconds) subtract the constant Logarithm 3 556302 (= Log. of 1° or 60' or 3600"), the Remainder will be the Logistical Logarithm of those Degrees, Min. &c.

The Reason of the above Rule is easily accounted for For supposing any Proportion, as 60' . 4' — 45" . . 44' — 23" 3' — 30" $\frac{197}{240}$; now reducing these to Seconds, it will be as 3600" 285" . : 2663" . 210" $\frac{197}{240}$; wherefore it is evident that these Proportions may be wrought by the common Logarithms, by subtracting the Log. of the first Term from the Sum of the Logs. of the second and third, the Remainder is the Log.

Sect. II.   ARITHMETIC.   63

Log. of the fourth Term; or otherwise, use the Complement Arithmetical of the first Term, and then the Whole may be added.

Now to shorten the Work, let the following Proportion, according to *Shakerly*'s Form, be made Use of, which by the Logarithms is thus

As the Logarithm of	$3600'$	$= 3556302$
To the Logarithm of	$285''$	$= 2454845$
So is the Log. of Radius	100000, &c.	$= 10000000$
To the Log. of	$\cdot 079166$, &c.	$= 8898543$

By the Nature of Proportion it is evident, that the two last Terms have the same Proportion one to the other as the two first, and likewise the same Properties, and consequently will in every Respect where Proportion is concerned, equally answer the same Purposes as the two first, and therefore the Logarithms of the two last may be put to represent the Logarithms of the two first Terms, that is, the Log. of Radius 10000000 is reputed the Logistical Logarithm of $3600''$ ($= 1°$) and the Log. $\cdot 8898543$ is the Logistical Logarithm of $285''$ ($= 4' - 45''$) And therefore it is plain, that the Logistical Logarithm of any Number of Degrees, Minutes, and Seconds may be found, by subtracting the constant Log. $3 \cdot 556302$ ($=$ Log of $1°$ in Seconds) from the Log. of the given Degrees, Minutes, and Seconds (reduc'd to Seconds), the Remainder will be the Logistical Log thereof.

Ex-

Example I.

Required the Logistical Logarithm of $53' - 21''$.

From the Log of $53' - 21'' = 3201'' = 3.505286$
Take the Log of $1° = 60' = 3600'' = 3.556302$

Rem is the Logist Log. $53' - 21'' = 3201 = 9.948984$

Example II.

Required the Logist. Log. of $3° - 10'$.

From the Log of $3° - 10' - 0'' = 11400'' = 4.056905$
Subt. the Log of $1° - 0' - 0'' = 3600 = 3.556302$

Rems. the Logist. Log $\rbrace$ $3° - 10' - 0'' = 11400 = 10.500603$

After this Method you may easily find the Logistical Log for any Degr. Min. and Sec. in *Shakerly*'s Form, and it is thus he hath compiled his Table

These Logarithms will serve equally as well in the Calculation of Time as Motion, as $60'$ or $3600''$ are equal to one Hour, as well as one Degree.

These Logistical Logarithms of Mr *Shakerly* consisting of a great many Places of Figures throughout the whole Table, gave Occasion to Mr *Street* to contrive a much more convenient and compendious Form of these Logarithms.

PROB.

Prob XVIII.

To find the Logistical Logarithm for any Number of Degrees, Minutes and Seconds, in Street's *Form.*

Rule.

Reduce the given Degrees, Minutes and Seconds into Seconds, subtract the common Logarithm of these Seconds from the constant common Logarithm 3.556302 (viz. the Log of 1° or 3600″) the Remainder is the Logistical Logarithm required.

The Reason of this Rule is evidently demonstrated thus. Suppose any Proportion in Sexagesimal Numbers, as that before made Use of in the last Prob. viz. as 3600″ 285″ . 2663″ : 210″ $\frac{197}{240}$, and according to Mr *Street*'s Method, let the two first Terms of the Analogy be inverted, then it will be as 285″ . 3600″ : . Unity a fourth Number, whose Logarithm is the Logistical Logarithm of the first Term 285″, as also is the Logarithm of Unity the Logistical Logarithm of the second Term 3600″. See the Work at large by the Logarithms.

As the Log. of   4′ 45″ = 285″ = 2.454845
To the Log. of   1° = 60′ = 3600″ = 3.556302
So is the Log. of Unity   ———   0.000000
                                    ———————
To the Logist. Log. of 4′ 45″ = 285″ = 1.101457

From the above Analogy it is apparent, that the Logiſtical Logarithm for any Number of Seconds is obtained, by ſubtracting the common Logarithm of thoſe Seconds from the conſtant common Logarithm of 3600″, the Remainder is the Logiſtical Logarithm required.

But if the Logiſtical Logarithm be required for any Number of Seconds greater than 3600′, then ſubtract the common Logarithm of 3600″ from the common Logarithm of the given Seconds; the Remainder is the Logiſtical Logarithm of thoſe Seconds. And thus may a Table of theſe Logiſtical Logarithms be continued to any Length; as that in Vol 2. of Mr *Leadbetter*'s *Complete Syſtem of Aſtronomy*, which is extended to 2 Degrees, or 120 Minutes.

From the above Analogy may be diſcovered, that the greater the Number of Seconds is, the leſs will be its Logiſtical Logarithm, till it arrive at 3600″, whoſe Logiſtical Logarithm will be nothing.

EXAMPLE I.

Required the Logiſtical Logarithm of 53′ 21″.

From the Logarithm of   3600″ = 3 556302
Subtract the Log of   53′ 21′ = 3201 = 3 505286
Remains Logiſt Log. of 53′ 21 = 3201″ =   51016

Ex-

Sect. III.   ARITHMETIC.   67

EXAMPLE II.

Required the Logistical Logarithm of 104′ 36″

From the Log. of   104′ 36″ = 6276″ = 3 797683
Take the constant Log. of   3600 = 3 556302

Remains the Logist. Log. of 104′ 36″ =   241381

Note, In forming these Logarithms it is to be observed, that the Index is never separated from the Logarithm by a Point, as is the Case in the common Logarithms, but the Whole (both Index and Logarithm) is accounted as one complete Logistical Logarithm. Also in Tables of these Sort of Logarithms, two Places of Figures are cut off on the right Hand of the Logarithms, the other being sufficient for any Purpose relating thereto.

The Table of Logistical Logarithms inserted at the End of the Tables of Logarithmic Sines and Tangents, I have continued to 60′ or 1°, that being sufficient for any Purpose thereof.

As to the Form of the Table, that is very easy to understand, being constructed upon the same Model with that of the Sines and Tangents. The first Column contains Degrees or Minutes, or Minutes and Seconds by Way of Tens, having the nine Digits running along in a Column on the Top, under which, in the several Columns, are the Logistical Logarithms abbreviated. The last Column contains the Numbers of the first reduced to Minutes or Seconds, which are to be com-

K 2   pleated

pleated by the Digits on the Top of the Table; and which are to be referr'd to, in finding the Logiſtical Logarithm for any Integral Number

This Table will likewiſe ſerve in the Computation of Time as well as Motion, by Means of the Table at the End thereof, which gives by Inſpection the Hours and Minutes correſponding to any Parts of Motion, and vice verſa Thus againſt 12 Min. in Time is 30 Min. in Motion; againſt $4^h\ 23'$ in Time is $10°\ 00' + 0°\ 58' = 10°\ 58'$ in Motion; alſo againſt $55°\ 43'$ in Motion $22^h + 17' = 22^h\ 17'$ in Time, &c.

The Method of conſtructing Logiſtical Logarithms being plainly and clearly demonſtrated, it remains now to ſhew their Uſe in Practical Aſtronomy, in which they are chiefly concerned. The following Examples will make all plain.

Example III.

Suppoſe the Sun's mean Anomaly be $5^s\ 10°\ 33'$ and $46''$; what is the true Equation and Logarithm of his Diſtance from the Earth?

Mean A-nomalies	$5^s\ 10°$ $5\ \ 11$	Equa-tions	$0°\ 40'\ 34''$ $0\ \ 38\ \ 37$	Lo-gar.	4.993055 4.993009
Differen.	$0\ \ \ 1 = 60'$		$1\ \ 57$		46

Then for the Proportional Parts of the Equation.

As one Degree, or	——	$60'\ 00'' =$	0
Is to the Diff Equat.	——	$1\ \ 57 =$	14881
So is the Anomaly	——	$33\ \ 46 =$	2497
To the Proportional Part		$1\ \ \ 6 =$	17378

Then

Sect. III.   ARITHMETIC.   69

Then 0° 40′ 34″ − 1′ 6″ (because the Equation is decreasing) = 0° 39′ 28″ = the true Equation required.

Then for the Proportional Part of the Logarithm, it will be

As one Degree, or ——— 60′ 00″ = 0
To Differ. Logarithms ——— 46 = 18935
So is the Anom. ——— 33 46 = 2497

To the Proportional Part ——— 26 = 21432

Then 4·993053 − 26 (because the Logarithm is decreasing) = 4·993027 = the true Logarithm of the Sun's Distance from the Earth, as required.

The Use of these Logarithms might be further shewn, in working Proportions relating to other Particulars in Practical Arithmetic; but as these are foreign to our present Purpose, I shall pass them by, and proceed to apply the Logistical Logarithms to the finding the common Logarithms of such Numbers as exceed the Verge of the Tables, as also the Logarithmic Sine, Tangent, &c. for any Number of Degrees, Minutes, Seconds, &c. and vice versa.

EXAMPLE IV.

Required the common Logarithm of 6438764.

Numbers $\begin{Bmatrix}6438000\\6439000\end{Bmatrix}$ Logarithms $\begin{Bmatrix}6·808751\\6·808818\end{Bmatrix}$

Differ.   1000   67

Then

Then say,

As Differ Numbers	——	1000 = 5563
To Differ. Logarithms	——	67 = 17302
So Number	—— ——	764 = 6732
		24034
To the Proportional Part		51 = 18471

Then 6·808751 + 51 = 6 808802 = the complete Log. of 6438764, as required.

EXAMPLE V.

Required the correspondent Number to the common Logarithm 6 808802.

Given Log.	—— ——	6 808802
Log next less is of	6438000 =	6 808751
Differ. of the Logs.	—— ——	51
The Log next less is of	6438000 =	6·808751
The Log next greater is of	6439000 =	6·808818
Differences	——	1000 = 67

Then say,

As Diff. lesser and greater Logs	67 =	17302
To Diff their correspondent Numb.	1000 =	5563
So Diff. given Log. and the next less	51 =	18471
		24034
To the Proportional Part	764 =	6732

Which

Sect. III.   ARITHMETIC.   71

Which being annexed to the four Figures 6438 before found, will be = 6438764 = the true Number belonging the given Logarithm.

Example VI.

Required the Log. Sine of 24° 48′ 51″ 43‴.

Sine of $\begin{Bmatrix}24° & 48′\\ 24 & 49\end{Bmatrix}$ Logarithms $\begin{Bmatrix}9\ 622682\\ 9\ 622956\end{Bmatrix}$

Differ.   0   1 = 60″   274

Then to find the Proportional Part of the Log. for the 51″ 43‴, it will be by the Logist Logarithms,

As 1 Minute, or   ———   60′ 00″ =   0
To Differ of the Logarithms   274 = 11186
So is   ———   ———   51″ 43‴ =   645

To the Propor Part of the Log.   236 = 11831

Then 9 622682 + 236 = 9·622918 = the Log. Sine of 24° 48′ 51″ 43‴.

Example VII.

Given the Log. Sine 9 622918, to find the Arc

The given Log Sine is   ———   9·622918
The Log. Sine next less is of 24° 48′ = 9·622682

Difference   ———   ———   236

Next greater Log. Sine is of 24° 49′ = 9·622956

Difference greater and less Logs. 0   1 = 60″   274

Then

Then

As Diff. greater and lefs Logs.   274 = 11186
To 1 Minute, or   ——   60ʺ =   0
So Diff. given Log. and the next lefs 236 = 11831

To the Proportional Part —— 51ʺ 43‴ = 645

Which added to 24° 48′ (firſt found) the Sum 24° 48′ 51ʺ 43‴ is the Quantity of the Arc.

SECT. IV

DUODECIMAL ARITHMETIC, *performed Numerically and Logarithmically.*

PROB XIX.

To multiply Duodecimal Numbers together.

RULE I.

FEET multiplied by Feet give Feet.
    Feet multiplied by Inches give Inches.
Feet multiplied by Seconds give Seconds.
Inches multiplied by Inches give Seconds.
Inches multiplied by Seconds give Thirds.
Seconds multiplied by Seconds give Fourths, &c.

Note, To work Examples of this Kind by the Logarithms, it is neceſſary to reduce Numbers of lower Denominations than Feet, to the Decimal Part thereof; and therefore

Sect. IV. ARITHMETIC. 73

therefore to avoid the Trouble of reducing, I have subjoined the following Table, which gives by Inspection the Decimal of any Number of Primes, Seconds, and Thirds, a Foot being the Integer.

The Duodecimal Table.

Duode- cimals.	Decimal Parts		
	Primes ′	Seconds ″	Thirds ‴
1	·083333	·006944	·000578
2	·166666	·013888	·001157
3	·25	·020833	·001736
4	·333333	·027777	·002314
5	·416666	·034722	·002893
6	·5	·041666	·003472
7	·583333	·048611	·004051
8	·666666	·055555	·004629
9	·75	·0625	·005208
10	·833333	·069444	·005787
11	·916666	·076388	·006365

EXAMPLE I.

Multiply 7^f 5′ by 4^f 6′ ′   8^f 3′ by 6^f 8′.

1. Numerically.

```
   7f 5′            8f 3′
   4  6             6  8
  ─────            ─────
  29  8            49  6
   3  8 6″          5  6
  ─────            ─────
  33  4  6         55  0
```

L 2. Lo-

2 Logarithmically

Add $\begin{cases} \text{The Log. of } 7^f\ 5' = 7\cdot 4166 = 0\cdot 870205 \\ \text{The Log of } 4\ 6 = 4\cdot 5\ \ \ = 0\cdot 653212 \end{cases}$

The Sum is the Log. of $\quad 33\cdot 375 = 1\cdot 523417$

The Log of $\quad\quad\quad 8^f\ 3' = 8\cdot 25\ \ = 0\cdot 916454$
The Log of $\quad\quad\quad 6\ 8 = 6\cdot 6666 = 0\cdot 823904$

The Sum is the Log. of $\quad\quad 55\quad\quad = 1\cdot 740358$

EXAMPLE II.

Multiply $10^f\ 11'\ 3''\ 5'''$ by $5^f\ 7'\ 4''\ 8'''$.

1 Numerically.

$$\begin{array}{r} 10^f\ 11'\ 3''\ 5'' \\ 5\ \ 7\ \ 4\ \ 8 \\ \hline 54\ \ 8\ \ 5\ \ 1\ \\ 6\ \ 4\ \ 6\ 11\ \ 11^{4''} \\ 3\ \ 7\ 9\ \ 1\ \ 8^5 \\ 7\ 3\ \ 6\ 3\ \ 4^6 \\ \hline 61\ \ 5\ \ 3\ \ 1\ \ 6\ 11\ \ 4^6 \end{array}$$

2. Logarithmically.

The Log of $10^f\ 11'\ 3''\ 5''' = 10\cdot 940 = 1\cdot 039017$
The Log. of $\ \ 5\ \ 7\ \ 4\ \ 8 = 5\cdot 6157 = 0\cdot 749404$

The Sum is the Log. of $\quad\quad 61\ 435 = 1\cdot 788421$

Note,

Sect. IV.   ARITHMETIC.   75

Note, If the Number of Feet in one or both of the Factors happen to be large, instead of multiplying by the Inches, Seconds, &c. take Parts and work therewith, as in the Rule of Practice.

EXAMPLE III, IV

	Multiply	68ᶠ 4′				84ᶠ 7′	
	By	46 9				58 10	
		3128 0				4872 0	
4 is ⅓	15 4		6 is ½	29 0
6 — ½	34 2		1 — ⅙	4 10
3 — ½	17 1		6 — ½	42 3 6
				4 — ⅓	28 2 4
	3194 7			4976 3 10

Logarithmically.

The Log. of   68ᶠ 4′ = 68.333 = 1.834630
The Log. of   46 9 = 46.75 = 1.669782
The Sum is the Log. of   3194.58 = 3.504412

The Log. of   84ᶠ 7′ = 84.583 = 1.927283
The Log. of   58 10 = 58.833 = 1.769621
The Sum is the Log. of   4976.32 = 3.696904

L 2   RULE

Rule II.

If Yards be introduced into the Question, the Work is the same as before, only when you are working with the Yards and Feet you must have Respect to Threes instead of Twelves, because three Feet are (in this Respect) to be reckoned equal to one Yard.

Example V, VI.

```
Multiply  3ʸ 2ᶠ 4′              43ʸ 1ᶠ 8′
By         2  1  3                6  2  5
          ─────────             ─────────
           7  1  8               261  1  0
1 is ⅓   1  0  9  4″   1 is ⅓   14  1  6  8′
3 — ¼    0  0 11  4    1 — ⅓   14  1  6  8
          ─────────    4 — ⅓    4  2  6  2  8′
           9  0  4  8  1 — ¼    1  0  7  6  8
                                ─────────────
                                296  1  3  1  4
```

Logarithmically.

The Log. of	3ʸ 2ᶠ 4′ =	3·7777 =	0·577227
The Log. of	2 1 3 =	2·4166 =	0·383205
The Sum is the Log. of		9·1292 =	0·960432
The Log of	43ʸ 1ᶠ 8′ =	43·555 =	1·639038
The Log of	6 2 5 =	6·8055 =	0·832860
The Sum is the Log of		296·41 =	2·471890

Sect. IV.   ARITHMETIC.   77

EXAMPLE VII, VIII.

Multiply 96ʸ 1ᶠ 6ʹ   64ʸ 2ᶠ 0ʹ
By   48 2 8   36 1 4
          ─────────   ─────────
          4608 0 0   2304 0 0
1 is ⅓   16   0 0   2 is ⅔ 24   0 0
6 — ½   8   0 0   1 — ⅓   21   1 8
1 — ⅓   32   0 6   4 — ⅓   7   0 6 8ʹ
1 — ⅓   32   0 6   ─────────────
4 — ⅓   10   2 2   2356 2 2 8
4 — ⅓   10   2 2
          ─────────
          4717 2 4

Logarithmically

The Log. of   96ʸ 1ᶠ 6ʹ = 96·5   = 1·984527
The Log. of   48 2 8 = 48·888 = 1·689202
                                      ─────────
The Sum is the Log. of   4717·7 = 3·673729

The Log. of   64ʸ 2ᶠ 0ʹ = 64·666 = 1·810676
The Log. of   36 1 4 = 36·444 = 1·561626
                                      ─────────
The Sum is the Log of   2356·6, &c. = 3·372302

PROB. XX

To divide Duodecimal Numbers one by another

RULE.

If the Dividend and Divisor be both compound Numbers, Division is most conveniently performed by the

the Logarithms, for otherwise the Numbers must be reduced into their least Terms; after which divide as in Division of simple Integers But if the Divisor be a simple Number, then divide your compound Dividend thereby, according to the Method of Compound Division of Integers. A few Examples will clear up all

Example I.

What is the Quote of 46ᶠ 3′ 8″ by 8?

1. By natural Numbers

8) 46ᶠ 3′ 8″
―――――――
  5 9 5 6″ the Quotient.

2. By the Logarithms.

From the Log. of   46ᶠ 3′ 8″ = 46 305 = 1·665628
Subtract the Log of   8   = 0 903090
―――――――――――――――――――――――――――――――
Remains the Quote   5 7881 = 0 762538

Example II.

Divide 14ᶠ 4′ 7″ by 3ᶠ 8′ 10″.

By the Logarithms.

From the Log. of   14ᶠ 4′ 7″ = 14 333 = 1·156337
Take the Log. of   3 8 10 = 3 7361 = 0 572418
―――――――――――――――――――――――――――――――
Remainder is the Quotient   = 3·8363 = 0·583919

Example III.

What is the Quote of 8′ 3″ by 3ᶠ 6′ 4″.

By the Logarithms.

From the Log of   8′ 3″ = 0·6875 = 1·837273
Subtract the Log. of 3ᶠ 6′ 4″ = 3 5277 = 0 547492

Remains the Log. Quote   0 019488 = 2 289781

Prob XXI

To involve Duodecimals to any Power.

Rule

' To perform this by natural Numbers is a most laborious and troublesome Piece of Work, I shall therefore omit that, and proceed to shew how completely Duodecimals may be involved by the Logarithms, and which is wholly effected by the Rule in Prob. 15.

Example I.

Involve 8ᶠ 4′ 6′ 7″ to the Square or 2d Power.

The Log of 8ᶠ 4′ 6″ 7″   = 8·3790 = 0·923192
Multiplied by the Index of the Power   2

The Product is the Log. of   70 208 = 1 846384

Example II.

Involve $2^f\ 3'\ 8''\ 5'''$ to the Cube or third Power.

The Log of $2^f\ 3'\ 8''\ 5'''$ $= 2{\cdot}3084 = 0{\cdot}363311$
Multiply by the Index of the Power $\qquad\qquad 3$

The Prod is the Log of the Cube $12{\cdot}301 = 1{\cdot}089933$

Then $12{\cdot}301 = 12^f\ 3'\ 7''\ 4'''$ the required Cube

Prob XXII.

To extract the Root of any Power of a Duodecimal.

Rule.

This is best performed by the Logarithms, according to the Rule in Prob 16.

Example I.

What is the Square Root of $70^f\ 2'\ 5''\ 11''' —$?

The Log of $70^f\ 2'\ 5''\ 11''' — = 70{\cdot}208 = 1{\cdot}846384$
Which divide by the Index $\qquad\qquad 2$

The Quote is the Log. of the Root $8{\cdot}379 = 0{\cdot}923192$

Then $8{\cdot}379 = 8^f\ 4'\ 6''\ 7'''$ the required Root.

Example II.

Required the Cube Root of $12^f\ 3'\ 7''\ 4''' —$.

The Log of $12^f\ 3'\ 7''\ 4''' — = 12{\cdot}301 = 1{\cdot}089933$
Which divided by $\qquad\qquad\qquad 3$

The Quote is the Log. of $\qquad 2{\cdot}3084 = 0{\cdot}363311$

Then $2{\cdot}3084 = 2^f\ 3'\ 8''\ 5'''$ the Root sought.

SECT.

SECT. V.

Mensuration *of* Superficies.

Prob. XXIII

To menfure a Square.

Rule I.

MULTIPLY the Side into itfelf, and the Product is the Area of the fame Name with the Dimenfions.

Now suppofe $a = BC = CD = BI = DI$. Then $a \times a = aa = a^2 =$ Area $\square\ BCDI$. (Fig. 29)

Example I.

Suppofe the Side of a Square be 12 Feet 6 Inches, required the Area thereof.

1. Arithmetically.

$12.5 \times 12.5 = 156.25 =$ the Area.

Or thus:

```
  12ᶠ   6ⁱ
  12    6
  ─────────
  156   3 = the Area as above.
```

M 2. Lo-

2. Logarithmically.

The Log. of the Side   12ᶠ 6ˡ 125 = 1·096910
Multiply by   ———   ———   2

The Prod is the Log of the Area 156·25 = 2·193820

3. By the Sliding Rule.

  A   B   A   B
As 1   12·5   125 . 15625 the Area.

Rule II.

When the Area is in square Links, to bring these into Acres divide them by 100000 (= the square Links in an Acre) which is only cutting off 5 Places of Figures on the left Hand, and the remaining Figures on the right will be Acres, and those cut off Decimal Parts of an Acre, whose Value find by multiplying them by 4 and 40, for the Roods and Poles.

Or thus, which is better:

When the Side of the Square is given in Links, multiply the Double of the Side by the Side, so is the Product the double Area, in which make a Point between the 4th and 5th, and 5th and 6th Places of Figures from the right Hand towards the left, then Half the Sum cut off on the left Hand of the last Point will be Acres, and the Remainder (if any) will be two Roods or Half an Acre, then observe, if the Figure between the Points be 5 or above, subtract 5 from it, which must be called a Rood more, and the Re-

Sect. V.   Of SUPERFICIES.

Remainder (if any) multiply by 8 (taking Care to carry to the Product the Increase from the Figures first cut off) is the Poles. Then to know the Value of the four Figures first cut off, multiply them by 8, so shall the Product (the Increase being carried forward, as before directed) be the Decimal Part of a Pole.

Note, The latter Part of this Rule can only be applied, when the first Product or double Area is in square Links, and then it is preferable to the first Method.

EXAMPLE II.

Suppose the Side of a square Field = 8 Chains 64 Links (= 864 Links), how many Acres are contained therein?

1. Arithmetically.

864 × 864 = 746496, which properly reduced is 7 Acres, 1 Rood, 34·39360 Poles, according to the first Part of the Rule.

Then 864 × 2 × 864 = 1492992 Links, which reduced according to the latter Part of the same Rule, will be = 7 Acres, 1 Rood, 34·3936 Poles, the same as before.

2. Logarithmically.

The Log. of 864	= 2·936514
Multiply by	2
Product is the Log of 746496	5·873028
The Log. of 100000 subtract	5·000000
Remains the Log. of 7·46496 Acres	0·873028

3. By the Sliding Rule.

$$\text{As } \begin{array}{cc} A & B \\ 10 . 8\cdot64 \end{array} :: \begin{array}{cc} A & B \\ 8\cdot64 & 7\cdot46 \end{array}, \&c. \text{ Acres.}$$

Prob. XXIV.

To measure a Parallelogram.

Rule I.

Multiply the Length and Breadth together, and the Product is the Area.

Suppose $a = CD$, and $b = DE$; then $a \times b = ab =$ the Area of the Parallelogram $CDEF$. (Fig 30)

Example I.

Suppose a Board 18 Feet 4 Inches long and 2 Feet 8 Inches broad; how many square or superficial Feet are therein?

1. Arithmetically.

$18\cdot33$, &c. $\times 2\cdot66$, &c. $= 48\cdot7578$ Feet the Area.

Or thus

$18^f\ 4^i \times 2^f\ 8^i = 48^f\ 10^i\ 8p$ the Area.

2. Logarithmically

The Log of	——	$18\cdot33 = 1\cdot263162$
The Log of	——	$2\cdot66 = 1\cdot424882$
The Sum is the Log. of		$48\cdot7578 = 2\cdot688044$

Then $48\cdot7578 = 48^f\ 10^i\ 8p$ the same as above

3. By

Sect V.   *Of* Superficies.   85

3. By the Sliding Rule.

    A   B   A   B
As 1   18·33 . . 2·66 : 48·75, &c. the Area.

Rule II.

Multiply the Length in Feet by the Breadth in Inches, or the Breadth in Feet by the Length in Inches, the Product divided by 12 is the Area in Feet.

Example II.

Suppose a Board 15 Feet 6 Inches long, and 9¼ Inches broad, how many Feet are therein?

1. Arithmetically.

$$\frac{15·5 \times 9·25}{12} = 11·948 + \text{Feet the Area.}$$

Or thus

$15^f\ 6^i \times 0^f\ 9^i\ 3p = 11^f\ 11^i\ 4p\ 6^\circ$ the Area

2. Logarithmically.

The Log of 15 Feet, 6 Inches, = 15·5 = 1·190332
The Log. of 9¼ Inches   = 9·25 = 0·966142
The Comp. Arith. of the Log. of = 12·0 = 8·920819

Sum is the Log. of   11·948 +, = 1·077293

3. By the Sliding Rule.

    A   B   A   B
As 12 : 15·5 : : 9·25 : 11·94, &c. Feet.

Rule

Rule III.

Multiply the Length in Inches by the Breadth in Inches, and divide the Product by 144 for Feet

Example III.

Suppose a Window $68\frac{1}{2}$ Inches long, and $38\frac{1}{4}$ high, how many Feet of Glass are therein?

1. Arithmetically.

$$\frac{68\frac{1}{2} \times 38\frac{1}{4}}{144} = 18\frac{25}{128} \text{ Feet, the Area}$$

2. Logarithmically.

The $\begin{cases} \text{Log of the Length} & 68\frac{1}{2} = 1\cdot835691 \\ \text{Log of the Breadth} & 38\frac{1}{4} = 1\cdot582631 \\ \text{Comp Arithmet. of} & 144 = 7\cdot841638 \end{cases}$

The Sum is the Log of the Area $= 18\frac{25}{128} = 1\cdot259960$

By the Sliding Rule

$$\begin{array}{cccc} A & B & A & B \\ \text{As } 144 : & 68\frac{1}{2} & 38\frac{1}{4} \cdot & 16\frac{1}{5} \end{array}$$ nearly, the Area.

Prob XXV.

To find the Length or Breadth of a Parallelogram, having the Area and Breadth, or the Area and Length respectively given.

Rule I.

The Area divided by the Breadth gives the Length.

Then

Sect. V.   *Of* Superficies.   87

Then suppose $x =$ the Area, $b =$ the Breadth, and $a =$ the Length; then is $\frac{x}{b} = a =$ the Length.

Example I.

Suppose the Breadth of a Board $= 9\frac{1}{4}$ Inches, and the Area $= 11'948$, &c. square Feet; required the Length in Feet.

1. Arithmetically.

$\frac{11'948}{0'77083} = 15'5 = 15$ Feet, 6 Inch. $=$ Length

2. Logarithmically.

The Log of the Area $= 11'948 = 1'077293$
The Log of the Breadth $9\frac{1}{4}$ Inches $= '77083 = \overline{\cdot 1'886961}$

Rem is the Log. of the Length $= 15'5 = 1'190332$

3. By the Sliding Rule.

A   B   A   B
As 0'77, &c. : 1 :: 11'948 : 15'5 the Length.

Rule II.

The Quote of the Area by the Length is the Breadth. For put $x =$ the Area, $a =$ the Length, and $b =$ the Breadth, then is $\frac{x}{a} = b =$ the Breadth

Ex-

Example II.

Suppose a Field 11 Chains, 46 Links long, what Breadth must be taken to make $2\frac{1}{2}$ Acres?

1. Arithmetically.

$\frac{250000}{1146}$ = 2 18 15 Links, = 2 Chains, 18 15 Links the required Breadth.

2. Logarithmically.

The Log. of $\begin{cases} 2\frac{1}{2} \text{ Acres} = 25^{ch} = 1\cdot397940 \\ 11 \text{ Ch. } 46\text{ Links} = 11\cdot46 = 1\cdot059185 \end{cases}$

Remainder is the Log. of $= 2\cdot1815 = 0\cdot338755$

3. By the Sliding Rule.

    A   B   A   B
As 11·46 . 1 . . 25 : 2·18 — Chains the Breadth.

Prob. XXVI.

To measure a Rhombus.

Rule.

Multiply the Length of one of its Sides by the Perpendicular let fall from the obtuse Angle upon the opposite Side, and the Product is the Area.

For making BC ($= CD = DE = EB$) $= a$, and the Perpendicular $BF = b$, then will $a \times b = ab =$ the Area of $BCDE$. (Fig. 11.)

Sect V.   *Of* SUPERFICIES.   89

EXAMPLE

Suppose the Side of a Rhombus = 12 Yards, 1 Foot, and 3 Inches, and the perpendicular Breadth = 4 Yards, 2 Feet, 7 Inches, how many Yards are therein?

1. Arithmetically

12 Yards, 1 Foot, 3 Inches, = 12.4166, &c Yards; also 4 Yards, 2 Feet, 7 Inches, = 4.8611, &c Yards. Then 12.4166 × 4.8611 = 60.35833426 Yards the Area.

Or thus

12^y 1^f 3^i × 4^y 2^f 7^i = 60^y 1^f 0^i 11^s the Area.

2. Logarithmically.

The Log. of $\begin{cases} 12\cdot416 \text{ is} \\ 4\cdot8611 \text{ is} \end{cases}$ = 1·093982
                                    = 0·686734

Sum is the Log. of 60.35, &c. Yds.   = 1.780716

3 By the Sliding Rule.

   A   B   A   B
A 1 : 12·416 :: 4·8611 : 60·35 Yards, the same as above.

PROB XXVII

To measure a Rhomboides, or an oblique-angled Parallelogram.

RULE.

Multiply one of its longest Sides by the Perpendicular

cular let fall from one of the obtuse Angles, and the Product is the Area thereof.

For put $a = AB (= CD)$ and $b = AE$, then $a \times b = ab =$ the Area. (FIG. 12.)

EXAMPLE.

Given the longest Side of a Rhomboides = 14 Chains, 35 Links, and the perpendicular Breadth = 6 Ch. 60 Links, how many Acres are therein?

1. Arithmetically.

1435 × 666 = 9 55711 Acres, = 9 Acres, 2 Roods, 9 136 Poles, = the Area.

2. Logarithmically.

The Log. of $\begin{cases} 14\ 35 \text{ Chains} & = 1\ 156852 \\ 6\ 66 \text{ Chains} & = 0\ 823474 \end{cases}$
The Comp. Arith. Log. 10 Chains $= 9\ 000000$

The Sum is the Log of 9 5571 Acres $= 0\ 980326$

3. By the Sliding Rule.

    A   B   A   B
As 10   14 35 . · 6 66   9 55, &c Acres.

PROB XXVIII.

To measure a plain Triangle.

RULE I.

Multiply Half the Base by the whole Perpendicular, or Half the Perpendicular by the whole Base, or multiply

Sect. V.   *Of* Superficies   91

multiply the Base and Perpendicular together, and take Half the Product, any of these will be the Area

Put $a = AB$ and $b = BC$, then $\frac{1}{2} a \times b = \frac{1}{2} b \times a = \frac{a \times b}{2} = \frac{a b}{2} = $ Area of the Triangle ABC (Fig 5)

Example I.

Given the Base of a Triangle 15 Feet 4 Inches, and the Perpendicular = 8 Feet 10 Inches, required the Area

1. Arithmetically.

$\frac{15^f 4^i}{2} \times 8^f 10^i = \frac{15\ 33^f}{2} \times 8\cdot83^f = \frac{8^f 10^i}{2} \times 15^f 4^i = \frac{8\ 83^f}{2} \times 15\cdot33^f = \frac{15^f 4^i \times 8^f 10^i}{2} = \frac{15\ 33^f \times 8\ 83^f}{2} = 67\ 6819^f = $ the Area $= 67^f\ 8^i\ 8^p = $ the Area of the Triangle.

2. Logarithmically.

The Log. of $\begin{cases} \text{Half the Base} & = 7\cdot67 = 0\cdot884795 \\ \text{the Perpendic.} & = 8\ 83 = 0\ 945961 \end{cases}$

The Sum is the Log of $67\cdot7 + = 1\cdot830756$

3. By the Sliding Rule.

   A   B   A   B
As 1   7 67 : 8 83   67 7 nearly = the Area of the Triangle.

Rule

Rule II.

From the Half-sum of the three Sides subtract each Side severally, the Square Root of the Product of the Half-sum and three Remainders is the Area.

Let $a = AB$, $b = BC$, and $c = AC$. (Fig 6)

Then $\frac{a+b+c}{2} - a =$ 1st Remainder; $\frac{a+b+c}{2} - b =$ 2d Remainder, and $\frac{a+b+c}{2} - c =$ 3d Remainder.

But $\frac{a+b+c}{2} - a \times \frac{a+b+c}{2} - b \times \frac{a+b+c}{2} - c : \times \frac{a+b+c}{2} = \frac{b+c-a}{2} \times \frac{a-b+c}{2} \times \frac{a+b-c}{2} \times \frac{a+b+c}{2}$

$= \frac{b+c-a \times a-b+c \times a+b-c \times a+b+c}{2 \times 2 \times 2 \times 2 = 16}$,

whose square Root

$\sqrt{\frac{b+c-a \times a-b+c \times a+b-c \times a+b+c}{2 \times 2 \times 2 \times 2 = 16}}$

$=$ the Area of the Triangle ABC.

Example II.

Suppose one Side of a Triangle $= 460$ Links, another Side $= 648$, and the third $= 850$, required the Area thereof in Acres.

1. Arithmetically.

$\sqrt{\frac{460+648+850}{2} - 460 \times \frac{460+648+850}{2} - 648}$

Sect. V.   *Of* Superficies.   93

$$\times \frac{460+648+850}{2} - 850 \times \frac{460+648+850}{2} := $$

$$\sqrt{\frac{648+850-460}{2} \times \frac{460-648+850}{2} \times \frac{460+648-850}{2}}$$

$$\times \frac{460+648+850}{2} . = \sqrt{519 \times 331 \times 129 \times 979} =$$

$\sqrt{21695404599} = 147293$ fquare Links $=$ 1 Acre, 1 Rood, 35,66880 Poles the Area.

2 Logarithmically.

The Log of the {
1ſt Remainder $519 = 5\cdot19 = 0\cdot715167$
2d $331 = 3\cdot31 = 0\cdot519828$
3d $129 = 1\cdot29 = 0\cdot110590$
Half-fum $979 = 9\cdot79 = 0\cdot990783$
}

Sum is the Log of 21695404599 Ch. $= 2\cdot336368$
Which divide by   2

The Quotient is the Log of $14\cdot7293$ Ch $= 1\cdot168184$
The Log. of 10 fubtract $= 1\cdot000000$

Remains the Log. of $1\cdot47293$ Acres $= 0\cdot168184$

3. By the Sliding Rule.

As {
A   B   A   B
1   5·19 ·· 3·31 · 17·1789
1   17·17 : 1·29 . 22·1608
A   D   A   D
9·79 9·79 · 22·1608 . 14·729 Ch. $= 1\cdot4729$
Acres.
}

Note, The Refult of the laſt Analogy is no more than a mean Proportion between 22·1608 (the Refult

of

of the second Analogy) and 9·79 (the Half-sum of the Sides). But Questions of this Kind are more conveniently solved arithmetically or logarithmically, than instrumentally.

Prob. XXIX.

To measure a Trapezium.

Rule I.

Multiply the Diagonal by Half the Sum of the Perpendiculars, and the Product is the Area.

For putting $a = DB$, $b = AE$, and $c = CF$, then $a \times \frac{b+c}{2} = \frac{ba+ca}{2} =$ the Area (Fig. 13.)

Example I.

Suppose the Diagonal of a Trapezium = 48, the one Perpendicular = 16 and the other = 24·5, required the Area.

1. Arithmetically.

$$\frac{16 + 24 \cdot 5}{2} \times 48 = \frac{\overline{16 + 24 \cdot 5} \times 48}{2} = 972 \text{ the Area.}$$

2. Logarithmically.

The Log. of $\begin{cases} \frac{16 + 24 \cdot 5}{2} & = 20\cdot 25 = 1\cdot 306425 \\ \text{Diagonal} & = 48 = 1\cdot 681241 \end{cases}$

The Sum is the Log. of the Area = 972 = 2·987666

By

Sect V.   *Of* Superficies.

3. By the Sliding Rule.

```
   A    B      A    B
As 2 · 40 5 . 48   972 = the Area
```

Rule II.

When the Dimensions are in Links, multiply the Diagonal by the Sum of the Perpendiculars, so will the Product be the double Area, which reduce by the latter Part of Rule 2, Prob. 23.

Example II.

Given the Diagonal = 1260 Links, the one Perpendicular = 584, and the other = 657, how many Acres are contained therein?

1. Arithmetically.

$\overline{584 + 657} \times 1260 = 1563660$ square Links the double Area, which reduced by Rule 2, Prob. 23, is = 7 Acres, 3 Roods, 10 9280 Poles, the true Area.

Note, The Logarithmical and Instrumental Performance hereof, being the same as that in the foregoing Example, is omitted as unnecessary.

Prob. XXX.

To measure an irregular Polygon.

Rule.

Reduce the Polygon into Triangles or Trapeziums, whose Area find by the Rules in Prob. 28, 29.

If

If therefore you put $a =$ the Base AC, $b =$ the $\perp r$ BF, $c =$ the Diagonal AD, $d =$ the $\perp r$ CG, and $e =$ the $\perp r$ EH, then $a \times \frac{b}{2} = \frac{ab}{2} =$ the Area of the $\triangle ABC$. Also $c \times \frac{d+e}{2} = \frac{cd+ce}{2} =$ Area of the Trapezium $ACDE$; then $\frac{ab}{2} + \frac{cd+ce}{2} = \frac{ab+cd+ce}{2}$ $=$ the Area of the Polygon $ABCDE$. (Fig 16)

Prob. XXXI.

To measure a regular Polygon.

Rule I.

Multiply the Perimeter (or Sum of the Sides) by the Perpendicular let fall from the Center of the Polygon to the Middle of one of its Sides, Half the Product is the Area Or, the Product of Half the Perimeter by the Perpendicular let fall from the Center, or Half the Perpendicular by the whole Perimeter, either of these will be the Area.

Now suppose $a = BC$ a Side of an Hexagon, $b = AD$ the Perpendicular let fall from the Center. (Fig 56)

Then $\frac{6a \times b}{2} = \frac{6ab}{2} = 3ab =$ Area of the Hexagon.

Example I.

Suppose the Side of a regular Hexagon to be 24 Yards,

Sect V.   *Of* S U P E R F I C I E S   97

Yards, and the Perpendicular let fall from the Center to the Middle of one of its Sides $= 16\frac{1}{2}$, required the Area.

1. Arithmetically.

$$\frac{24 \times 6 \times 16\frac{1}{2}}{2} = 24 \times 3 \times 16\frac{1}{2} = 1188 \text{ Yards, the Area}$$

2. Logarithmically.

The Log of $\begin{cases} 24 \times 3 \quad\quad\quad = 72 = 1\cdot857332 \\ 16\frac{1}{2} \quad\quad\quad\quad = 16\cdot5 = 1\cdot217484 \end{cases}$

The Sum is the Log of the Area $= 1188 = 3\cdot074816$

3. By the Sliding Rule.

$\quad$ A $\quad$ B $\quad\quad$ A $\quad$ B
As 2 . 144 : $16\frac{1}{2}$: 1188 Yards, the Area.

When the Side is only given, the Perpendicular must be found before the Area can be obtained; now if we suppose the Side BC of a regular Hexagon $= 1$, then in the right-angled plain Triangle BDA we have $BD\ (=\frac{1}{2}BC) = 0\cdot5$ and the $\angle BAD\ (=\frac{1}{2}\angle BAC$ at the Center$) = 30°$, from whence the Perpendicular AD (by Case 3 of right-angled plain Triangles) is found $= 0\cdot8660254$, and consequently the Area of the Hexagon will be $= 2\cdot59807$. Thus are the several Areas calculated in the following Table. (Fig. 56)

O   Names

Names of the Polygons.	Number of Sides	Half the ∠s at the Center.	Areas, the Sides being Unity.	Multipliers turn'd to Divisors.
Trigon	3	60° 00′	433013	2 3094
Square	4	45 00	1 000000	1 0000
Pentagon	5	36 00	1·72047	·5812
Hexagon	6	30 00	2 59807	3849
Heptagon	7	25 42	3 6340	2752
Octagon	8	22 30	4 8284	2071
Nonagon	9	20 00	6 1818	·1617
Decagon	10	18 00	7 6942	1299
Endecagon	11	16 21	8 5142	1174
Dodecagon	12	15 00	9 3301	·1071

RULE II.

Multiply the Square of the Side by the tabular Area belonging the Polygon, or divide it by the tabular Divisor, the Product or Quotient is the Area.

EXAMPLE II

Suppose the Side of a regular Octagon 40, required the Area.

1 Arithmetically.

$$40 \times 40 \times 4\,8284 = \frac{40 \times 40}{\cdot 2071} = 7725\,44, \text{ the Area.}$$

2 Logarith-

Sect. V.   *Of* Superficies.   99

2. Logarithmically.

The Log of the Side —   = 40 = 1·602060
Multiply by   2
───
The Prod is the Log. of the □ Side 1600 = 3·204120
The Log of 4 8284 (= the Tab. Mul) = 0·683803
───
The Sum is the Log of the Area 7725 44 = 3 887923

3. By the Sliding Rule

D.   B.   D.   B.
As 1   4 82 ·   40   7722 44 = the Area as above.

Prob XXXII.

Having the Diameter of a Circle given to find the Periphery, or the Periphery to find the Diameter.

Rule I.

Multiply the Diameter by 3·14159, or divide the Circumference by 3 14159, the Product in the former Case, and the Quote in the latter, will be the Circumference or Diameter.

Put d = the Diameter AC, and c = the Periphery $ABCD$. Then $d \times 3·14159 = 3 14159\, d$ = Periphery. (Fig 57)

Also $\dfrac{c}{3\ 14159}$ = the Diameter.

Exampll I.

Suppose the Diameter of a Circle = 20, required the Periphery.   1. Arith‒

1. Arithmetically

3.14159 × 20 = 62.8318 the Periphery.

2. Logarithmically

The Log of $\begin{cases} \text{the Diameter} = 20 = 1.301030 \\ \text{the Multip.} = 3.14159 = 0.497149 \end{cases}$

The Sum is the Log. of Periph. 62.8318 = 1.798179

Also,

The Log. of the $\begin{cases} \text{Periphery} \\ \text{Divisor} \end{cases}$ $\begin{matrix} 62.8318 = 1.798179 \\ 3.14159 = 0.497149 \end{matrix}$

Remains the Log. of the Diameter = 20 = 1.301030

3. By the Sliding Rule.

$\quad\quad$ A $\quad\quad$ B $\quad\quad$ A $\quad\quad\quad$ B

As $\begin{cases} 1 \quad\; 3.14159 : 20 : 62.8318 \text{ the Periph} \\ 3.14159 \;.\; 1 : 62.8318 : 20 \text{ the Diameter.} \end{cases}$

RULE II.

Multiply the Diameter by $\frac{22}{7}$ (= $3\frac{1}{7}$ = 3.1428—) or divide by $\frac{7}{22}$ (= 0.3181—), the Product or Quotient is the Periphery or Circumference. That is $d \times \frac{22}{7} = \frac{22d}{7} = 3\frac{1}{7}d = 3.1428\,d = $ the Periphery. Or $\frac{d}{.3181} = $ the Periphery the same as before.

Note, This Rule will not give as accurate an Answer as the last, though sufficient in many Cases.

EXAMPLE II.

Suppose the Diameter the same as before, required the Periphery.

1. Arith-

Sect. V.   *Of* SUPERFICIES.   101

1 Arithmetically.

$$20 \times \tfrac{22}{7} = \tfrac{20 \times 22}{7} = \tfrac{440}{7} = 62\tfrac{6}{7} = 62.8571 =\text{ the}$$

Periphery. Or $20 \div \tfrac{7}{22} = \tfrac{20}{.3181} = 62.8371$

2. Logarithmically.

The Log of the $\begin{cases}\text{Diameter } 20 \\ \text{Multiplier } \tfrac{22}{7}\end{cases}\begin{matrix}= 1.301030 \\ = 0.497125\end{matrix}$

The Sum is the Log. Periph. 62.85 &c. = 1.798355

3. By the Sliding Rule.

A.   B.   A.   B.
As 7   22   20   62.85, &c. the Periphery.

RULE III.

Divide the Periphery by $\tfrac{22}{7}$ ($= 3\tfrac{1}{7} = 3.1428-$) or multiply by $\tfrac{7}{22}$ ($= 0.3181-$), for the Diameter.

This being the Reverse of Rule II. Examples are unnecessary.

RULE IV.

Multiply the Diameter by $\tfrac{355}{113}$ ($= 3\tfrac{16}{113} = 3.1416+$), or divide by $\tfrac{113}{355}$ ($= 0.31831+$), the Product or Quote is the Periphery.

Therefore $d \times \tfrac{355}{113} = \tfrac{355d}{113} = 3\tfrac{16}{113}d = 3.1416\,d.$
$=$ the Periphery. Also $d \div \tfrac{113}{355} = \tfrac{d}{.31831} = $ the Periph.

EXAMPLE III.

Suppose the Diameter the same as before; required the Periphery.   1. Arith-

1 Arithmetically.

$$20 \times \frac{355}{113} = \frac{20 \times 355}{113} = \frac{7100}{113} = 62\frac{94}{113} = 62\cdot 8318$$

= the Periphery   Or $20 \div \frac{113}{355} = \frac{20}{0\cdot31831+} = 62\cdot 8318$
= the Periphery as above.

By what goes before it is evident, that Rules 1 and 4 give out exactly the same Answer, and differ a little from the Result of Rule 2, but the Difference is a Trifle, the former being 62.8318, and the latter 62.8571, the Difference is only 0.0253.

2 Logarithmically.

The Log of the $\begin{cases}\text{Diameter} & 20 = 1\cdot 301030 \\ \text{Multiplier} & \frac{355}{113} = 0\cdot 497150\end{cases}$

The Sum is the Log. Periph   62.8318 = 1.798180

3. By the Sliding Rule.

$\quad$ A $\quad$ B $\quad\quad$ A. $\quad$ B.
As 113 . 355 :   20 . 62.8318 the Periphery.

RULE V.

Divide the Periphery by $\frac{355}{113}$ (= $3\frac{16}{113}$ = 3.1416), or multiply by $\frac{113}{355}$ (= 0.31831 +), the Quote or Product is the Diameter. *Note*, As this is just the Reverse of the last Rule, Examples are needless.

PROB.

Sect. V.   *Of* Superficies.   103

Prob XXXIII

To find the Area of a Circle, by having the Diameter and Periphery given.

Rule

Multiply half the Periphery by half the Diameter, or multiply the Periphery and Diameter together and divide the Product by 4, either of these will give the Area.

Put $d = AC =$ the Diameter, and $p = ABCD =$ the Periphery or Circumference, then $\frac{d}{2} \times \frac{p}{2} = \frac{d \times p}{4} = \frac{dp}{4} =$ the Area. (Fig 57)

Example

Suppose the Diameter of a Circle $= 24$, and the Periphery $= 75\frac{3}{7}$, required the Area.

1. Arithmetically.

$$\frac{75\frac{3}{7}}{2} \times \frac{24}{2} = \frac{377}{10} \times \frac{24}{2} = \frac{377 \times 24}{20} = \frac{9048}{20} = 452\frac{2}{5} =$$
the Area.

2. Logarithmically.

The Log of $\begin{cases} \text{Half the Diam. } \left(\frac{24}{2}\right) & = 1{\cdot}079181 \\ \text{Half the Perip } \left(\frac{75\frac{3}{7}}{2}\right) & = 1{\cdot}576341 \end{cases}$

The Sum is the Log. of the Area $452\frac{2}{5} = 2{\cdot}655522$

By

3. By the Sliding Rule.

```
 A.   B     A.     B.
As 4 : 24 ·· 75·4   452·4 = the Area.
```

Prob. XXXIV

The Diameter of a Circle given, to find the Area.

Rule I

Multiply the Square of the Diameter by 0·7854 (= the Area of a Circle whose Diameter is 1), or divide it by 1·2732, the Product or Quote is the Area.

That is, put d = the Diameter AC; then $dd \times 0{\cdot}7854 = 0{\cdot}7854\, dd = \dfrac{dd}{1{\cdot}2732} =$ Area (Fig 57.)

Example I

Suppose the Diameter 24, as before, required the Area or superficial Content.

1. Arithmetically.

$$24 \times 24 \times 0{\cdot}7854 = 24^2 \times 0{\cdot}7854 = \dfrac{24^2}{1{\cdot}2732} = 452{\cdot}4 =$$ the Area.

2. Logarithmically.

The Log of the Diameter 24	= 1·380211
Multiply by	2
Product is the Log. of 24^2	= 2·760422
The Log of 0·7854	= 1·895091
Sum is the Log of 452·4 = Area	= 2·655513

3. By

Sect V.   *Of* SUPERFICIES.   105

3. By the Sliding Rule.

$$\begin{array}{cccc} A & B & A & B \\ \end{array}$$
As 1·2732 : 24 ∷ 24 : 4524 the Area.

Or,

$$\begin{array}{cccc} D & B & D & B \\ \end{array}$$
As 1 · 07854 : 24 ∷ 4524.

RULE II

Multiply the Square of the Diameter by $\frac{11}{14}$, or divide by $1\frac{3}{11}$ $(= \frac{14}{11})$; the Product or Quote is the Area. That is $\frac{11dd}{14} = \frac{dd}{1\frac{3}{11}}$ = Area.

EXAMPLE II.

Given the Diameter as before, required the Area.

1. Arithmetically.

$\frac{24^2 \times 11}{14} = \frac{24^2}{1\frac{3}{11}} = 452\frac{4}{7}$ = Area, which differs a little from the first.

2. Logarithmically.

The Log of the Diameter	24	= 1·380211
Multiply by	——	2
Product is the Log of 24^2	——	= 2·760422
The Log. of Multiplier 11	——	= 1·041393
The Comp. Arith. Log. of 14	——	= 8·853872
Sum is the Log. of 452·57	——	= 2·655687

P   3 By

3. *By the Sliding Rule.*

$$\text{As } 1\tfrac{9}{14} \overset{A}{.} 24 \overset{B}{.} : 24 \overset{A}{.} 452\tfrac{4}{7} \overset{B}{=} \text{ the Area.}$$

Or,

$$\text{As } 1 \overset{D}{:} \tfrac{14}{9} \overset{B}{:} : 24 \overset{D}{:} 452\tfrac{4}{7} \overset{B}{=} \text{ Area as above.}$$

RULE III.

Multiply the Square of the Diameter by $\frac{355}{452}$ or divide by $\frac{452}{355}$ ($= 1\frac{97}{355} = 1\cdot2732$), the Product or Quotient is the Area. That is $\frac{355 dd}{452} = \frac{dd}{1\frac{97}{355}} = \frac{dd}{1\cdot2732} =$ the Area.

EXAMPLE III.

Suppose the Diameter the same as before, required the Area.

1. *Arithmetically,*

$$\frac{24^2 \times 355}{452} = \frac{24^2}{1\cdot27} = 452 \frac{44}{113} = 452\cdot4 = \text{the Area the}$$

same as by Rule I.

2. *Logarith-*

Sect. V.   *Of* Superficies.   107

2. Logarithmically.

The Log. of 24^2	$= 2\cdot 760422$
The Log. of 355	$= 2\cdot 550228$
The Comp. Arithmet. Log. 452	$= 7\cdot 344862$
Sum is the Log of 452·4	$= 2\cdot 655512$

3. By the Sliding Rule.

$$\begin{array}{cccc} A & B & A & B \end{array}$$

As $1\frac{97}{355} : 24 :: 24 : 452\cdot 4 = $ the Area

Prob. XXXV.

The Periphery of a Circle being given, to find the Area.

Rule.

Multiply the Square of the Circumference or Periphery by ·07958, (= the Area of a Circle whose Periphery is 1), or divide it by 12·566; the Product or Quotient is the Area. That is, put $p = $ the Periphery $ABCD$, then $pp \times \cdot 07958 = \frac{pp}{12\cdot 566} = $ the Area. (Fig. 57)

Example.

Suppose the Periphery of a Circle $= 75\cdot 4$; required the Area

P 2   1. Arith.

1. Arithmetically.

$$75.4^2 \times .07958 = \frac{75.4^2}{12.566} = 452.4 \text{ the Area.}$$

2. Logarithmically.

The Logarithm of 75.4^2 — $= 3.754743$
The Logarithm of $.07958$ — $= \overline{.2}.900804$
Sum is the Log of 452.4 — $= 2.655546$

3. By the Sliding Rule.

   D   B   D   B
As 1 : .079 :: 75.4 : 452.4 = the Area.

Or,

   A   B   A   B
As 12.56 : 75.4 :: 75.4 : 452.4 = the Area.

Prob. XXXVI

The Diameter of a Circle being given, to find the Side of a Square equal in Area thereto.

Rule.

Multiply the Diameter by 0.8862 $(= \sqrt{.7854})$ or divide by 1.1284, the Product or Quote is the Side of the Square. Put $d = AC$, then $d \times 0.8862 = \frac{d}{1.1284} =$ the Side of a Square equal (Fig. 58.)

Example.

Suppose the Diameter of a Circle = 36, required the Side of a Square equal in Area to the Area of the given Circle.   1. Arith-

Sect. V.   *Of* Superficies.   109

1. Arithmetically.

$$36 \times 0.8862 = \frac{36}{1.1284} = 31.9\text{---} = \text{Side of Square.}$$

2. Logarithmically

The Log. of $\begin{cases} \text{the Diameter } 36 & = 1.556302 \\ \text{the Factor } 0.8862 & = \overline{1}.947532 \end{cases}$

The Sum is the Log. Side of the □ 31.9 = 1.503834

3. By the Sliding Rule.

  A   B   A   B
As 1 . 36 . . ·88 . 31.9 = Side of the Square
Or,
As 1.12 . 1 : 36 . 31·9 the same as above.

Prob. XXXVII.

Having the Periphery of a Circle given, to find the Area of a Square whose Area is equal to that of the given Circle

Rule.

Multiply the Periphery by 0·2821 ($\sqrt{.07958}$), or divide by 3.5448; the Product or Quote is the Side of the Square equal

Then putting p = the Periphery $ABCD$, $p \times \sqrt{.07958} = p \sqrt{.07958} = \frac{p}{3.5448}$ = Side of the Square equal. (Fig. 58)

Example

Example.

Given the Periphery 72, required the Side of the Square equal.

1. Arithmetically.

$$72 \times \sqrt{\cdot 07958} = \frac{72}{3\cdot5448} = 20\cdot31 = \text{Side of } \square.$$

2. Logarithmically.

The Log. of $\begin{cases} \text{the Periphery } 72 & = 1\cdot857332 \\ \text{the Multip. } \sqrt{\cdot 07958} & = \overline{1}\cdot450402 \end{cases}$

Sum is the Log. of the Side of Square $20\cdot31 = 1\cdot307734$

3. By the Sliding Rule.

$$\begin{array}{cccc} A & B & A & B \\ \text{As } 1 & \cdot 28 \text{ \&c.} & : 72 & \cdot 20\cdot 31 \end{array} = \text{Side of the Square.}$$

Or,

$$\text{As } 3\cdot54 \quad 1 \quad .72 \quad 20\cdot31 = \text{the same as above}$$

Prob. XXXVIII.

The Diameter of a Circle given, to find the Side of its greatest inscribed Square.

Rule.

Multiply the Diameter by $0\cdot7071$, or divide it by $1\cdot4142$, the Product or Quote is the Side of the inscribed Square

Suppose

Sect V.   *Of* Superficies.   111

Suppose $AC = 1$, then $AE\; (= EB) = .5 =$ the Length of the Legs of the right angled plain $\triangle AEB$. Then (by Theorem 17) the Hypothenuse $AB = \sqrt{AE^2 + EB^2} = \sqrt{.5^2 + .5^2} = \sqrt{.25 + .25} = \sqrt{.50} = 0.7071 =$ the Side of the inscribed Square of that Circle whose Diameter is 1   (Fig 58)

Then put $d = AB$, so will $d \times 0.7071 = \dfrac{d}{1.4142} = AB =$ the Side of the inscribed Square

Example.

Given the Diameter of a Circle $= 36$; required the Side of its greatest inscribed Square.

1. Arithmetically.

$36 \times 0.7071 = \dfrac{36}{1.4142} = 25.45 =$ Side of the inscribed Square required.

2 Logarithmically.

The Log. of $\begin{cases} \text{the Diameter } 36 & = 1.556302 \\ \text{the Multiplier } 0.7071 & = \overline{1.849481} \end{cases}$

The Sum is the Log. of $25.45\quad —\quad = 1.405783$

3. By the Sliding Rule.

A   B   A   B
As $1 : 36 :: .70 : 25.45$ as above.

Prob.

Prob XXXIX

Having the Circumference of a Circle given, to find the Side of its greatest inscribed Square.

Rule.

Multiply the Circumference by 0·2251, or divide by 4·4424, the Product or Quote is the Side of the inscribed Square.

Put c = the Circumference $ABCD$, then $c \times 0{\cdot}2251 = 0{\cdot}2251\,c = \dfrac{c}{4{\cdot}4424}$ = the Side of the inscribed Square (Fig. 58.)

Example.

Suppose the Circumference = 72, required the Side of its greatest inscribed Square.

1. Arithmetically.

$$72 \times 0{\cdot}2251 = \dfrac{72}{4{\cdot}4424} = 16{\cdot}2 \text{ the Side of the } \square.$$

2. Logarithmically.

The Log of { the Circumference 72 = 1·857332
{ the Multiplier 0·2251 = 1·352375

The Sum is the Log 16·2 = Side of the □ = 1·209707

3. By the Sliding Rule.

A	B	A	B
As 1	72	2·2	16·2, as above.

Sect. V.   *Of* SUPERFICIES.   113

PROB XL.

To measure a Sector of a Circle, Semicircle, or Quadrant.

RULE.

Multiply the Radius and Arch together, and take Half the Product for the Area Or multiply Half the Radius into the Arch, or Half the Arch by the Radius, either of which will give the Area

Put a = Arch XY, and r = the Radius $AX = AY$, then $\frac{ra}{2} = \frac{a}{2} \times r = \frac{r}{2} \times a$ = Area of the Sector AXY. (FIG. 17.)

EXAMPLE.

If the Radius be = 40, and the Arch = 15; required the Area of the Sector.

1 Arithmetically

$\frac{40 \times 15}{2} = \frac{40}{2} \times 15 = \frac{15}{2} \times 40 = 300$ = Area of the Sector.

2 Logarithmically.

The Log. of the Radius 40 ——	= 1 602060
The Log of the Arch 15 ——	= 1 176091
The Comp. Arithmet. Log. 2 ——	= 9 698970
Sum is the Log. of the Area = 300	= 2 477121

Q 3   By

3. By the Sliding Rule.

A   B   A   B
A. 2 . 40   15 · 300 = Area of the Sector.

Prob. XLI

To measure the Segment of a Circle

Rule.

Find the Area of the Sector $ABCD$ by the last Problem, then it is evident, if from the Area of the Sector $ABCD$ you take the Area of the $\triangle ADC$, the Remainder will be the Area of the Segment ABC.

Put $r = AD (= DC)$, $c = AC$, $a =$ Arch ABC, $v =$ versed Sine EB, and $x = DB - EB = DE$. Then $\frac{ra}{2} =$ Area Sector $ABCD$, and $\frac{cx}{2} =$ Area of the $\triangle ADC$, then $\frac{ra}{2} - \frac{cx}{2} = \frac{ra - cx}{2} =$ Area of the Segment ABC. (Fig 59)

Example

Suppose the Chord of a Segment = 48, and versed Sine = 6, also the Length of the Arch = 48.72, required the Area.

1. Arithmetically

$\frac{48^2}{6} + 6 = \frac{48^2 + 36}{6} = 102$ the Diameter of the Circle, whose Half 51 is the Radius. Then $\frac{51 \times 48.72}{2} = 1242.36 =$ Area of the Sector. Also $\frac{51 - 6}{2} \times 48 = 1080$ the Area of the $\triangle$, then $1242.36 - 1080 = 162.36$ the Area of the Segment.   Where

Sect. V   *Of* Superficies.   115

Where very great Exactness is not required, if you multiply the Chord by $\frac{2}{3}$ of the versed Sine, the Product is the Area

2. Logarithmically

The Log of $\frac{51-6}{2}$ — — = 1.352182
The Log of 48 — — = 1.681241
Sum is the Log 1080 = Area of the △ = 3.033423

Also,

The Log. of 51 — — = 1.707570
The Log of 48.72 — = 1.687703
The Comp. Arithmet. Log. 2 — = 9.698970
Sum is Log. of 1242.36 = Area of Sector = 3.094242

Then 1242.36 − 1080 = 162.36 = Area of the Segment as before.

3 By the Sliding Rule.

A   B   A   B
As 1 : 22.5   48   1080 = Area of the △.
As 1   48.72   51 . 1242.36 = Area of the Sector

Prob. XLII.

To measure a Parabola.

Rule.

Multiply $\frac{2}{3}$ of the Axis by the Ordinate, or $\frac{2}{3}$ of the Ordinate by the Axis, or take $\frac{2}{3}$ of the Product of the Axis and Ordinate; any of these will be the Area.

Q 2   Put

Put $x =$ Ordinate AB, and $v =$ the Axis CD; then $\frac{2x}{3} \times v = \frac{2xv}{3} = \frac{2v}{3} \times x =$ Area of the Parabola ACB. (Fig. 39)

Example.

Given the Axis of a Parabola $= 12\cdot5$, and its greatest Ordinate $= 18$, required the Area.

1 Arithmetically.

$\frac{12\cdot5 \times 2}{3} \times 18 = \frac{12\cdot5 \times 36}{3} = 150 =$ Area of the Parabola

2. Logarithmically

The Log of $\begin{cases} \text{the Axis } 12\cdot5 & = 1\cdot096910 \\ \text{the Multiplier } \frac{2}{3} & = 1\cdot823909 \\ \text{the Ordinate } 18 & = 1\cdot255272 \end{cases}$

Sum is the Log of the Area 150 — $= 2\cdot176091$

3 By the Sliding Rule.

As $\begin{matrix} A & B & A & B \\ 1\cdot5 & . & 12\cdot5 & 18 & . & 150 \end{matrix}=$ Area.

Prob. XLIII.

To measure an Oval or Ellipsis.

Rule.

Multiply the Product of the two Diameters by ⋅7854, or divide it by 1⋅2732; the Product or Quote is the Area.

Ex-

Sect. V. *Of* Superficies. 117

Put $b = AC$ = Transverse Diameter, and $c = BD$ = the Conjugate; then $bc \times .7854 = \dfrac{bc}{1.2732}$ = Area of the Oval or Ellipsis $ABCD$. (Fig. 18.)

Example.

If the transverse Axis be 24.5, and the Conjugate 16, required the Area of the Ellipsis.

1. *Arithmetically.*

$24.5 \times 16 \times .7854 = \dfrac{24.5 \times 16}{1.2732} = 307.87$ = Area.

2. *Logarithmically.*

The Log of the $\begin{cases} \text{Transf. Diam. } 24.5 & = 1.389166 \\ \text{Conjug. Diam } 16 & = 1.204120 \\ \text{Multiplier } 7854 & = .895091 \end{cases}$

Sum is the Log of the Area 307.87 $= 2.488377$

3. *By the Sliding Rule.*

$\begin{array}{cccc} A & B & A & B \end{array}$
As 1.27 : 24.5 :: 16 : 307.87 = Area.

Prob XLIV

To measure an Hyperbola

The Rule for this being (in Words) so intricate, I have therefore contracted the same into a Theorem, by which the Solution will be more easily attained.

Put t = transverse Axis, c = the conjugate Axis, and a = the Abscissa

THE-

Theorem.

$\overline{80\,t + 39\,a} \times \sqrt{a\,t} \times 4\,a\,c = x =$ the Dividend. $\overline{16\,t + 3\,a} \times 15\,t = z =$ the Divisor; then $\frac{x}{z} =$ the Area.

Example.

Given the transverse Axis $BD \times 34$, the Conjugate 20, and the Abscissa or Height $BG = 12$; required the Area.

1. Arithmetically.

$\overline{34 \times 80} \times \overline{12 \times 39} \times \sqrt{\overline{21 \times 34} \times 4 \times 12 \times 20}$
$= 60658176 =$ Dividend. Then $\overline{34 \times 16 + 3 \times 12}$
$\times \overline{15 \times 34} = 295800 =$ Divisor. Then $\frac{60658176}{295800} =$
20506 = Area of the Hyperbola.

Prob XLV.

To find the Area of any Curve-lined Space ABC.

Rule.

Measure in a direct Line AB from one End of the Curve to the other, and, as often as convenient, take Breadths perpendicular to AB, as DE, FC, GH. Then to find the Area, add the several Breadths together, and divide the Sum by the Number of Breadths,

fo

Sect V   *Of* Superficies.   119

so shall the Quotient be the mean Breath, which multiplied into the whole Length AB, the Product will be the Area   (Fig 60)

Or more accurately thus;

Multiply the half Sum of every two Breadths by the intermediate Length, the Sum of the several Products is the Area. The several Lengths and Breadths are as below.

	Lengths			Breadths	
		L			L
1	A	= 0	A		= 0
2	AD	= 110	DE		= 80
3	AF	= 200	FC		= 110
4	AG	= 275	GH		= 95
5	AB	= 410	B		= 0

$$\frac{0+80+110+95+0}{5} \times 410 = 0\,23370 \text{ Acres}$$

by the first Method.

$$\frac{0+80}{2} \times 110 + \frac{80+110}{2} \times \overline{200-110} + \frac{110+95}{2}$$

$$\times \overline{275-200} + \frac{95+0}{2} \times \overline{410-275} = 0\,27049$$

Acres by the second Method.

But the common and practical Method of finding the Area of any irregular curve-lined Superficies, is to take a Breadth in the Middle of every one, two, three, &c Chains, Yards, Feet, &c. which Breadth multiplied by its respective Length will give the Area of that particular Part, then the Sum of the several Areas will be the Area of the Whole.

SECT. VI

MENSURATION of the SUPERFICIES of SOLIDS.

PROB. XLVI.

To find the Area of the Surface of any Cube, Prism, Cylinder, &c.

RULE.

MUltiply the Periphery of the Base by the Length of the Solid, to that Product add the Area of the Base or Bases, the Sum is the Area of the whole Solid.

Put $a = AB = BC = CD = DA$, &c. Then $\overline{4a \times a} + \overline{2a \times a} = 4aa + 2aa = 6aa =$ Area of the Superficies of the Cube ABC, &c. (FIG. 61.)

Also put $x =$ the Side of the Base AB of a triangular Prism, and $v = CD =$ its Height, then $\overline{3 x \times v} + 2 x^2 \times 0.433013$ ($=$ tabular Number for a Trigon) $= 3 v x + .866026 v^2 =$ Area of the Whole. (FIG 62.)

Also put $a = ABCD =$ the Periphery of a Cylinder, and $b = CE =$ its Length, then $a b + .15916 a^2 =$ Area of the Surface of a Cylinder (FIG 63.)

EXAMPLE I.

Suppose each Side of a Cube $= 14.5$; required the superficial Content.

1. Arith-

Sect VI.   *Of* Solids.   121

1. Arithmetically.

$$\overline{14\cdot 5 \times 4 \times 14\cdot 5} + \overline{14\cdot 5 \times 2 \times 14\cdot 5} = 841 + 420$$
$$= 1261 = \text{Area}$$

2. Logarithmically.

Because a Cube consists of six equal Sides, therefore the Area of one Side multiplied by 6 or divided by $\frac{1}{6}$, will be the Area of the Whole

The Log $14\cdot 5^2$ + Log. 6 = Log 1261 = the Area of the Superficies.

3. By the Sliding Rule.

    A   B   A   B

As ·166 . 14·5 :: 14·5 · 1261 = the Area the same as above

Example II.

If each Side of the Base of a triangular Prism be 8, and the Length 30, required the superficial Content.

1. Arithmetically.

$$\overline{8 \times 3 \times 30} + \overline{8^2 \times 0.866026} = 720 + 55\cdot 42 =$$
$$775\cdot 42 = \text{Area}.$$

2. Logarithmically

The Log. $\overline{8 \times 3}$ + Log 30 = Log 720. The Log. 8^2 + Log. 0·866026 = Log. 55·42.

R

3. By

122   SUPERFICIAL MEASURE   Book II.

3. By the Sliding Rule

   A   B   A   B
As 1 24   30 720 = Area of the upper Part.
   D   B   D   B
As 1 : 086   30 55·42 = Area of the two Bases.

EXAMPLE III.

Suppose the Circumference of a Cylinder = 48, and the Length 130, required the superficial Content.

1. Arithmetically

$$\overline{48 \times 130} + 48^2 \times \cdot 15916 (= 07958 \times 2) = 66067$$
$$= \text{Area.}$$

2. Logarithmically

The Log of 48 + Log. of 130 = Log of 6240
The Log of 48^2 + Log. of ·15916 = Log of 3667

3. By the Sliding Rule.

   A   **B**   **A**   **B**
As 12 56 48   96 3667 = Area of the Bases.
As 1   ·48 130. 6240 = Area curve Super.

PROB XLVII.

To find the superficial Content of any Cone or Pyramid

RULE.

Multiply half the Periphery of the Base by the slant Height, or half the slant Height by the Periphery of the

Sect. VI.   *Of* SOLIDS.   123

the Base, or take half the Product of the Periphery of the Base into the slant Height; any of these three Ways will give the superficial Content, to which add the Area of the Base.

Put $a = AB = BC = CD = DA =$ the Side of a square Pyramid, and $b = EA =$ its slant Height. Then $\frac{4a}{2} \times b + a^2 = \frac{b}{2} \times 4a + a^2 = \frac{4ab}{2} + a^2 = \frac{4ab + 2a^2}{2}$ = superficial Content   (FIG 64)

Also put $p =$ the Periphery $ABCD$, and $a = EA$ = the slant Height of a Cone or round Pyramid, then $\frac{a}{2} \times p + \cdot 07958\ pp = \frac{p}{2} \times a + \cdot 07958\ pp = \frac{ap}{2} + \cdot 07958\ pp = \frac{ap + \cdot 15916\ pp}{2}$ = superficial Content.

EXAMPLE I.

Suppose each Side of a square Pyramid $= 15\ 5$ and its slant Height $= 40$, required the superficial Content.

1 Arithmetically.

$\frac{15\ 5 \times 4}{2} \times 40 + 15\cdot5^2 = 1480\cdot25 =$ superficial Content

2. Logarithmically.

The Log. of $\frac{15\ 5 \times 4}{2}$ + Log. of $40 =$ Log. of 1240. The Log. of $15\cdot5^2$ is $=$ Log. $240\ 25$. Then $1240 + 240\cdot25 = 1480\ 25 =$ superficial Content as above

3. *By the Sliding Rule.*

$$\text{As} \begin{cases} 2 \cdot 62 & 40 \quad 1240 = \text{curve Surface.} \\ 1 \quad 15\,5 & 15\,5 \cdot 240\cdot 25 = \text{Area of the Base.} \end{cases}$$

whose Sum $1240 + 240\,25 = 1480\,25$, is the same as above

EXAMPLE II.

If the Periphery of the Base of a Cone or Pyramid be 60, and its slant Height 350, required the superficial Content.

1. *Arithmetically.*

$$\frac{60}{2} \times 350 + 60^2 \times \cdot 07958 = \frac{60 \times 350}{2} + 60^2 \times \cdot 07958$$
$$= 1078\,649 = \text{superficial Content.}$$

2. *Logarithmically.*

The Log. of $\frac{60}{2}$ + Log of 350 = Log of 10500 = convex Superficies   Also the Log. of 60^2 + Log. of $\cdot 07958$ = Log of $286\cdot 49$ = Area of the Base

3 *By the Sliding Rule.*

$$\text{As} \begin{cases} 2 \quad \cdot 60 : & 350 : 10500 = \text{curve Superficies.} \\ 12\cdot 56 \cdot 60 \ . & 60 : 286\,49 = \text{Area of Base.} \end{cases}$$

PROB.

Sect VI.   *Of* SOLIDS.   125

PROB. XLVIII.

To find the superficial Content of the Frustum of any Cone or Pyramid.

RULE.

Multiply Half the Sum of the Peripheries of the Bases by the slant Height, or Half the slant Height by the Sum of the Peripheries, or Half the Product of the slant Height by the Sum of the Peripheries; any of these three Ways will give the Area of the curve Surface, to which add the Areas of the two Bases, the Sum is the whole superficial Content.

Suppose $p =$ the Periphery at the greater Base AC, $r =$ the Periphery at the lesser Base FG, and $v =$ the slant Height $AF = CG$, then $\frac{p+r}{2} \times v + \cdot 07958\, pp + \cdot 07958\, rr = \frac{vp + vr}{2} + \cdot 07958\, pp + \cdot 07958\, rr =$ the superficial Content of the Frustum $AFGC$ (FIG 65)

EXAMPLE

There is a conical Frustum, the Periphery of whose greater Base is 64 and the Periphery of the less 38, and the slant Height or Length is 46; required the superficial Content thereof

1. *Arithmetically.*

$\frac{64 + 38}{2} \times 46 + 64^2 \times \cdot 07958 : + 38^2 \times \cdot 07958 .$
$= 2786\,8732 =$ superficial Content.

2. Loga-

2 Logarithmically.

The Log $\frac{64+38}{2}$ + Log of 46 = Log. of 2346 = curve Superficies. The Log of 38^2 + Log. 07958 = Log of 1149'1352 = Area of the lesser Base, also the Log of 64 + Log. of 07958 = Log. of 325'95968 = Area of the greater Base.

3 By the Sliding Rule.

```
    A   B     A   B
As  2  102   46  2346 = curve Superficies.
```
Then,
```
     D   B      D    B
As { 1  07958  64  325'95  = Area greater B.
   { 1  07958  38  114'91  = Area lesser B.
```

PROB XLIX.

To find the Area of the Superficies of any Globe or Sphere

RULE

The Area of a Globe being equal to four Times the Area of its greatest Circle, therefore the Square of the Axis multiplied by 3'1416 (= 4 × 0'7854), or the Square of the Periphery by 31832 (= 4 × 07958), either of these will give the Area

Or thus,

Divide the Square of the Axis by 0'3183, or the Square of the Periphery by 3'1414, the Quotients shall be the superficial Content, according as you use the Axis or Periphery.　　　　　　　　　　Put

Sect. VI   *Of* S o l i d s   127

Put x = the Axis AC, add p = the Periphery $ABCD$ of a Globe or Sphere, then $x^2 \times 3.1416 = \dfrac{x^2}{.3183}$ = superficial Content when the Axis is given. Also $p^2 \times .31832 = \dfrac{p^2}{3.1414}$ = Superficies when the Periphery is given. (Fig 66)

E x a m p l e.

Given the Axis of a Globe or Sphere = 12; what is the superficial Content?

1. Arithmetically

$12^2 \times 3.1416 = \dfrac{12^2}{.3183} = 452.39$ = super. Content.

2. Logarithmically.

The Log of 12^2 + Log of 3.1416 = Log. 452.39 = superficial Content.

3. By the Sliding Rule.

   A   B   A   B
As .3183 : 12   12 452.39 = super. Content.

P r o b L
To find the Area of any spheric Triangle.

R u l e.

Subtract 180 from the Sum of the three Angles, multiply the Superficies of the whole Globe by this Remainder

mainder, the Product multiply or divide by ·0014 or 720, and the Product or Quotient will be the superficial Content.

Suppose, a, b, c the 3 Angles and $x =$ the Axis of the Globe, then $3·1416\ x^2 =$ superficial Content of the whole Globe, by the last Problem (Fig 67)

Then $\overline{a+b+c-180} \times 3·1416\ x^2 \times ·0014 = \dfrac{\overline{a+b+c-180} \times 3·1416}{720} x^2 =$ superficial Content of Triangle

EXAMPLE.

Suppose the Axis of a Globe be 17 Inches, what is the Area of a spherical △ thereon, whose 3 Angles are $35°, 10'$, $48° 16'$, and $108° 00'$?

1. Arithmetically.

$\overline{35·166 + 48·266 + 108 - 180} \times 907·9224$ (the Superficies of the Globe as by the last Problem) $\times ·0014$ $= 14·53 =$ the superficial Content of the spheric Triangle

2 Logarithmically.

The Log. of $\overline{35·166 + 48·266 + 108 - 180} +$ Log. of $907·9224 +$ Log of $·0014 =$ Log of $14·53 =$ Area.

PROB. LI.

To find the superficial Content of any irregular Solid.

RULE.

Divide the irregular Solid into as many regular Ones as it will admit of, whose Areas find by some or other of the foregoing Rules. But

Sect VI.   *Of* SOLIDS.   129

But the common practical Method of finding the Superficies of all such Solids, is to take a Periphery in the Middle of every 1, 2, 3, &c. Yards, Feet, &c. which multiply by each respective intercepted Length, the Sum of the several Products will be the superficial Content of the whole Solid. *Note*, The more Peripheries you take, the nearer the Truth will the Work be, and will give out an Answer sufficiently exact.

Put $a = AD$, $b = GH$, $c = EF$, $d = IK$ and $e = BC$, (the several Peripheries), also let $v = DH = AG$, $x = HF = GE$, $y = FK = EI$, and $z = KC = IB$ (the several intercepted slant Heights or Lengths, Then $\frac{a+c}{2} \times \overline{v+x}$ = superficial Content of the Frustum $AEFD$ by the former Part of the Rule. Also $\frac{c+e}{2} \times \overline{y+z}$ = the Superficies of the Frustum $EBCF$ by the same Part of the Rule, then $\frac{a+c}{2} \times \overline{v+x} + . \frac{c+e}{2} \times \overline{y+z}$ = superficial Content of $ABCD$. (Fig. 68.)

Again ;

$b \times \overline{v+x}$ = Superficies of $AEFD$ by the latter Part of the Rule, and $d \times \overline{y+z}$ = the Superficies of $EBCF$ by the same Method, then $b \times \overline{v+x} + .d \times \overline{y+z} = bv + bx + dy + dz$ = Superficies of $ABCD$.

EXAMPLE.

Let $ABCD$ be a Piece of Timber, whose several Peripheries $AD = 4.5$ Feet, $GH = 5$, $EF = 6.25$,

S IK

130   Superficial Measure, &c.   Book II.

$IK = 3.75$, and $BC = 2$; and the intercepted Lengths are $DH = 3$, $HF = 3.5$, $FK = 4$, and $KC = 3.25$, required the superficial Content of the Whole. (Fig. 68)

1. Arithmetically.

$$\frac{4.5 + 6.25}{2} \times 6.5 + \frac{6.25 + 2}{2} \times 7.25 = 64.84375$$

Feet = superficial Content of $ABCD$ according to the former Part of the Rule

Also,

$$\overline{6.5 \times 5} + \overline{7.25 \times 3.75} = 59.6875 = \text{superficial Content}$$

by the latter Part of the Rule, which differs from the other just 5.15625.

2. Logarithmically.

The Log. of $\frac{4.5 + 6.25}{2}$ + Log. of 6.5 = Log. of 34.9375, also the Log of $\frac{6.25 + 2}{2}$ + Log of 7.25 = Log. of 29.90625, whose Sum 64.84375 is the superficial Content as above.

3. By the Sliding Rule.

$$\text{As } \begin{cases} \text{A} \quad \text{B} \quad\quad \text{A} \quad\quad \text{B} \\ 2 \,.\, 10.75 \,:\, 6.5 \,.\, 34.93. \\ 2 \,.\, 8.25 \,:\, 7.25 \,:\, 29.9. \end{cases}$$

SECT

SECT. VII
MENSURATION of SOLIDS

PROB. LII.

To find the Solidity of a Cube.

RULE.

Multiply one Side into its Square, and the Product is the Solidity

That is, put $a = AB$, then $aa \times a = aaa = a^3 =$ the Solidity. (FIG 61.)

EXAMPLE.

Let the Side of a Cube be 14'5; required the Solidity.

1. Arithmetically.

$14'5^2 \times 14'5 = 14'5^3 = 3048\,625 =$ Solidity.

2. Logarithmically.

The Log of 14'5 multiply by 3, Product is the Log. of 3048 625 = the Solidity.

3. By the Sliding Rule.

$$\text{As } 1 \overset{D}{} \overset{B}{14'5} \,.\, \overset{D}{} 14'5 \,.\, \overset{B}{3048\,6} = \text{Solidity}$$

132 MENSURATION Book II.

PROB. LIII.

To find the Solidity of any Parallelopipedon, Prism, or Cylinder.

RULE.

Multiply the Area of the Base by the Length, the Product is the solid Content.

Put $x = AB = $ a Side of a Base of a square Prism, and $v = AC = BD = $ its Length, then $x^2 \times v = v x^2$ = the solid Content of $ACDB$. (FIG. 69)

Also if $a = AC$ the Diameter of the Base of a Cylinder, and $b = CE = $ its Length, then $\cdot 7854\, a^2 \times b = \cdot 7854\, a^2 b = $ Solidity of the Cylinder $AGEC$. (FIG 63)

EXAMPLE I.

Suppose a Piece of Timber in Form of a Parallelopipedon, 20 Feet long, 18 Inches broad, and 10 Inches deep, how many solid Feet are contained therein?

1. Arithmetically

$20 \times 1.5 \times 0.833 -, = \dfrac{20 \times 18 \times 10}{144} = 25$ Feet = the Solidity

2. Logarithmically

The Log of 20 + Log of 1.5 + Log. of 0.833 = Log of 25 Feet = the Solidity.

Or thus,

The Log of 20 + Log. 18 + Log 10 + Comp Arith. Log of 144 = Log of 25 the Solidity as above.

3 By

Sect VI.   *Of* Solids.

3. By the Sliding Rule.

$$\begin{array}{cccc} B & D & B & D \end{array}$$
As 18   18 :   10 . 13·4 a mean Proportion between the Breadth and Depth

Then,
$$\begin{array}{cccc} D & B & D & B \end{array}$$
As 12   20 . 13·4 : 25 = Solidity.

Example II.

Suppose the Diameter of the Base of a Cylinder be 3·4, and its Length = 12, required the Solidity.

1. Arithmetically.

$3·4^2 \times ·7854 \times 12 = 108·950688 =$ the Solidity.

2. Logarithmically.

The Log. of $3·4^2$ + Log of ·7854 + Log. of 12 = Log of 108·95 = Solidity.

3. By the Sliding Rule.

·7854 turn'd to a Divisor is 1·2732, whose square Root is 1·128, therefore,
$$\begin{array}{cccc} D & B & D & B \end{array}$$
As 1·128   12 :   3·4 : 108·95 = solid Content.

Example III

Given the Periphery of the Base of a Cylinder = 65, and the Length of the Cylinder = 14; required the Solidity.   1. Arith-

1. Arithmetically.

$65^2 \times \cdot 07958 \times 14 = 47 07157 =$ solid Content

2. Logarithmically.

The Log. of 65^2 + Log. of $\cdot 07958$ + Log. of 14 = Log. of $47\,07157$ = solid Content.

3. By the Sliding Rule

$\cdot 07958$ turn'd to a Divisor is $12\,566$, the square Root of which is $3\,54$, then,

```
   D     B     D     B
As 3 54  14    65   47 07
```
= the solid Content of the given Cylinder

PROB LIV

To find the Solidity of any Cone or Pyramid.

RULE

Multiply the Area of the Base (of whatever Form) by ⅓ of the perpendicular Height or Axis, and the Product is the solid Content

Put $a = AB =$ one of the Sides of a square Pyramid, and $b = EB$ its Axis then $a^2 \times \dfrac{b}{3} = \dfrac{a^2 b}{3} =$ Solidity of AEC (FIG. 64)

Also put $x = AC =$ Diameter of a Cone, and $v = EB$ its Axis, then $7854\, x^2 \times \dfrac{v}{3} = \dfrac{7854\, x^2 v}{3} =$ the solid Content of AEC. (FIG. 65)

Ex-

Sect VI.   *Of* SOLIDS.   135

EXAMPLE I

Let each Side of the Base of a square Pyramid be 15 Inches, and its perpendicular Height 14 Feet, required the solid Content.

1. Arithmetically.

$$15^2 \times \tfrac{14}{3} \div 144 = 1\cdot25^2 \times \tfrac{14}{3} = \frac{1\cdot25^2 \times 14}{3} = 7\cdot29 = \text{Solidity}$$

2. Logarithmically.

The Log. of 15^2 + Log. of $\tfrac{14}{3}$ + Comp. Arith. Log. of 144 = Log of $7\cdot29$ = the Solidity as above.

3. By the Sliding Rule.

$$\begin{array}{cccc} D & B & D & B \end{array}$$

As $12 \cdot 4\cdot66 :: 15 : 7\cdot29$ = the Solidity.

EXAMPLE II.

If the Diameter of the Base of a Cone be 15, and its Axis = 64, required the solid Content.

1. Arithmetically.

$$15^2 \times \cdot7854 \times \tfrac{64}{3} = \frac{15^2 \times \cdot7854 \times 64}{3} = 11309\cdot76 = \text{the solid Content.}$$

2. Logarithmically

The Log of 15^2 + Log of $\cdot7854$ + Log. $\tfrac{64}{3}$ = Log. of $11309\cdot76$ = the Solidity.   3. By

3. By the Sliding Rule.

As 1 $\overset{D}{128}$ $\overset{B}{21\cdot 33}$: 1 $\overset{D}{5}$ $\overset{B}{11309\cdot 76}$ = Solidity.

PROB. LV.
To find the Solidity of the Frustum of any Cone or Pyramid.

RULE

Find the Area in the middle of the Solid, which Area multiply by 4, and add to the Product the Area of each Base, that Sum multiplied by one sixth Part of the Frustum's Length, will be the Solidity.

Note, The middle Area is easily found in straight-sided Solids, for Half the Sum of the Sides of any two similar Bases is equal to the Side of a similar Base in the Middle.

Put $a = AB$ a Side of the greater Base of a square Pyramid, $b = GI$ a Side of the lesser Base, and $x = pB =$ its Axis, then $\overline{\frac{a+b}{2}}\Big|^2 \times 4 + a^2 + b^2 \times \frac{1}{6} x = \overline{\frac{a+b}{2}}\Big|^2 \times \frac{x}{6} + \frac{a^2 + b^2 x}{6} =$ Solidity of $AGHC$. (FIG. 64)

Also put $x = AC =$ Diameter of the greater Base of a Cone, $v = FG =$ Diameter of the lesser Base, and $r = pB =$ its Axis, then $\overline{\frac{x+v}{2}}\Big|^2 \times 4 + x^2 + v^2 \times$ $\cdot 7854 \times \frac{1}{6} r = \frac{r}{6} \times \overline{\frac{x+v}{2}}\Big|^2 \times 4 + \frac{x^2 r + v^2 r}{6} \times \cdot 7854$ = Solidity of $AFGC$. (FIG. 65.)

Or thus;

$\overline{a+b}\Big|^2 + a^2 + b^2 \times \frac{1}{6} x = \frac{x}{6} \times \overline{a \times b}\Big|^2 + \frac{a^2 x + b^2 x}{6}$ = the Solidity of the Frustum $AGHC$. Also

Sect VI.   *Of* Solids   137

Also $\overline{x+v}^2 + x^2 + v^2 \times \cdot 7854 \times \frac{1}{6} r = \overline{x+v}^2 \times \frac{1}{6} r + \frac{x^2 r + v^2 r}{6} \times 7854 =$ the Solidity of the conical Frustum $AFGC$.

Example I

There is a Frustum of a square Pyramid, a Side of whose greater Base is 24 Inches, a Side of the lesser Base 8 Inches, and the Axis 15 Feet, required the Solidity.

1. Arithmetically.

$2 + 0.6666^2 + 2^2 + 0.6666^2 \times \frac{1}{6} = 2.6666^2 + 2^2 + 0.6666^2 \times 2.5 = 28.8877 =$ the Solidity.

2. Logarithmically

The Log. of $2.6666^2 + 2^2 + 0.6666^2$ + Log. of $2.5 =$ Log. of $28.8877 =$ the Solidity.

3. By the Sliding Rule

As 1 on D 2.5 ($= \frac{1}{6}$ of 15) on B 2.6666 ($= 2 + 0.6666$) on D 17.8 on B .2 on D 10 on B .66, &c on D . 1.1 on B, whose Sum $17.8 + 10 + 1.1 = 28.9 =$ the Solidity.

Example II.

Suppose the Diameter of the greater Base of the Frustum of a Cone $= 14$, the Diameter of the lesser Base $= 6$, and the perpendicular Height or Length $= 18$, required the solid Content thereof.

T   1. Arith-

1. Arithmetically.

$\overline{14 + 6^2 + 14^2 + 6^2} \times .7854 \times \frac{1}{6} = \overline{14 + 6^2 + 14^2 + 6^2} \times .7854 \times 3 = 1489\,1184 =$ the folid Content.

2. Logarithmically.

The Log. of $\overline{14 + 6^2 + 14^2 + 6^2}$ + Log of .7854 + Log of 3 = Log of 1489 1184 = the Solidity.

3. By the Sliding Rule.

$.7854 \times \frac{1}{6} = \frac{.7854}{6}$ whofe Reciprocal is $\frac{6}{.7854} = 7\,639$ whofe fquare Root 2 76 is a conftant Gauge Point for conical Fruftums when the Diameters of their Bafes are ufed, fo

As 2 76 on D 18 on B 20 on D 943 on B
14 on D 461 on B .6 on D 85 1 on B, then
943 + 461 + 85·1 = 1489 1 = Solidity as above.

EXAMPLE III.

Suppofe the Periphery of the greater Bafe of a conical Fruftum = 48, the Periphery of the leffer Bafe = 15, and the Length or Height = 24; the Solidity thereof is required.

1. Arithmetically.

$\overline{48 + 15}|^2 + 48^2 + 15^2 \times .07958 \times \frac{24}{6} = \overline{48 + 15}|^2 + 48^2 + 15^2 \times .07958 \times 4 = 2068\,44336 =$ Solidity

2. Loga-

Sect. VII.   *Of* Solids

2. Logarithmically.

The Log. of $\overline{48+15|^2}+48^2+15^2$ + Log of $\cdot 07958$ + Log of 4 = Log. of $2068\cdot 44336$ = the Solidity.

3. By the Sliding Rule.

The $\sqrt{\frac{6}{\cdot 07958}}$ is nearly 8·7, a constant Guage Point for conical Frustums, when the Peripheries of their Bases are given. Then

As 8·7 on D 24 on B .   63 on D : 1263·9 on B
· 48 on D . 732·8 on B 15 on D 71·7 on B, whose Sum 2068·4 = the Solidity as above.

Prob. LVI.

To find the solid Content of any irregular Solid.

Rule

Divide the irregular Solid into as many regular Ones as it is possible, whose Solidities may be all found by the Rule in the last Problem. But the practical Method of measuring such Solids, is to take a Periphery in the middle of every 1, 2, 3, &c. Yards, Feet, &c. that is to divide the Solid so, as that the Sides shall be straight from one divisional Mark to the next, then shall a Periphery taken in the middle of every such Part be a

T 2   mean

mean Periphery, and equal to the Periphery of a Cylinder of equal Dimensions therewith, whose Area multiplied by its respective perpendicular Height or Length, will give the Solidity thereof. In like Manner find the Solidity of every Part, whose Sum shall be the Solidity of the Whole.

Note, The more Peripheries you take, or the more Parts you divide the Solid into, the truer will your Work be.

Let $a =$ the Periphery $c\,d$, $b =$ Periphery $g\,h$, $c =$ the Periphery $l\,m$, and $d =$ the Periphery $n\,o$, also put $r = \perp r$ Altitude $D\,E$, $v = E\,F$, $x = F\,G$, and $z = G\,B$. (Fig. 70.)

Then $.07958\,a^2\,r =$ the Solidity of $A\,a\,b\,c$, also $.07958\,b^2\,v =$ the Solidity of $a\,e\,f\,b$, also $.07958\,c^2\,x =$ the Solidity of $e\,i\,k\,f$, and lastly, $.07958\,d^2\,z =$ the Solidity of $i\,B\,k$, then $.07958\,a^2\,r + .07958\,b^2\,v + .07958\,c^2\,x + .07958\,d^2\,z = A\,a\,b\,c + a\,e\,f\,b + e\,i\,k\,f + i\,B\,k =$ the Solidity of $A\,B\,C$.

Or shorter thus,

$\overline{a^2\,r + b^2\,v + c^2\,x + d^2\,z} \times .7854 =$ Solidity of $A\,B\,C$.

Sect VII.   *Of* S o l i d s   141

Example.

Suppose an irregular Solid, as a Stack of Hay, &c. whose several Dimensions taken, are as below

Periph	Altitudes.	Contents.
20 5	1·5	50 1652
24 25	2 75	128 6942
16·2	1 00	20 8850
8 5	1 4	8 0496
	Content	207 7940

$20 5^2 \times 1\cdot 5 + 24 25^2 \times 2 75 + 16 2^2 + 8 5^2 \times 1\cdot 4 \times 07958 = 207 7942 =$ the Solidity, the same as above.

2 Logarithmically

The Log. of $20 5^2$ + Log. of $1\cdot 5$ = Log. of $630 3750$, the Log of $24 25^2$ + Log of $2\cdot 75$ = Log of $1617\cdot 1719$, the Log of $16 2^2$ = Log of $262\cdot 44$, the Log of $8 5^2$ + Log of $1 4$ = Log. of $101 15$, then the Log of $630\cdot 375 + 1617 1719 + 262\cdot 44 + 101\cdot 15$. + Log. of 07958 = the Log of $207 794$ = the solid Content, as above.

3 By the Sliding Rule.

As 3·54 on *D* · 1 5 on *B*   20 5 on *D*   50·4 on *B*, as 3·54 on *D* 2·75 on *B*   24 25 on *D* . 128 5 on *B*, as 3·54 on *D*   1 on *B* : 16 2 on *D*   21 on *B*, and as 3·54 on *D*   1 4 on *B* : 8 5 on *D*   8 on *B*, then 50 4 + 128 5 + 21 + 8 = 207 9 as above.

Prob.

142　　　Mensuration　　　Book II.

Prob. LVII.

To find the solid Content of the Hoof of a Cone or Pyramid.

Rule

Multiply the square Root of the Product of the two Diameters by the less Diameter, that Product subtract from the Square of the Diameter of the Hoof's Base, multiply the Remainder by that Diameter, its Height, and 0.2618, divide the last Product by the Difference of the two Diameters, and the Quotient is the solid Content of the greater elliptic Hoof. From the Product of the square Root of the Product of the two Diameters by the greater Diameter, take the Square of the Diameter of the Hoof's Base, the Remainder multiply by the Diameter of the Hoof's Base, its Height, and 0.2618, that Product divide by the Difference of the two Diameters, and the Quotient is the Solidity of the lesser Hoof.

Put $x = AB$ the greater Diameter, $v = CD =$ the lesser Diameter, and $z = CF =$ their Height, then

$$\frac{\sqrt{x v} \times v \times 0.2618 \times z}{x - v} =$$

the Solidity of the greater elliptic Hoof ABC. Also $\frac{\sqrt{x v} \times x - v^2 \times 0.2618 \times z}{x - v} =$ the Solidity of the lesser Hoof CDB.

Ex-

Sect VII.   *Of* SOLIDS.   143

EXAMPLE.

Suppose the Diameters of two elliptic Hoofs be, the greater, equal to 14, the lesser equal to 9, and their Heights equal to 25, required the Solidities of each

First, for the greater Hoof.

$$\dfrac{14^2 - \sqrt{14 \times 9} \;\; \times 9 \times \cdot 2618 \times 14 \times 25}{5} = 1740\,6768 =$$

the Solidity of the greater Hoof

Secondly, for the lesser Hoof

$$\dfrac{\sqrt{14 \times 9} \times \overline{14 - 9^2} \;\; \times 9 \times 25 \times \cdot 2618}{5} = 896\,9582 =$$

the Solidity of the lesser Hoof.

The Solution of this Example, as also of others of the like Kind, is more conveniently performed arithmetically than either by the Logarithms or the Sliding Rule.

Note, The Solidity of the elliptic, parabolic, hyperbolic, or any other Hoof may be nearly obtained by the Rule in Prob. 55. But as Hoofs of all Kinds (except the Elliptic which are used in finding the Drip of a Tun) are of little Use, I shall forbear to treat any further thereon.

PROB LVIII.

To find the solid Content of any Globe or Sphere.

RULE.

Multiply the Cube of the Axis by 0·5236 or divide it by 1·909, the Product or Quotient is the solid Content

Or,

Multiply the Cube of the Axis by $\frac{11}{21}$ and the Product is the Solidity.   Put

144 MENSURATION Book II.

Put $x = DE =$ the Axis; then $x^3 \times 0.5236 = 0.5236\, x^3 = \frac{x^3}{1.909} = \frac{11\, x^3}{21} =$ the Solidity of the Globe or Sphere $DBEO$. (Fig. 72.)

EXAMPLE.

Let the Axis of a Globe or Sphere be $= 12$ required the solid Content thereof.

1. Arithmetically

$12^3 \times 0.5236 = \frac{12^3}{1.909} = 12^3 \times \frac{11}{21} = \frac{12^3 \times 11}{21} = 905.1428 =$ the solid Content.

2. Logarithmically.

The Log of 12^3 + Log of $0.5236 =$ Log. of 905.14.

3. By the Sliding Rule.

The $\sqrt{\frac{1}{5236}} = 1.382$ a constant Guage Point.

    D B D B
Then as 1.382 $20 \mathrel{..} 20$ 905.14 as above.

PROB. LIX.

To find the Solidity of any Segment of a Globe.

RULE.

Add three Times the Square of the Semi-diameter of the Segment's Base to the Square of the Segment's
Height

Sect VII.   *Of* SOLIDS.   145

Height, that Sum multiplied by the Height of the Segment, and by ·5236, the Product is the Solidity of the Segment. But if the Axis of the Sphere and Height of the Segment be given, then subtract twice the Segment's Height from thrice the Axis, that Remainder multiply by the Square of the Height of the Segment, and by ·5236, the last Product is the solid Content.

Put $x = AC$ the Diameter of the Segment's Base, $v = BQ$ its Height, and $z = BO$ the Axis of the Globe. (FIG. 72.)

Then $\frac{3x^2}{4} + v^2 \times v \times \cdot5236 = \frac{3x^2}{4} + v^2 \times \cdot5236\, v$
$= \frac{3x^2 + 4v^2 \times \cdot5236\, v}{4} = \frac{1\cdot5708\, x^2 v + 2\cdot0944\, v^3}{4} =$
$\cdot3927\, x^2 v + \cdot5236\, v^3 =$ the Solidity of the Segment ABC by the former Part of the Rule.

Also $3z - 2v \times v^2 \times \cdot5236 = 3z - 2v \times \cdot5236\, v^2$
$= 1\cdot5708\, v^2 z - 1\cdot0472\, v^3 =$ the Solidity of ABC according to the latter Part of the Rule.

EXAMPLE.

There is a Segment of a Globe, the Diameter of whose Base is 18, its Height = 6, and the Globe's Axis = 19·5; required the Solidity thereof.

1. Arithmetically

$\cdot 18^2 \times 6 \times \cdot 3927 : + \cdot 6^3 \times \cdot 5236 = 876\,5054$
= the solid Content.

2. Logr.

2. Logarithmically.

The Log. of 18^2 + Log of 6 + Log of ·3927 = Log. 763 4088, also the Log. of 6^3 + Log of ·5236 = Log of 113·0976; then 763 4088 + 113 0976 = 876 5064 = the Solidity of the Segment

3. By the Sliding Rule

As 1·382 on D 6 on B : 6 on D 113 09 — on B .. 9 on D . 254·46 — on B then 254 46 — × 3 = 763·4088.

By the latter Part of the Rule.

·6^2 × 19 5 × 1 5708 + : 6^3 × 1 0472 : = 876 5064 = the Solidity.

Note, The Operation by the Logarithms, as also by the Sliding Rule I have omitted, being much the same as above.

Prob. LX.

To find the solid Content of a Frustum or middle Zone of a Globe.

Rule I

Add the Square of the least Diameter to twice the Square of the Axis or greatest Diameter, that Sum multiply by the Length of the Zone, and by 0 2618, the last Product is the Solidity.

Put

Sect VII.   Of Solids.

Put $a = FG = HI =$ the Diameter of the Frustum's Base, $b = DE =$ the Axis of the Globe, and $v = KL =$ the Length of the Zone, $2b^2 + a^2 \times v \times 0.2618 = 2b^2 + a^2 \times 0.2618\, v = 0.5236\, b^2 v + 0.2618\, a^2 v =$ the Solidity of the Zone $FGHI$.

Example I.

Required the Solidity of a middle Zone, whose Length is 12, the Diameter of its Base $= 20$, and the Axis of the Globe $= 24$.

1. Arithmetically.

$24^2 \times 12 \times 0.5236 + 20^2 \times 12 \times 0.2618 = 4875.7632 =$ the solid Content of the middle Zone.

2. Logarithmically.

The Log. of 24^2 + Log of 12 + Log. of 0.5236 = Log of 3619.1232, also the Log. of 24^2 + Log of 12 + Log of 0.2618 = Log of 1256.64, then $3619.1232 + 1256.64 = 4875.7632 =$ the Solidity as above.

3. By the Sliding Rule.

The $\sqrt{\frac{1}{0.2618}}$ is 1.954. Then, is 1.954 on D. 12 on B $33.9 (= \sqrt{24^2 \times 2})$ on D $3619.12 -$ on B 20 on D 1256.4 — on B.

Note, The Solidity of the middle Frustum or Zone of a Spheroid may be had by this Rule.

Rule II.

When the Solid is less than an half Zone, as $HIMN$, then add $\frac{2}{3}$ of the Square of the Zone's Height to Half the Sum of the Squares of its two Diameters, that Sum multiplied by the Height of the Zone, and by 0.7854, the last Product will be the Solidity. But if it be a like Part of a Spheroid, multiply $\frac{2}{3}$ of the Square of the Height by the Square of the Spheroid's greatest Diameter, that Product divide by the Square of the Spheroid's Axis, and then add the Quotient and work as directed in the fore Part of the Rule. (Fig. 72.)

Let $a = BO$ the Axis of a Spheroid, $b = DE$, its greatest Diameter, $x = HI$ the greatest Diameter of the Part $HIMN$ to be measured, $v = MN$ its least Diameter, and $z = LP$ its Height. (Fig. 73.)

Then,

$$\frac{2 z^2}{3} \times \overline{b^2 - a^2} = \frac{2 z^2 v^2}{3 a^2}, \text{ also } \frac{x^2 + v^2}{2} + \frac{2 z^2 b^2}{3 a^2} \times$$

$0.7854\, z$ = the Solidity of the Zone $HIMN$.

Example II.

Suppose the Axis of a Spheroid = 40, its greatest Diameter = 30, the greatest Diameter of the Zone or Part to be measured = 20, the least Diameter = 15, and Height = 10, required the Solidity thereof.

1. Arith-

Sect. **VII.**   Of SOLIDS.   149

Arithmetically.

$$\frac{10^2 \times 2 \times 30^2}{40^2 \times 3} + \frac{20^2 + 15^2}{2} \times 10 \times 0.7854 =$$

$$\frac{10^2 \times 2 \times 30^2}{40 \times 3} + \frac{20^2 + 15^2}{2} \times 7.8540 = 2748.9 = \text{the}$$

Solidity of the Zone or Part given to be measured

Note, Examples of this Kind are more conveniently wrought by the Pen than by any other Method.

EXAMPLE III.

Suppose the Part or Zone be that of a Globe, and Dimensions the same as in the last Example, required the solid Content thereof.

1 Arithmetically.

$$\frac{20^2 + 15^2}{2} \times \frac{2 \times 10^2}{3} \times 7854 = 2977.92264 = \text{the}$$

Solidity

2. Logarithmically.

The Log. of $\frac{20^2 + 15^2}{2}$ = Log of 312.5, the Log. $\frac{2 \times 10^2}{3}$ = Log. of 66.666, then the Log. of 312.5 + 66.666 + Log. 7854 = Log of 2977.92264 = the Solidity as above.

3 By the Sliding Rule.

As 1 128 on *D* 10 on *B*. 20, 15, and 10 on *D* 3 such Numbers on *A*, as that if to ½ the Sum of the two first be added ⅔ of the Last, the Sum shall be the solid Content of the Zone = 2977.92264   PROB.

Prob. LXI.

To find the Solidity of any right or oblate Spheroid.

Rule.

Multiply the Square of the Spheroid's greatest Diameter by the Axis, that Product multiply by 0.5236, or divide by 1.909, the Product or Quotient is the Solidity.

That is put $a = BO$ the Axis of a right Spheroid, and $b = DE$ its greatest Diameter; also put $b = DE$ the Axis of an oblate Speroid, and $a = BO$ the greatest Diameter thereof. Then $b^2 a \times 0.5236 = 0.5236\, b^2 a = \dfrac{b^2 a}{1.909} =$ the Solidity of the right Spheroid: Also $a^2 b \times 0.5236 = 0.5236\, a^2 b = \dfrac{a^2 b}{1.909} =$ the Solidity of the oblate Spheroid. (Fig. 73)

Example.

Suppose the Axis of a right Spheroid = 40, and the Diameter of its greatest Circle = 30, or the Axis of an oblate Spheroid = 30, and its greatest Diameter = 40; required the solid Content of each.

First, for the right Spheroid.

1 Arithmetically.

$$30^2 \times 40 \times 0.5236 = \dfrac{30^2 \times 40}{1.909} = 18849.6 \text{ Solidity.}$$

2. Loga-

Sect. VII. *Of* SOLIDS 151

2. Logarithmically

The Log. of 30^2 + Log of 40 + Comp. Arith. Log of 1·909 = Log of 188496 = the Solidity

3. By the Sliding Rule.

```
  D      B     D        B
```
As 1·382 · 40 · 30 : 188496 = Solidity.

Secondly, for the oblate Spheroid

1. Arithmetically

$$40^2 \times 30 \times 0·5236 = \frac{40^2 \times 30}{1·909} = 25132·8 = \text{Solidity}.$$

2. Logarithmically.

The Log. of 40^2 + Log. of 30 + Comp Arith of the Log of 1·909 = Log. of 25132·8 = Solidity.

3. By the Sliding Rule

```
  D     B    D      B
```
As 1·382 . 30 · : 40 25132·8 = the Solidity.

PROB LXII

To find the Solidity of the Segment of a Spheroid (F 73)

RULE.

By Prob 59, find the Solidity very exactly, by having the Spheroid's Axis and Height of the Segment given, and then it will be, as the Square of the said Axis

Axis : Segment thus found ∷ the Square of the Spheroid's greatest Diameter : the Solidity of the Segment required.

Put $x = AC =$ Diam. spheroidal Segment's Base, $v = BQ$, its Height, and $z = BO$ the Axis, also let $r = DE =$ the greatest Diameter of the Spheroid. (Fig. 73.)

Then $1.5708 \, v^2 z - 1.0472 \, v^3 =$ the Solidity of the Segment, if it was globular; then as z^2 : $1.5708 v^2 z - 1.0472 v^3$ :: r^2 : $\frac{1.5708 v^2 z r^2 - 1.0472 v^3 r^2}{z^2}$ = the Solidity.

Example.

Let the Diameter of the Segment of a Spheroid either right or oblate, be 18, its Height 6, and Axis of the Spheroid 19.5, also let the greatest Diameter of the Spheroid be 14, required the Solidity of the spheroidal Segment.

1. Arithmetically.

According to the Example in Prob. 59, the Solidity of the Segment (provided it was globular) is 876.5; then as 19.5^2 : 876.5 :: 14^2 : $\frac{876.5 \times 14^2}{19.5^2}$ = 451.79 = the Solidity of the spheroidal Segment.

2. Logarithmically.

The Log. of 876.5 + Log of 14^2 + Comp. Arith Log of 19.5^2 = Log of 451.79 = the Solidity.

Sect. VII.   *Of* S o l i d s.   153

3 By the Sliding Rule.

As
$$\begin{array}{cccc} D & B & D & B \\ 195 & 8765 & 14\cdot45179 \end{array} = \text{Solidity.}$$

P r o b. LXIII.

To find the Solidity of a parabolic Conoid.

R u l e

Multiply the Area of the Base by Half the Axis, the Product is the solid Content.

Put $x = AC =$ Diameter of its Base, and $v = BD =$ the Axis, then $0.7854\, x^2 \times \frac{v}{2} = \frac{0.7854\, x^2\, v}{2} =$ the Solidity of the parabolic Conoid ABC. (Fig 74.)

E x a m p l e.

Let the Diameter of the Base of a parabolic Conoid be 30, and Axis 50, required the Solidity.

1. Arithmetically.

$$\frac{0.7854 \times 30^2 \times 50}{2} = 17671.5 = \text{Solidity.}$$

2. Logarithmically.

The Log. of 0.7854 + Log. 30^2 + Log. of 50 + Comp. Arith. Log. of 2 = Log. of 17671.5.

3. By the Sliding Rule.

As
$$\begin{array}{cccc} D & B & D & B \\ 1\cdot128 & 25 & 30 & 17671\cdot5 \end{array} = \text{Solidity as above}$$

154   MENSURATION   Book II.

PROB. LXIV.

To find the Solidity of the Frustum of a parabolic Conoid.

RULE

Multiply the Sum of the Squares of the two Diameters by the Frustum's Height, that Product multiplied by 0.3927 or divided by 2.5464, will give the Solidity of the Frustum.

Suppose $x =$ the greater Diameter AC, $v =$ lesser Diameter EF, and $a =$ the Height of the Frustum $= DG$ (FIG. 74.)

Then $ax^2 + av^2 \times 0.3927 = \dfrac{ax^2 + av^2}{2.5464} =$ Solidity of the Frustum $AEFC$.

EXAMPLE

Let the Diameter of the greater Base be $= 45$, the Diameter of the lesser Base $= 30$, and the Height of the Frustum $= 42$; required the Solidity.

1 Arithmetically.

$45^2 + 30^2 \times 42 \times 0.3927 = \dfrac{45^2 + 30^2 \times 42}{2.5464} =$ 48243.195 $=$ Solidity of the Frustum

2 Logarithmically

The Log of $45^2 + 30^2$. $+$ Log of 42 $+$ Log. of 0.3927 $=$ Log. of 48243·195 $=$ Solidity as above.

3. By

Sect. VII.   *Of* SOLIDS   155

3. By the Sliding Rule.

As $1595 \left(= \sqrt{\frac{1}{3827}}\right)$ on D 42 on B 45 and 30 on D 33399 and 14844 on B whose Sum 48243 is the Answer

PROB LXV

To find the Solidity of an hyperbolic Conoid

RULE.

Every hyperbolic Conoid being $\frac{5}{12}$ of its circumscribing Cylinder, therefore multiply the Square of the Diameter of the Base by the Height, that Product multiply by 0·3272 ($= \frac{5}{12}$ of 7854) or divide by 3·05, the Product or Quotient is the solid Content

That is, put $a = BD =$ the Altitude, and $x = AC =$ the Diameter of its Base, then $x^2 a \times 0·3272 = \frac{x^2 a}{3·05} =$ the Solidity of the hyperbolic Conoid ABC (FIG 75.)

EXAMPLE

Suppose the Diameter of the Base $= 50$, and its Height $= 60$; required the Solidity of the Hyperbolic Conoid.

1. Arithmetically.

$$50^2 \times 60 \times 0·3272 = \frac{50^2 \times 60}{3·05} = 49080 =$$ the solid Content required

2. Logarithmically.

The Log. of 50^2 + Log. of 60 + Comp Arithmet. of the Log. of 3·05 = Log of 49080 = Solidity.

X 2   3. By

3 By the Sliding Rule.

As D : B   D : B
   1·74 : 60   50 : 49080 the same as above.

Prob. LXVI.

To find the Solidity of a parabolic Spindle.

Rule.

Every parabolic Spindle is $\frac{8}{15}$ of its circumscribing Cylinder; therefore multiply the Square of the greatest Diameter by the Axis, that Product multiplied by 0·41888 ($=\frac{8}{15}$ of 0·7854,) or divided by 2·3873, will give the solid Content.

Put $x = AB$ the Diameter of its greatest Circle, and $v = CD$ its Axis. Then $vx^2 \times 0\cdot41888 = \frac{vx^2}{2\cdot3873}$ = the Solidity of the parabolic Spindle $ACBD$ (Fig. 76).

Example

Let the greatest Diameter of a parabolic Spindle be = 40, and its Axis or Length = 60, required the Solidity.

1. Arithmetically.

$40^2 \times 60 \times 0\cdot41888 = \frac{40^2 \times 60}{2\cdot3873} = 40212\cdot48 =$ the solid Content.

2. Logarithmically.

The Log of 40^2 + Log of 60 + Log of 0·41888 = the Log. of 40212·48 as above.

3 By

Sect VII.   *Of* Solids.   157

3. *By the Sliding Rule.*

As 1545 ($= \sqrt{2\cdot3873}$) on D 60 on B ∴ 40 on D 4021248 on B = the Solidity

Prob LXVII.

To find the Solidity of the Frustum of a parabolic Spindle

Rule

Add the Square of the least Diameter to two Times the Square of the greatest Diameter, multiply the Difference between that Sum and $\frac{4}{10}$ of the Square of the Difference of the two Diameters by the Length, that Product multiply by 0.2618, or divide by 3.819, and the Product or Quotient is the Solidity

For put $v = EF = GH =$ the least Diameter, $\lambda = BD =$ the greatest Diameter, and $z = mn =$ its Length.

Then $2\lambda^2 + v^2 - \dfrac{4 \times \overline{\lambda - v}^2}{10} \times 0.2618 \times z =$
$\dfrac{2\lambda^2 z + v^2 z - 4 \times \overline{\lambda - v}^2 z}{3.819} =$ the Solidity.

Example.

Suppose the middle Frustum of a parabolic Spindle, whose greatest Diameter is 34, least Diameter 26 and Length or Height = 50; required the solid Content thereof.

1. Arith-

1. Arithmetically.

$$34^2 \times 2 + 26^2 - \overline{\frac{4 \times \overline{34-26}^2}{10}} \times 50 \times 0{\cdot}2618 =$$

$$\frac{34^2 \times 2 + 26^2 - 4 \times \overline{34-26}^2 \cdot \times 50}{3\,819} = 38777{\cdot}8 =$$

the folid Content.

2. Logarithmically

The Log of $34^2 \times 2 + 26^2 - {\cdot}4 \times \overline{34-26}^2$ ∶ + Log. of 50 + Comp. Aritmet. Log. 3 819 − = Log of 38777·8 = the Solidity.

3. By the Sliding Rule

As 1·954 on D 50 on B ∶ 34, 26, and 8 on D ∶ 15132, 8848·8, and 83·7·8 on B, then 15132 × 2 + 8848·8 − $\frac{4}{10}$ of 8·37·8 = 38777·68 = Solidity as above.

Note, The Rule in Prob. 54, being general for finding the Solidities of all Solids, the Content of the laft mentioned Fruftum may be found thereby, by finding a Diameter in the Middle between the two given Diameters, which mean Diameter may be obtained either by actual Meafuring, or by the following

RULE

To three Times the greater Diameter add the lefs Diameter, the Quote of that Sum divided by 4 will give a Diameter in the Middle. Or becaufe Diameters are as their Peripheries, you may ufe the Cucumferences or Girths inftead of the Diameters.   Put

Sect. VII. *Of* Solids. 159

For putting (as before) $x = BD$ and $v = EF$ or GH, then $\frac{3x+v}{4}$ = the Diameter in the Middle. (F. 77.)

1. Arithmetically.

$\frac{34 \times 3 + 26}{4} = 32 =$ the Diameter in the Middle. Then by Prob. 54. $32^2 \times 4 + 34^2 + 26^2 \times \cdot 7854 \times \frac{5\circ}{6}$ $= \overline{32 \times 2}|^2 + 34^2 + 26^2 = 1309 \; (= \frac{1}{6} \text{ of } 7854) \times$ $50 = \frac{\overline{32 \times 2}^2 + 34^2 + 26^2 \times 50}{7\;6395 +} = 38795,$ which differs from the Content found by the particular Rule just 17 2.

3. By the Sliding Rule.

As 2·764 on D : the Height 50 on B : 64 (= twice 32), and 34, and 26 on D . three Numbers on B, whose Sum is the Content.

SECT. VIII.

Mensuration *of* Solid Timber.

Prob. LXVIII

Any Piece of solid Timber being given, whose Bases or Ends are equal, parallel, and similar, to find the Length, Breadth, Depth, or Thickness required to make any proposed Content.

Rule

RULE.

Divide the propofed Content by the Area of the Bafe or Side of the Solid, and the Quotient will be the Length, Breadth, Depth or Thicknefs required.

EXAMPLE I.

Suppofe a Piece of Timber 10 Inches broad, and 4 Inches deep; what Length muft be taken to make 2 folid Feet,

$$\frac{2}{\cdot 8333 \times \cdot 3333} = \frac{144 \times 2}{10 \times 4} = \frac{1728 \times 2}{10 \times 4 \times 12} = 72 \text{ Feet}$$

the required Length.

2. Logarithmically.

The Log. of $\cdot 144 \times 2 : -$ Log. of $. 10 \times 4 := $ Log. of $72 = $ Anf.

3 By the Sliding-Rule.

As ·8333 on B . ·8333 on D . . 3333 on B . ·524 on D, a mean Proportion between the Breadth and Depth. Then, as ·524 on D : 2 on B . . 1 on D . 72 on $B = $ the Anfwer.

EXAMPLE II.

Suppofe the Depth $= 4$ Inches and Length $= 72$ Feet, what Breadth is required to make 2 cubic Feet.

1. Arith-

Sect VIII.   *Of* Solid Timber.

1. Arithmetically.

$$\frac{2}{7\frac{2}{15} \times \frac{1}{4}} = \frac{144 \times 2}{7\cdot 2 \times 4} = \frac{1728 \times 2}{7\cdot 2 \times 4 \times 12} = 10 \text{ Inch the required Breadth}$$

2. Logarithmically

The Log of 2 + Comp. Arith Log. of $7\frac{2}{15} \times \frac{1}{4}$ = 10 Inches the Breadth

3 By the Sliding Rule.

As 1·54 (a mean Proportion between 7·2 and 0·33, &c.) on *D*   2 on *A*   . 1 on *D*   0·833— on *A*, = 10 Inches the Breadth

Example III

Let the Length be 7·2 Feet and Breadth = 10 Inches, required the Depth or Thickness to make 2 solid Feet.

1. Arithmetically.

$$\frac{2}{7\frac{2}{10} \times \frac{10}{12}} = \frac{144 \times 2}{7\cdot 2 \times 10} = \frac{1728 \times 2}{7\cdot 2 \times 10 \times 12} = 4 \text{ Inches the required Depth.}$$

2. Logarithmically.

The Log of . 1728×2 · — Log. of $7\cdot 2 \times 10 \times 12$ = Log of 4 Inches.

3. By

3. *By the Sliding Rule.*

As 2·45 (a mean Proportion between 7 2 and 0·83 —) on $\mathcal{D}$ · 2 on $\mathcal{A}$ 1 on $\mathcal{D}$ 0·33 — (= 4 Inches) on $\mathcal{A}$, the Answer.

Example IV.

Suppose a Cylindrical Solid, the Diameter of whose Base is 1½ Foot, what Length thereof is required to make up 5½ solid Feet?

1. *Arithmetically.*

The Area of the Base (by Prob. 34) is 1·7672 Then $\frac{5\cdot 5}{1\cdot 7672}$ = 3·112 — Feet = the Length required.

2. *Logarithmically.*

The Log of 5·5 — the Log. of 1·7672 = Log. of 3·112 Feet the Length required to make up 5½ solid Feet.

3. *By the Sliding Rule.*

As 1·7672 (= Area of the Base) on $\mathcal{A}$ 1 on B · 5·5 on $\mathcal{A}$ 3·112 on B = the Length required, as above.

Prob. LXIX.

To find the Solidity of equal-sided Timber, whose Bases are equal and parallel.

Rule.

Multiply the Square of one of its Sides by the Length, for the Solidity.   There

Sect. VIII.   *Of* Solid Timber.

Example.

There is a Piece of Timber 14 Inches square, and 18 Feet long, how many solid Feet are contained therein?

1. Arithmetically

$$\overline{1\tfrac{1}{6}}|^2 \times 18 = \tfrac{282}{36} = \frac{14^2 \times 18}{144} = \frac{14^2 \times 18 \times 12}{144 \times 12} = 24\tfrac{1}{2}$$

Feet the Solidity.

2. Logarithmically.

The Log of 14^2 + Log of 18 + Comp Arith. Log. of 144 = Log of $24\tfrac{1}{2}$ Feet, the Solidity.

3. By the Sliding Rule.

As 12 on D 18 on B 14 on D $24\tfrac{1}{2}$ Feet on A = the Solidity.

Or,

As 1 on D . 18 on B . 1166 on D 245 on B, as above.

Prob LXX

To find the Solidity of unequal-sided Timber, having the same equal and parallel Bases

Rule

The Product of the Length, Breadth and Depth is the Content.

Example.

How many solid Feet are contained in a Piece of Timber 13 Inches broad, $9\tfrac{1}{4}$ deep, and 20 Feet long?

1. Arith-

1. Arithmetically

$$1\tfrac{1}{12} \times \tfrac{7}{18} \;(= 9\tfrac{1}{4} \text{ Inches}) \times 20 = \frac{13 \times 37 \times 20}{12 \times 18} =$$

$$\frac{13 \times 9\cdot 25 \times 20}{144} = \frac{13 \times 9\cdot 25 \times 240}{1728} = 16\tfrac{101}{144} = 16\cdot 7014$$

Feet the Solidity.

2. Logarithmically

The Log of $1\tfrac{1}{12}$ + Log $\tfrac{7}{18}$ + Log. of 20 = Log. of $16\tfrac{101}{144} = 16\cdot 7014$ Feet

3. By the Sliding Rule.

As 12 on D 20 on B 10·94 (a mean Proportion between 13 and $9\tfrac{1}{4}$) on D 16·7 on B = the Solidity the same as above.

Prob. LXXI

To find the Solidity of Timber whose Sides and Bases are unequal, viz. the Solidity of tapering Timber.

Rule.

Take the Breadth and Depth in the Middle of the Solid, or take Half the Sum of the Breadths, and also Half the Sum of the Depths at the two Ends for a mean Breadth and Depth, (or a Breadth and Depth in the Middle) which multiplied into the Length, will give the folid Content. Or you may find the Solidity by Prob. 55

E x-

Sect. VIII. *Of* Solid Timber. 165

EXAMPLE.

How many solid Feet are contained in a Piece of Timber 15 Inches broad, and $10\frac{1}{4}$ Inches deep at one End, 9 Inches broad and $4\frac{3}{4}$ deep at the other End, and $18\frac{1}{2}$ Feet long?

1. Arithmetically

$$\frac{1\frac{1}{4}+\frac{3}{4}}{2} \times \frac{10\frac{1}{4}+4\frac{3}{4}}{2} \times 18\frac{1}{2} = \frac{15+9}{2 \times 2 \times 144 \ (=576)} \times \frac{10\ 25+4\ 75 \times 18\ 5}{}$$

$$= \frac{24 \times 15 \times 18\frac{1}{2} \times 12}{576 \times 12} = 11\frac{27}{36} = 11\ 562 \text{ Feet the Solidity}$$

2. Logarithmically

The Log of $\frac{1\frac{1}{4}+\frac{3}{4}}{2}$ + Log of $\frac{10\frac{1}{4}+4\frac{3}{4}}{2}$ + Log. $18\frac{1}{2}$ = Log of $13\frac{1}{128}$ = 11·562 Feet the Solidity.

3. By the Sliding Rule

As 12 on *D* 18 5 on *B* 9 5 (a mean Proportion between $\frac{15+9}{2}$ and $\frac{10\ 25+4\ 75}{2}$) on *D*. 11 56 — on *B*, as above.

PROB LXXII.

To find the Solidity of round Timber whose Bases are equal and parallel

RULE.

The common Method of measuring Timber of this Sort, is to take $\frac{1}{4}$th Part of the Circumference for a Side

166   MENSURATION   Book II.

Side of a mean Square, which squar'd, and multiplied by the Length, the Product is the solid Content.

But that this Method is false, is proved thus: Suppose the Circumference to be 1, one fourth thereof is 25, which squar'd is 0625 = the Area according to this false customary Method, but we know from other Principles, that the Area of a Circle whose Circumference is 1, is 07958, therefore the true Area will be to the false, as 07958 is to 0625, which is nearly as 5 is to 4; and hence the true Content will be to the false, in the Proportion of 5 to 4, or very near it; which makes it evident, that the false Content is less than the true, by upwards of a fifth Part

And therefore in measuring Timber, &c. according to this false, customary Method, there is always ⅕ Part of the true Content lost or rejected. The true Content of Solids of this Form, is had from Prob. 53.

EXAMPLE.

How many solid Feet are contained in a Piece of Timber whose Circumference is 56 Inches, and Length 14 Feet?

1. Arithmetically

$$\overline{\tfrac{56}{4}}\Big|^2 \times 14 = \frac{\overline{56}|^2 \times 14}{144} = \frac{\overline{56}|^2 \times 14 \times 12}{1728} = 19\tfrac{1}{18} =$$

19 055 Feet, the solid Content according to the false Method. But the true Content by Prob. 53, is 24 25 Feet, which exceeds the other by 5 2 Feet.

2. Loga-

Sect. VIII. *Of* Solid Timber.

2. Logarithmically.

The Log. of $\overline{\tfrac{4\frac{3}{4}}{4}}\Big|^{2}$ + Log. of 14 = Log. of 19·055 Feet = Solidity according to the common Method.

3 By the Sliding Rule

As 12 on $\mathcal{D}$ · 14 on B . 14 (= ¼ of 56) on $\mathcal{D}$. 19 05 on B.

Prob LXXIII.

To find the Solidity of round Timber whose Bases are unequal.

Rule.

Take the Circumference in the Middle, either by measuring, or by taking Half the Sum of the Peripheries of the two Ends for a mean Periphery (or a Pephery in the Middle of the Solid), one fourth Part of which multiplied by the Length, will give the Solidity. This is the common Method used by Carpenters, Joiners, &c. and is likewise liable to the same Error as before. The true Content is obtained by Prob 55, by considering it as a Frustum of a Cone, which it really is

Example.

There is a Piece of Timber of a tapering Form, whose mean Circumference is 42·5 Inches and Length 8 Feet, required the Solidity.

1. Arith-

1. Arithmetically

$$\overline{\tfrac{3\cdot5}{4}}\Big|^2 \times 8 = \overline{\tfrac{42\cdot5}{4}}\Big|^2 < 8 - 144 = \frac{\overline{\tfrac{1\cdot5}{4}}\Big|^2 \times 8 \times 12}{1729} = 6\cdot125$$

Feet = the folid Content according to the cuftomary Method

2 Logarithmically.

The Log of $\overline{\tfrac{3\cdot5}{4}}\Big|^2$ + Log of 8 = Log. of 6 125 folid Feet as above

3 By the Sliding Rule.

As 12 on D 8 on B 10 6·25 (= ¼ of 42·5) on D · 6125 Feet on B, = the Solidity, and the fame as above

---

BOOK III.

Plain Trigonometry, or *the* Doctrine *of* Plain Triangles.

Definitions.

1. By plain Trigonometry we find the Quantity of the Sides and Angles of plain Triangles, either right or oblique angled.

2. The Chord of an Arch is a Line drawn from one End of the Arch to the other, as EB is the Chord of the Arch BE Fig. 78. 3. The

Sect. I.   Plain Trigonometry.   169

3. The Sine of an Arch is Half a Chord of double the Arch, as DE is the Sine of the Arch BE, and is perpendicular to CB.

4. The Cosine of an Arch is the Distance of the Sine from C the Center of the Circle, as CD (= GE) is the Cosine of the Arch BE, or the Sine of the Arch BE, or the Sine of the Arch AE.

5. The Complement of an Arch is what it wants of a Quadrant or 90 Degrees, as AE is the Complement of the Arch BE, (the Arch AEB being a Quadrant.)

6. The Supplement of an Arch is what it wants of a Semicircle or 180 Degrees, as the Arch IAE is the Supplement of the Arch BE.

7. The versed Sine of an Arch is the Distance between the Sine and the Periphery, as DB is the versed Sine of the Arch BE.

8. The coversed Sine of an Arch is the versed Sine of its Complement, as GA is the coversed Sine of the Arch BE, or the versed Sine of its Complement AE.

9. The Tangent of an Arch is a Line drawn to touch the Arch at one of its Ends, and is perpendicular to a Line drawn from the Center of the Circle to the Point of Contact, which tangential Line is cut by another Line drawn from the Center, and passing through the other End of the Arch, as BF is a Tangent to the Arch BE, being cut by the Line CE passing through E, in the Point F.

10. The Cotangent of an Arch is the Tangent of that Arch's Complement, as AK is the Cotangent of the Arch BE, or the Tangent of its Complement AE.

Z.   11. The

11. The Semitangent of an Arch is the Tangent of Half that Arch, as CH is the Semitangent of the Arch BE For a Line IE being drawn from I to E, (the Extremity of the Arch BE) will intersect AC in H, so is CH the Tangent of the $\angle CIH$, which (by the 20. Euc. 3) is Half the $\angle BCF$.

12. The Secant of an Arch is a Line drawn from the Center of the Circle through the extreme Part of the Arch, and continued 'till it intersect the tangential Line thereof, as CF is the Secant of the Arch BE (FIG 78.)

13 The Cosecant of an Arch is the Secant of its Complement, as CK is the Cosecant of the Arch BE, or the Secant of its Complement AE.

14 A Degree is the 360th Part of the Periphery of a Circle, for all Circles great or small are understood to have their Peripheries divided into 360 equal Parts or Divisions called Degrees, and each of these Degrees is supposed to be subdivided into 60 equal Parts called Minutes, and each Minute into 60 other equal Parts called Seconds, and each Second into 60 equal Parts called Thirds, &c

SECT I.

PROPORTIONS for solving the several Cases of right and oblique angled plain TRIANGLES

PROP. I

In any right angled Triangle ABC, if the Hypothenuse AC be made the Radius of a Circle, then will the Legs

Legs *A B* and *B C* be the Sines of their opposite Angles C and A, but if one Leg *A B* be Radius, the Hypothenuse *A C* will be Secant, and the other Leg *B C* the Tangent of the opposite Angle A and what Proportion soever the Side made Radius hath to Radius, the same Proportion hath the other Sides to the Sines, Tangents, or Secants by them represented. Therefore it will be,

AS Radius
To the Hypothenuse *A C* ·
So is the S of the ∠ C :
To the Base *A B* :
So is the Cof. of the ∠ C
To the Perpendicular *B C*   (Fig 79.)

By inverting the Terms of the Analogy, you will will gain the Quantity of the Angles *A* and *C*.

Again, making the Base *A B* Radius it will be,
As Radius
To the Base *A B* :
So is the Tan of the ∠ *A* ·
To the Perpendicular *B C*
So is the Sec. of the ∠ *A*
To the Hypothenuse *A C*.

The Terms of this Analogy being inverted, the Quantity of the Angles will be discovered the same as before.

Prop. II.

In any Triangle ABC, *the Sides are proportional to the the Sines of their opposite Angles, and therefore it is,*

As the Side or Base AB.
To the $S.$ of its opposite $\angle C$. :
So is the Side AC
To the S of its opposite $\angle B$:
So is the Side BC.
To the Sine of its opposite $\angle A$

Prop III

In any Triangle ABC.

As the Sums of any two Sides $AB + AC$.
To their Difference $AB - AC$
Tan Half the Sum of their op Angles, Tan $\frac{C+B}{2}$
Tan Half their Difference, Tan $\frac{C-B}{2}$

Then the half Difference of the Angles added to and subtracted from the Half Sum, the Sum in the first Case and Difference in the latter, will give the greater and lesser of the required Angles, that is $\frac{C+B}{2} + \frac{C-B}{2}$ = greater $\angle C$, and $\frac{C+B}{2} - \frac{C-B}{2}$ = lesser $\angle B$

Or the Cotangent of Half the included Angle may be used instead of the Tangent of Half the Sum of the opposite Angles, for the Complement of Half an Arch is equal to Half the Supplement of the whole Arch, and therefore it will be.

As Sum of the Sides $AB + AC$
To their Difference $AB - AC$
Cotan of Half the included Angle, Cotan $\frac{1}{2} \angle A$.
Tan. Half the Difference $\angle \frac{C-B}{2}$.

Prop

Sect. I.   PLAIN TRIGONOMETRY.   173

PROP. IV.

In all right lined Triangles whatsoever,

As the longest Side or Base AB
Sum of the other two Sides $AC + BC$.
Difference of the said Sides $AC - BC$
Differ of the Seg of the Base $AD - BD = AE$.
Then $\frac{AB}{2} + \frac{AE}{2} =$ greater Segment AD, and $\frac{AB}{2} - \frac{AE}{2} =$ the lesser Segment BD. (FIG 81.)

SECT II.

The Solution of the several CASES *of plain* TRIANGLES *both right and oblique angled.*

BY the foregoing Propositions, the several Cases of plain Triangles may be solved, and as every Triangle consists of 6 Parts, viz 3 Sides and 3 Angles, therefore any three Parts (except the 3 Angles) being given, the other 3 may be found, for if the three Angles were alone given without a Side, an infinite Number of Triangles might be formed, all having the same Angles Therefore to have a determinate Answer, it is necessary always to have a Side (at least) given. The several Cases of both right and oblique Triangles are resolved three Ways, viz Geometrically, Logarithmically, and Algebraically   In the Algebraic Solutions, the natural

Sines

Sines, Tangents, &c. muſt be uſed, which you muſt actually work with, as you do with common Numbers, always making the Radius = to 1

Note, In all right angled Triangles if one acute Angle is given, the other is eaſily known, being its Complement, for by ſubtracting the given Angle from 90°, there will remain the Quantity of the Angle required

Alſo in oblique Triangles, if 2 Angles are given the 3d is found by ſubtracting their Sum from 180°, or if one Angle be taken from 180, the Remainder will be the Sum of the other two

In ſolving the following Caſes, let given Things be marked thus ('), and required Things thus (°)

Right angled plain Triangles.

CASE I

Given the Hypothenuſe BC = 450, *and the Angle* C = 50° 30', *to find the Side* BA (FIG 82.)

I. Geometrically

Draw *AC* at Pleaſure, and from *C* draw *CB* to make an Angle with *AC* = 50° 30', make *CB* = 450, and from *B* draw *BA* perpendicular to *AC* Then *BA* meaſured is 347·2.

Sect. II.   PLAIN TRIGONOMETRY.   175

2. Logarithmically.

As Radius — — 10 000000
To Hypothenuse $BC = 450$ — 2 653212
So is $S \angle C = 50° 30'$ — 9 887406

To the Side $BA = 347\cdot 2$ — 2 540618

3. Algebraically, by the Table of nat. Sines, &c.

Put $b =$ Hyp BC, $s =$ nat. of Sine $\angle C$, and $1 =$ Radius, then $1 : h :: s : sb = 347\cdot 2 = BA$

CASE II

The Angl. $C = 50° 30'$, and the Leg $AC = 286\cdot 2$ being given, to find the Hypothenuse BC (FIG 82)

1. Geometrically.

Draw AC and BC to make an Angle at C of $50° 30'$, also make $AC = 286\cdot 2$, at A erect a Perpendicular AB to interfect CB in B, then is BC measured $= 450 =$ the Hypothenuse.

2. Logarithmically

As Cof. $\angle C = 50° 30'$ Leg. $AC = 286\cdot 2$ Rad
Hypoth. $BC = 450$.

3. Algebraically.

Let $c =$ Cof. $\angle C$, and $p = AC$, then $\frac{p}{c} =$ Hyp.
$BC = 450$.

CASE

CASE III.

Given the Angle C = 50° 30′, *and the adjacent Leg* A C = 286·2, *to find the opposite Leg* A B (FIG 82.)

1 Geometrically.

Draw the Triangle as in the laſt Caſe, ſo will AB be = 347·2.

2. Logarithmically.

As Rad · Leg CA = 286·2 Tan $\angle C$ = 50° 30′ : Leg AB = 347·2, as required.

3. Algebraically.

Put $s = S. \angle C$, $c = $ Coſ. $\angle C$ (= $S. \angle B$), $t = $ Tan $\angle C$, and $p = CA$, then $pt = AB$, or $\frac{ps}{c}$ = Leg AB 347·2.

CASE IV.

Given the Hypothenuſe B C = 450, *and the Leg* C A = 286·2, *to find the Angles* B, C. (FIG 82.)

1. Geometrically

Draw CA and AB perpendicular to each other at the Point A, and make CA = 286·2, then with the Diſtance 450, and one Foot in C, with the other croſs the

Sect. II.   PLAIN TRIGONOMETRY.   175

the indefinite Line AB in B, compleating the $\triangle$ ABC; then the $\angle B$ measured is $39^\circ\ 30'$, whose Complement $50\ 30'$ is the $\angle C$.

2. Logarithmically

As Hyp. BC 450 . Rad $\cdot\cdot$ Leg CA 286 2 S. $\angle B$ 39° 30′, whose Complement 50° 30′ is the other acute $\angle C$.

3. Algebraically.

Put h = Hyp. BC, p = Leg CA, then $\frac{p}{h}$ = S. $\angle B$ = 39° 30′.

CASE V.

Given the Hypothenuse $BC = 450$, *the Leg* $CA = 286\cdot2$, *to find the other Leg* AB (FIG. 82)

1. Geometrically

Construct the $\triangle\ ABC$ (by Case 4), then is AB found = 347·2.

2. Logarithmically

Find the Angles, by Case 4, and then the Leg AB, by Case 1.
               Or thus;

Find the Logarithms of the Sum and Difference of the Hypothenuse BC and given Leg CA, viz. the

A a   Log.

Log. of $450 + 286.2$ and the Log. of $450 - 286.2$: Half the Sum of these Logarithms is the Logarithm of the required Side $AB = 347.2$.

3. Algebraically

Let $BC = h$, $CA = p$, then $\sqrt{bb - pp} = AB = 347.2$.
Or let $z = BC + CA$, $x = BC - CA$, then $\sqrt{xz} = AB$.

CASE VI.

Given the Leg $AB = 347.2$, *the Leg* $CA = 286.2$; *to find the Angles* C, B. (Fig. 82.)

1. Geometrically.

Draw AC perpendicular to AB; make $AB = 347.2$, $AC = 286.2$, and draw the Hypothenuse BC then the $\angle B$ measured is $39° 30'$, whose Complement $50° 30'$ is the $\angle C$.

2 Logarithmically.

As Leg $AB = 347.2 \cdot$ Rad. Leg $CA = 286.2$: Tan $\angle B = 39° 30'$; then $90° - 39° 30' = 50° 30'$ = the Angle C

3 Algebraically

Put $b = $ Leg AB, and $p = $ Perp. CA, then $\dfrac{b}{p} = $ Tan $\angle B$ $39° 30'$ or $\dfrac{p}{\sqrt{bb + pp}} = $ S. $\sqrt{} B$ $39° 30'$ as before.

CASE

CASE VII.

Given the Leg A B = 347·2, *the Leg* C A = 286·2 ; *to find the Hypothenuse* B C.   (FIG. 82.)

1. Geometrically.

Draw the Triangle *A B C*, by the laſt Caſe, then will the Meaſure of the Hypothenuſe *B C* be = 450

2. Logarithmically.

Find either of the Angles *B*, *C*, by Caſe 6, after which find the Hypothenuſe *B C* = 450 by Caſe 2 or 3.

3. Algebraically.

Put b = Leg *A B*, p = Leg *C A*, then $\sqrt{bb + pp}$ = 450 = the Hypothenuſe *B C*.

Oblique plain Triangles.

CASE I.

Given the Angle D = 34° 30′, *the Angle* E = 54° 30′, *and the oppoſite Side* D F = 259·8 ; *to find the other oppoſite Side* E F.   (FIG. 83.)

1. Geometrically.

Draw *D E* at Pleaſure, from *D* draw *D F* to make an Angle with *D E* of 34° 30′, and make *D F* = 259·8, from *F* draw *F E* to make an Angle of 91° 00′ (the Supplement of the √s 34° 30′ + 54° 30′) with

178 PLAIN TRIGONOMETRY.   Book III.

FD, which will interfect DE in E. then EF meafured is 180.

2. Logarithmically.

As S ∠ $E = 54° 30'$ Comp. Arith. 0.089314
To its oppofite Side $DF = 258.7$ 2.412796
So S. ∠ $D = 34° 30'$ ——   9.753128
                                         ————————
To oppofite Side $EF = 180$ —   2.255238

3. Algebraically.

Put $s = S. ∠ E$, $x = S ∠ D$, $b =$ op. Side DF, then $\frac{bx}{s} = 180 =$ oppofite Side EF.

CASE II.

Given the Side $EF = 180$, *the Side* $DF = 258.7$, *and an oppofite Angle* $E = 54° 30'$, *to find the other oppofite Angle* D. (FIG. 83)

This is called an ambiguous Cafe, for if the given Angle E be obtufe, or its oppofite Side DF be greater than the other Side EF, then the required Angle D is acute, otherwife it is ambiguous or doubtful.

1. Geometrically.

Draw DE at Pleafure, and from E draw EF to make an Angle with DE of $54° 30'$, alfo make $EF = 180$, then with the Diftance 258.7 (and one Foot in F), with the other crofs ED in D; then the Angle D meafured on the Chords is $34° 30'$.

2 Loga-

Sect. II. PLAIN TRIGONOMETRY. 179

2. Logarithmically.

As Side DF 258·7 . S. opp. $\angle E$ 54° 30′ : Side EF 180 S opp. $\angle D$ 34° 30′, which is acute because DF is greater than EF

3. Algebraically.

Let $b = DF$, $s = S \angle E$, $c = EF$, then $\frac{cs}{b} = S$ opp $\angle D = S.$ 34° 30′.

CASE III.

Given the Sides EF *and* DF *the same as before, with the same opposite Angle* E, *to find the third Side* DE. (FIG 83.)

1. Geometrically

Draw the Triangle according to Case 2, so will DE measure 317·7.

2. Logarithmically.

Find the Angle D by Case 2, from whence the Angle F is known. Then find the Side DE 317·7 by Case 1.

3. Algebraically.

Put $b = DF$, $c = EF$, $s = S \angle E$, $m = \text{Cos} \angle E$, Then $cm \pm \sqrt{bb - sscc} = DE$ 317·7, + if $\angle D$ is acute, and − if obtuse, where now, if E be obtuse m will be negative. This is *Linsor*'s Rule.

CASE

180   PLAIN TRIGONOMETRY.   Book III

CASE IV.

Given the Side DF = 2587, *the Side* EF = 180, *and the included Angle* F = 91° 00', *to find the Angles* D *and* E   (Fig. 83)

1. Geometrically.

Draw DF and EF to make an Angle at $F = 91°\ 00'$, make $DF = 2587$, $EF = 180$, and join the Points E, D, then the Angle D measured on the Chords is 34° 30', and the Angle E 54° 30'. Or the Quantity of either of the Angles D or E being found as above, if to it be added the Angle F (which is given), and that Sum subtracted from 180° (= Sum of the 3 Angles), the Remainder will be the other Angle.

2. Logarithmically.

As Sum of Sides $DF + EF\ (= 2587 + 180)$. Diff Sides $DF - EF\ (= 2587 - 180)$ Tan. ½ Sum of Angles $\frac{E+D}{2}\ (= \frac{54°\ 30' + 34°\ 30'}{2})$ Tan. ½ their Differ $\frac{E-D}{2}\ (= \frac{54°\ 30' - 34°\ 30'}{2}) = 10°$, then $\frac{E+D}{2} + \frac{E-D}{2}\ (= \frac{89° + 20°}{2}) = 54°\ 30' = $ the greater Angle E, and $\frac{E+D}{2} - \frac{E-D}{2}\ (= \frac{89° - 20°}{2}) = 34°\ 30' = $ the lesser Angle D

3. Algebraically.

Put $b = DF$, $c = EF$, $v = $ Tan. $\frac{E+D}{2}$, then $v + bv$

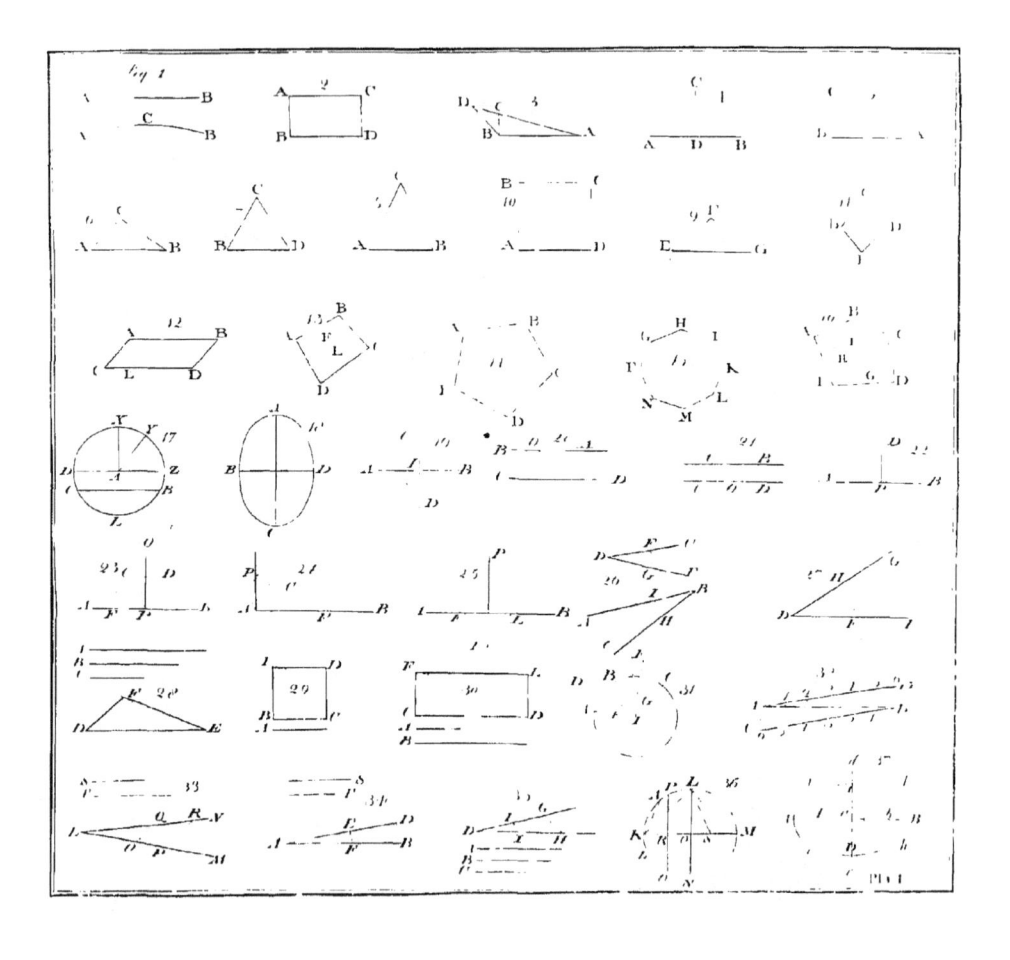

Pl. II.

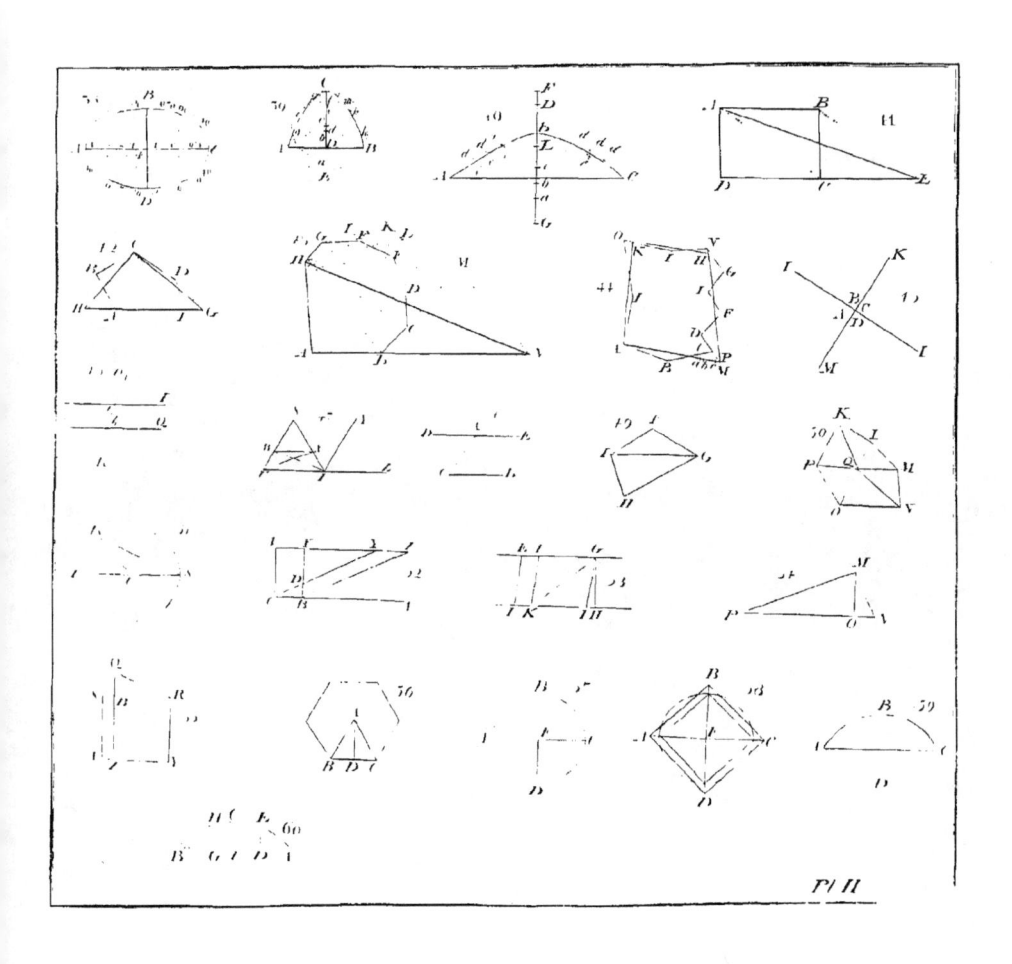

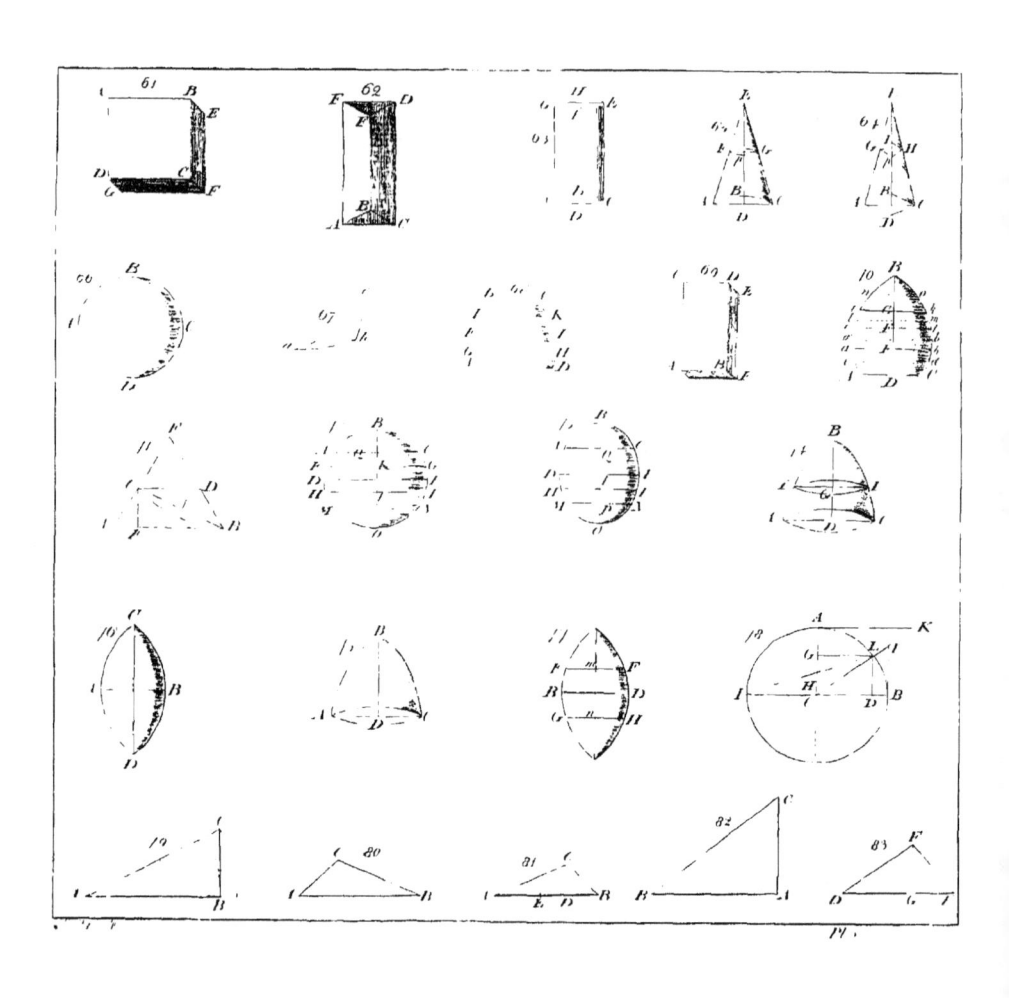

$+\dfrac{bv-cv}{b+c}=\dfrac{2bv}{b+c}=$ greater $\angle E$, and $v-\dfrac{bv+cv}{b+c}=\dfrac{2cv}{b+c}$
$=$ lesser $\angle D$.

CASE V.

Given two Sides D F, E F, *and the included Angle* F, *as before; to find the third Side* D E. (Fig. 83)

1. Geometrically.

Draw the Triangle by Case 4. Then DE measured is 317.7.

2. Logarithmically.

Find D or E by Case 4, and $DE = 317.7$ by Case 1.

3. Algebraically.

Put $b = DF$, $c = EF$, $y = $ Cof $\angle F$. Then $\sqrt{bb + cc - 2bcy} = DE$. This is *Emerson*'s Theorem.

CASE VI.

Given three Sides D F $= 258.7$, E F $= 180$, and D E $= 317.7$; *to find an Angle* D. (Fig. 83)

1 Geometrically.

Make $DE = 317.7$, then with the Distances 258.7, and 180, on D and E describe Arcs to cut each other in F, and join the Points D, F, E, so will the $\angle D$ measured be $= 34° \; 30'$.

2. Logarithmically.

Let fall a Perp. FG on a Side adjoining a required Angle, then as Base DE (317.7) . Sum Sides $DF + EF$

EF (438.7) . : their Diff. $DF - EF$ (78.7) . $DG - GE$ (= 108.6) the Diff Segments Base; then ½ Base DE + ½ Diff. = greater Segment, and ½ Base DE − ½ Diff = lesser Segment. Then there is given DF, DG, to find $\angle D$, which by Case 4, of right angled Triangles is 34° 30′.

3 Algebraically.

Put $b = DF$, $c = EF$, $d = DE$; then $\frac{2dd + bb - cc}{2bd}$ = Cos $\angle D$ = 34° 30′.

BOOK IV.

The PROJECTION *of the* SPHERE, ORTHOGRAPHIC *and* STEREOGRAPHIC, *on the* PLANES *of the* MERIDIAN, *the* SOLSTITIAL COLURE, *and the* HORIZON.

DEFINITIONS

1. THE Projection of the Sphere, is the Delineation of the Circles thereof upon the Plane of one of its Circles.

2. The primitive Circle, is the Plane upon which the Projection is made, and therefore called the Plane of Projection

3 Orthographic Projection, is the drawing the Circles of the Sphere upon the Plane of one of its Circles, by Lines or Rays let fall from every Part of the Circle

to

to be projected, perpendicular to the Plane of Projection.

4. Stereographic Projection, is the delineating the Circles of the Sphere upon the Plane of some of its Circles, by Lines or Rays passing from the Pole of the Circle of Projection to every Part of the Circle to be projected.

5. The projecting Point, is the Point from whence the Rays or projecting Lines flow to every Part of the Circle to be projected

6. The Line of Measures of any Circle, is a Line passing through the Poles of the primitive and projected Circles, or it is a Line parallel thereto; being the Intersection of the Plane passing through the Pole of the Circle to be projected, and the Plane of Projection, and is perpendicular to both.

7 The Pole of a Circle is a Point every Way 90 Degrees distant from it.

8. A great Circle of the Sphere, is that which divides the Globe or Sphere into two equal Parts or Hemispheres.

9. A right Circle is that whose Plane stands at right Angles with the Plane of Projection, and in the Stereographic Projection passeth through the Eye, and is a Diameter to the Primitive.

10. An oblique Circle has its Plane inclining to the Plane of Projection, making an oblique Angle therewith

11. Parallel Circles, are Circles parallel to some great Circle of the Sphere, having their Planes parallel to one another.

SECT I

Theorems *of the* Orthographic Projection *of the* Sphere.

Prop I

The optic or visual Angle of any Object A B, *always decreases or increases according to the different Distances of the Eye therefrom* (Fig 1)

FOR suppose AB an Object viewed by an Eye at C, then is the $\angle ACB$ = the optic or visual Angle. But suppose the Eye removed to D, the $\angle ADB$ becomes then the visual Angle, which Angle by 21 Euc. 1. is less than the $\angle ACB$, and therefore the farther any Object AB is removed from the Eye, the less will the visual Angle be found to be, and if infinitely extended, the Rays passing from the Eye to it, will differ infinitely little from the parallel Lines EA, FB. Q E D.

Prop. II.

Any right Line AB *or* CD *is projected into another right line* cd, *different from the former in proportion as* Radius Cof *of the Line's Inclination above the Plane of Projection* (Fig. 2)

From the Ends of the Line A, B, let fall the Perpendiculars Ac, Bd, or from C and D let fall the Perpendiculars Cc, Dd, so is cd the Projection of the Lines AB, CD. From A let fall the Perpendicular
Ao,

Sect. I.   *Of the* Sphere   185

Ao, then by Cafe 4, of right angled plain Triangles $AB \cdot Ao$ Radius : Cos $\angle BAo =$ Cof of its inclination above the Plane. *Q. E. D.*

Prop. III

A Circle standing at right Angles to the Plane of Projection, is projected into a right Line on the said Plane, equal in Length to its Diameter

Let ABC be the given Circle to be projected, from the Points A, B, C, D in the Periphery let fall the Perpendiculars AL, BH, CK, DG upon the Plane, then becaufe the given Circle, by Hypothefis, is at right Angles to the Plane, therefore the Perpendiculars are fo too, and fo all the Parts of the Periphery of the given Circle will be projected into the Diameter $FI\ Q\ E\ D$ (3)

Cor.   Hence it follows, that a Semicircle standing perpendicular to the Plane of Projection, is projected into a Diameter equal to that of itfelf.

Prop. IV.

A Circle parallel to the Plane of Projection, is projected into a Circle equal to itfelf on the faid Plane

Let $ABCD$ be the given Circle and E its Center, which is projected into the Circle FGI, the Center E into the Center H, for the Parallelogram $AFHE$ is equal to the Parellelogram $EHIC$. *Q. E. D.* (Fig 4)

Prop. V

A Circle oblique to the Plane of Projection, is projected into an Ellipfis on the faid Plane.

For let $ABCD$ be the given Circle to be projected
B b 2   upon

upon the Plane *F I*, from *A, B, C, D*, let fall the Perpendiculars *Aa, Bb, Cc, Dd, Kk*, so is *a bcd* the true Projection of the Circle *ABCD*, being a true elliptial Curve. For a further Demonstration, see *Emerson*'s Projection of the Sphere, Page 5, where the Curious may meet with Satisfaction. (Fig. 5.)

SECT. II.

Problems *of the* Orthographic Projection *of the* Sphere.

Prop. VI. Prob.

To project a Circle parallel to the Primitive, at any proposed Distance from it.

Example I.

TO draw a Circle parallel to the Primitive *ABCD*, at the Distance of 35° 40' from it, or 54° 30' from *E* its Pole. (Fig. 6)

Rule.

Set 54° 30' (the Parallel's Distance from the Primitive) from *B* to *F*, or its Complement 35° 30' from *A* to *F*, and draw *FG* parallel to *AC*, to cut *BD* in *G*; with the Radius *EG*, and Center *E*, describe the Circle *GIK* the Parallel required.

By

Sect. II. *Of the* Sphere. 187

By the Sector.

Take the parallel Sine of 35° 30' (the Parallel's Distance from the Pole of the Primitive), and describe therewith on E, the parallel Circle GIK as before.

Prop. VII. Prob.

To project a Circle parallel to a right Circle, or one perpendicular to the Plane of Projection.

Example II

Let it be required to draw a Circle parallel to the right Circle AB, at 23° 30' Distance from it. (Fig. 7.)

Rule.

Set the Parallel's Distance from the given right Circle AB, from A and B to D and E, and draw the Parallel DE, which is ∥ to AB, and perpendicular to the Plane of Projection $AFBG$.

By the Sector.

Set the Sine of 23° 30' from C to H, through H draw the Parallel DE.

Prop. VIII. Prob.

To project a Circle which is oblique to the Plane of Projection.

Ex-

Example III.

Required the Projection of the parallel oblique Circle DE, whose nearest Distance from the Primitive is $17° 30'$, and greatest Distance $45° 30'$.

Rule.

Through the Center C draw the Line of Measures AB, set the Circle, nearest Distance from the Primitive (viz $17° 30'$) from B upwards to E, if it be above the Primitive, or downwards if it be below, also set its greatest Distance ($= 45° 30'$) from A to D, and draw DE, from E and D let fall the Perpendiculars EG, DF, so is DE projected into $FG =$ the conjugate Diameter of an Ellipsis. Bissect FG in H, and through H draw IK perpendicular to FG, which make $= DE =$ the transvese Diameter, upon the two Diameters IK, FG describe the Ellipsis $FIGK$ by Prop 18, B. 1 which will represent the given oblique Circle.

By the Sector.

Set the Cosine of $45° 30'$ from C (the Center of the Primitive), to F, as also the Cosine of $17° 30'$ from C to G (viz both Ways, if the Circle incompass the Pole C, but the same Way if it lye on one Side of C) bissect FG in H, and draw IK perpendicular to FG, also make HI, HK each equal to the Radius of the given Circle, or the Sine of its Distance from its own Pole, on these Diameters describe an Ellipsis, and it is done.

Prop. IX Prob.

To find the Pole of any Ellipsis.

Example IV

Given an Ellipsis *KGHI*; the Pole thereof is required. (Fig 9)

Rule

Draw the conjugate Diameter *HK* through *C* the Center of the primitive Circle, from *K* and *H* draw *DK* and *HE* ⊥ *HK*, or make *DE* = *GI*, and bisect *DE* in *F*, from *F* draw *FP* parallel to *GI* to cut *HE* in *P* the Pole required

By the Sector

Measure *CK*, *CH* on the Sines, then take the Sine of Half their Difference, and set from *C* to *P*, if *C* lye between *K* and *H*, but if *K* and *H* be on the same Side of *C*, then the Sine of their half Sum must be set from *C* to *P* the required Pole

Prop. X. Prob.

To measure any Part of a parallel Circle, or to lay any Number of Degrees thereon

Example V.

Required the Measure of the Part *KI* of the Parallel *GIK*, or to lay any Degrees, &c. thereon

Rule

RULE.

Through the Extremities of the Arch K, I, draw the Radii EC, EH, and draw the primitive Circle $ABCD$, then the Arch CH is 30° 15′ = the Arch KI, or 30° 15′ set from C to H, and Lines drawn therefrom to E, will cut off an Arch KI = 30° 15′. (F. 6.)

PROP. XI. PROB.

To measure any Part of a right Circle, or to lay any Number of Degrees thereon.

EXAMPLE VI.

Let it be required to find the Measure of the Part AB of the right Circle DE. (FIG. 10.)

RULE.

Upon the Diameter DE describe the Semicircle DFE, draw AF perpendicular to DE, also from B draw BH parallel to AF, so is FH = 20° = the Measure of AB; or if 20° be set from F to H, and HB be drawn parallel to AF, it will give the Part AB = 20°.

If the right Circle pass through the Center C of the Primitive, as KI, and the Part CG is to be measured; then Cc being drawn perpendicular to KI, from G draw Gd parallel to Cc to cut the Primitive in d, so is cd the Measure of CG; the Reverse of this will make CG = any proposed Number of Degrees.

By

By the Sector.

Make $AD (= AE = AF) = $ the parallel Sine of 90; then will AB be $=$ the Sine of 20°. Or 20° being taken from the Sines, and set from A towards E, will give AB. In like Manner is CG measured, by making $CK (= CI = Cc)$ a Radius of 90° on the Sines, and then CG measured thereon, will give the Degrees, &c. thereof; or the Sine of those Degrees being set from C, will give G.

Prop XII. Prob.

To measure any Arch of an Ellipsis.

Example VII.

Let ADF be a given Ellipsis, to find the Measure of the Arch DE. (Fig. 11.)

Rule.

Upon the transverse Axis AF describe the Circle ABF; through the extream Parts of the Arch DE, draw GB and HC perpendicular to the Axis AF, to cut the Circle ABF in B, C; then the Arch BC is the Measure of the Arch $DE = 30°\ 10'$

Prop. XIII. Prob.

To set any Number of Degrees upon the Arch of an Ellipsis.

Example VIII.

Let it be required to set 30° 10′ upon the elliptical Arch ADF, from D towards F. (Fig. 11.)

Rule.

Upon the tranfverſe Axis AF draw the Circle ABF, as in the laſt Prop. and through D draw GB perpendicular to AF, which will cut the Arch ABF, in B. Make $BC = 30°\ 10'$, and from C draw CH parallel to GB, to cut the Arch of the Elliplis in E, making $DE = 30°\ 10'$, as was required.

Sect. III.

Theorems *of the* Stereographic Projection *of the* Sphere.

Prop. I.

Any Point on the Surface of the Sphere is projected into a Point on the Plane of Projection, diſtant from the Center, the Semitangent of its Diſtance from the Point oppoſite to the projecting Point. (Fig 12)

LET P be the projecting Point, H the Point oppoſite to it, A, and G two Points on the Sphere's Surface to be projected, from the projecting Point P draw the Rays PA, PG, which will cut the Plane of Projection DF, in B and F; then is CB the Tangent of the

the Angle *CPB*, or the Semitangent of the ∠ *ACH*, which is = the Arch *AH*, also *CF* is the Semitangent of the Arch *HG*. Q. E. D.

P R O P. II.

A right Line in the remote Hemisphere is projected into a right Line less than itself, but in the contiguous Hemisphere it is projected into a Line greater than itself

For let *DE*, *FG* be the two right Lines, from *P* draw *PD*, *PE*, to cut the Plane of Projection *AB* in *K*, *L*, so is *KL* the Projection of *DE*, also from *P* draw *PF*, *PG* to cut *AB* extended, in *H*, *I*, then *HI* is the Projection of the right Line *FG* Q. E. D. (F 13)

P R O P. III.

The Diameters of all Circles great or little, are projected into the Line of Measures, the Extremities of whose projected Diameters are distant from the Center of the Primitive, the Semitangents of their nearest and greatest Distances from the Pole opposite the projecting Point.

Let *FG* be the Diameter of the given Circle, whose projected Diameter is *HK*, on whose Center *L* describe the Circle *HKG*, or *HKE*; now *EF* being drawn, *GH* is the Tangent of the ∠ *CEH*, but the ∠ *CEH* (by the Elements) is = ½ ∠ *DCF*, therefore *CH* is = Tangent of ½ ∠ *DCF*, or the Semitangent of the Arch *DF* In like Manner is the Tangent of the ∠ *CEK* equal to *CK*, and as the ∠ *CEK* is (by the Elements) = ½ ∠ *DCG*, therefore *CK* is = the Tangent of Half the ∠ *DCG*, or the Semitangent of the Arch *DG*. Q. E. D (Fig. 14, 15)

COR. 1. The Points of Interſection between the Line of Meaſures and the Periphery of any oblique great Circle, within and without the Primitive, are diſtant from the Center of the primitive Circle, the Tangent and Co-tangent of Half the Complement of the Circle's Inclination to the Primitive. For CH is = the Tangent of $\frac{1}{2}$ the $\angle FCD$.

COR. 2. Hence may be gathered, that the Centers of all projected Circles are in the Line of Meaſures, and diſtant from the Center of the primitive Circle, Half the Difference of the Semitangents of their neareſt and greateſt Diſtance from the Pole oppoſite the projecting Point, if the ſaid Pole lie within the Circles; but if the Pole be without, Half the Sum of the Semitangents will give the Center.

PROP. IV.

The projected Center of any leſſer Circle perpendicular to the Plane of Projection, is in the Line of Meaſures, diſtant from the Center of the Primitive, the Secant of the leſſer Circle's Diſtance from its own Pole, and its Radius is the Tangent of the ſaid Diſtance.

Let E be the projecting Point, FG the Diameter thereof which is projected into HK, and being biſſected in L, is Center of the projected Circle. Draw $GL =$ the Tangent of the Arch $BG =$ Diſtance of the parallel Circle from its Pole B, which is likewiſe = the Radius, as CL is = the Secant, for in the right angled Triangle CGL, right angled at G, if CG be made a Radius, it is evident that GL is the Radius and CL the Secant of the

Arch

Arch $BG = BF =$ the Parallel's Distance from its own Pole. Q. E. D.

Prop V.

The Center of a great Circle when projected, is in the Line of Measures, distant from the Center of the primitive Circle, the Tangent of its Inclination to the Primitive, and its Radius is the Secant of that Inclination

Let E be the projecting Point, FG a great Circle projected in HK the Diameter thereof, whose Center is L, draw EL, and from E let fall the Perpendicular EC, so is the Angle HEK a right Angle, being in a Semicircle, and the $\angle HEC$ is $= \angle HLE$, also their Double $FCD = CLE$, whose Complement FCA is $= CEL$, whose Tangent CL is the Radius, and EL the Secant of the Arch AF. Q. E. D. (Fig 14.)

Cor. 1 If upon its Center L the great oblique Circle DHE be actually described, it will cut the Line of Measures without the Primitive in K, and therefore if the great oblique Circle DHE be now considered as the primitive Circle, whose Center is L, all great Circles passing through H and K will have their Centers in the Line NO which now becomes the Line of Measures, being perpendicular to AK. (Fig 16.)

Cor. 2 Hence it is evident, that one great oblique Circle may be drawn to make with another great Circle any certain proposed Angle; as suppose a Circle HIK be to be projected, which is to make some given Angle with another great oblique Circle HEK at a certain Point H, through L the Center of the given great Circle

Circle HEK, from the given Point H draw the Diameter HLK, and NLO perpendicular to it, which is the Line of Measures, then the Tangent of the proposed $\angle EHI$ being set from L upon the Line of Measures, will give the Point M, the Center of the required Circle HIK.

Also if an oblique Circle NrI be drawn to cut the great oblique Circle NHg at N or g, the Center of that Circle will be at x in the Line rq, and as N, g are not opposite Points of the Circle NHg, therefore any Circle Nrg passing through these Points, will be a lesser Circle, except the Circle NHg.

Prop. VI.

The Poles of any Circle great or little, are projected into the Line of Measures, within and without the Primitive, and distant from its Center, the Tangent and Co-tangent of Half its Inclination to the Primitive.

Let P, p be the Poles of the Circle AB, which are projected into the Line of Measures HI in K and s, therefore K, s are the Poles of the Circle AB. The $\angle GCP$ ($= \angle DCH$) is the Inclination of the Circle AB to the Primitive, and CK is $=$ the Tangent of the $\angle CFK$, and as CFK is $= \frac{1}{2} GCP$, by the Elements, therefore CK is $=$ Tangent of $\frac{1}{2} \angle GCP =$ Tangent of Half the Circle's Inclination to the Primitive. In like Manner Cs is the Tangent of the $\angle CFs$, or the Co-tangent of the $\angle CFK$, that is the Cotangent of Half the Inclination. (Fig. 17.)

Cor. The Pole of the Primitive Circle is its Center,

also

also the Pole of any right Circle is in the Primitive. The projected Centers of all Circles lie between the projected Poles.

SECT. IV.

Problems *of the* Stereographic Projection *of the* Sphere

Prop. I. Prob

To find the Pole of the primitive Circle ABCD.

Rule

Quarter the Circle, by drawing the Diameters *AC* and *BD* perpendicular to each other; their Point of Interfection *E* is the Pole required. (Fig. 18.)

Prop. II. Prob.

To find the Poles of a right Circle BED

Rule.

Through *E* the Center of the Primitive draw *AEC* perpendicular to *BD*, to cut the Primitive in *A* and *C* the required Poles.

By the Sector.

Set the Chord of 90° from *B* or *D* both Ways to *A* and *C*, the Poles of the right Circle *BED*. (F. 18.)

Prop III. Prob.

To find the Poles of an oblique Circle BLD.

Rule.

Draw DL to cut the Primitive in M, make $BG = AM$, draw GFD to cut the Line of Measures rI in F, so is F the interior Pole of the oblique Circle BLD. Then to find the external Pole, through E draw GEQ to cut the Primitive in Q, through which from D draw DQr to cut rI in r, so is r the external Pole required (Fig 19)

If it be a lesser Circle FHI, draw the Line of Measures rI, and from D draw DFG, DKI to cut the Primitive in G and K, bisect the Arch GK in P, and from P draw PpD to cut rI in p, the internal Pole of the lesser Circle FHI, also draw PEN, and from D draw DNq to cut rI in q the exterior Pole required

By the Sector.

Measure EL on the half Tangents, set the Tangent of Half its Complement from E to the internal Pole F, as also the Tangent of that Complement from F to the external Pole r (Fig 19)

If it be a lesser Circle as FHI, find the Degrees in EF and EI, the Semitangent of Half their Sum (if the Circle lie all on one Side E, the Pole of Projection) set from E, will give the internal Pole p, or the Semitangent of Half their Difference (if the Circle encompass the Pole E) will give the same Pole p; and the

Semi-

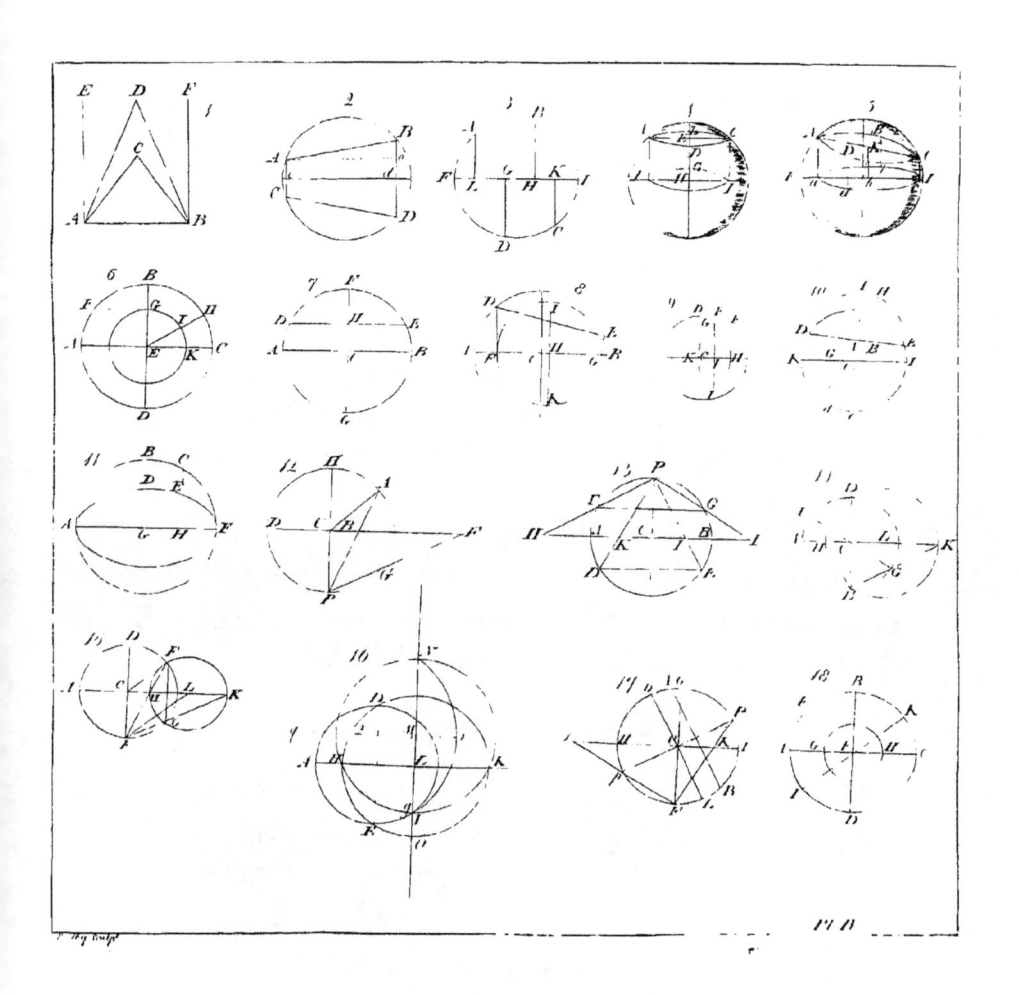

tangent of their Supplement will give the external Pole *q*.

PROP. IV. PROB.

To draw a Circle parallel to the Primitive ABCD, *at* 40° *Distance from it, or* 50° *from its Pole* E. (FIG. 18.)

RULE.

Make $AF = 40°$ = the Parallel's Distance from the Primitive, and draw AC and BD perpendicular to each other, or make $BF = 50°$ = the Parallel's Distance from the Pole of the Primitive, and draw DF to cut the Diameter AC in G, then with the Radius EG, and Center E, describe the Circle GH the Parallel required.

By the Sector.

With the half Tangent of 50°, (the Parallel's Distance from the Pole of the Primitive) on the Center E describe the Circle GH the required Parallel

PROP. V. PROB.

To draw a lesser Circle perpendicular to the Primitive, and parallel to the right Circle BD, *at the Distance of* 40° *from its own Pole, or* 50° *from its parallel great Circle.*

RULE.

Through the Pole E draw the Line of Measures Ah, make $CF = CH = 40°$ the Parallel's Distance from its own

own Pole, and draw DF, DK to cut AK in I and K, bissect IK in G, on the Center G, with the Radius GI ($= GK$) describe the parallel Circle FH Or EF being drawn, from F draw $FG \perp$ to EF to cut AK in G, on the Center G, with the Radius GF ($=$ the Tangent of $40°$ $=$ the Parallel's Distance from its Pole) describe the Circle FH as before   (Fig 20.)

By the Sector.

Make $CF = 40° =$ the Parallel's Distance from its Pole, with the Tangent thereof, and one Foot in F, with the other cross the Line of Measures AK in G the Center of the Parallel, or set the Secant of $40°$ from the Pole E to G, then with the Radius GF, or the Tangent of $40°$, and Center G, describe the Parallel FH. (Fig. 20)

Prop VI. Prob.

To draw a Circle about a given Pole p, *at* $40°$ *Distance from it, or* $50°$ *from its parallel great Circle* BRD.

Rule.

Through the Center E and the given Pole p draw the Line of Measures rI, draw DpP to cut the Primitive in P, and make $PG = PI = 40° =$ the Parallel's Distance from its Pole, or set $50°$ (the Circles Distance from its Parallel great Circle CRD) from B to G, and make $GP = PI = 40°$ as before, then from D draw DG, DI, which will cut rI in F and I, so will FI be
the

Sect. IV.   *Of the* Sphere   201

the Diameter of the Parallel, which bisect in *c* the Center, on which with the Radius $cF = cI$ describe the Circle *FHI* which will be distant 40° from its Pole *p*, and 50° from its Parallel great Circle *CRD*, as was required (Fig 21)

By the Sector.

Measure *Ep* on the Semitangents (= 70°), then set the half Tangent of $\overline{70° - 40°} = 30°$ from *E* to *F*, as also the half Tangent of $\overline{70° + 30°} = 100°$ from *E* to *I*, round the Diameter *FI* describe the Circle *FHI* the Parallel required.

Note, If the Circle lie all on one Side *E*, these half Tangents are set the same Way from *E* upon the Line *rI*, but if the Circle encompass the Pole, each is set its own Way.

Prop. VII. Prob.

To draw a great Circle through any two Points **A**, **B** *within the primitive Circle* **DEGH**.

Rule.

Through *A* (the Point farthest distant from the Center of the Primitive) draw the Diameter *DL*, at right Angles to which through the Center *C* draw another Diameter *EH*, draw *AE*, and from *E* erect the Perpendicular *EK*, to cut *DL* continued in a third Point *K*. Through the two given Points *A*, *B*, and this last third Point *K*, draw the great Circle *IBK*, cutting the Primitive in opposite Points *I*, *G*. (Fig. 22.)

By the Sector.

Find the Degrees in CA, the Semitangent of whose Supplement set from C to K, so is K a third Point, through which draw a great Circle IBK as before.

Or thus;

Measure CA on the Tangents, set the Tangent of its Complement from C to K.

Prop VIII. Prob.

To draw a great Circle round a given Pole F.

Rule.

Through the given Pole F draw the Line of Measures AH, at right Angles to which through the Center E of the Primitive draw the Diameter BD; through the Pole F draw DFP, and make $PH = BP$, also from H draw HD, which will give the Point H, the Center of the oblique Circle required, on which with the Radius HB or HD describe the great Circle BFD. (Fig. 23.)

By the Sector.

Apply EF to the Semitangents, set the Tangent of these Degrees from E to H, the Center of the required great Circle BFD.

Prop IX. Prob.

To draw a Circle round a given Pole A, *to pass through a given Point* B. (Fig. 24.)

Rule

Sect. IV.   *Of the* Sphere.

Rule.

Through the given Pole *A*, from the Center *C* draw the Line of Measures *CAH*, also through *A*, *B* describe a great Circle *EBF* whose Center is *G*, draw *GB*, and from *B* draw *BD* perpendicular to *GB*, to cut *CAH* in *D*, on the Center *D*, with the Radius *DB* describe the Circle *BKHI*, and it is done. For by the Conditions of the Prob. the Arch *AB* is the required Circle's Distance from its Pole *A*, and as *GB* is the Radius of the Arch *AB*, therefore *BD* being erected perpendicular to *GB*, at *B* in the Periphery, will be a Tangent Line to the Arch *AB*, which tangential Line cutting *CAH* in *D*, will (by Prop 4) be the Radius of the required Circle.

Prop. X. Prob.

To draw a great Circle perpendicular to the Primitive, to make an Angle of any Number of Degrees (suppose 50°) at the Center of the Primitive

Rule

Let *ABCD* be the primitive Circle, whose Pole is *E*; through *E* draw *AEC* and *BED* perpendicular to each other, make *BK* = *DI* = 50° = the Quantity of the proposed Angle, and from *K*, through the Pole *E* draw the right Circle *KEI*, which will make an ∠ *BEK* = *DEI* at the Center of the Primitive = 50°, as was required. (Fig. 18.)

Prop.

Prop. XI. Prob.

To draw a great Circle to make an Angle with the Primitive, of any Number of Degrees, &c. (suppose 50°).

Rule.

Quarter the Primitive, by drawing the Diameters *AFC*, *BFD*, then supposing *AFL* the Line of Measures, make *AK* = 50° = the Quantity of the proposed Angle, and *DM* = 2 *KB* = twice the Complement of the Inclination = 80°, or *BM* = 2 *AK* = twice the Inclination = 100°, draw *DEK*, *DML* to cut the Line of Measures in *E* and *L*, on the Center *L*, with the Radius *LE* describe the great oblique Circle *BED*, making an Angle at *B* with the Primitive of 50° (F.25.)

By the Sector.

Draw the Line of Measures *AL*, set the half Tangent of 40° (the Complement of the Circle's Inclination to the Primitive) from *F* to *E*, as also the Tangent of 50° (the Quantity of the Inclination) from *F* to *L*; with the Radius *LE* and Center *L*, describe the great oblique Circle *BED* which will cut the Primitive in *B* and *D*, and make therewith an Angle of 50°, as was required.

Or thus,

Set the Tangent of the Inclination (50°) from *F* to *L*, with the Secant thereof, and Center *L*, sweep the Circle *BED*, and it is done.

Prop.

Prop. XII. Prob.

To draw a great Circle through a given Point P, *to make a given Angle (suppose* 30°) *with the Primitive* ABCD. (Fig 26.)

Rule.

Through the given Point *P* and Center *E* draw the Diameter *AEC*; make *AG* = twice the propofed Angle = 60°, and draw *CHG*, to cut *BED* in *H*, fo *EH* is the Tangent of the propofed Angle, or Tangent of 30°, with which as a Radius, on the Center *E* defcribe the Circle *HIK*, in fome Part of which, the Center of the required Circle will be found, as the Centers of all great Circles (by Prop. 5) are diftant from the Center of the Primitive, the Tangents of their Inclinations to the Primitive, and their Radii the Secants of thefe Inclinations. Now as *CH* is evidently the Secant of the ∠ *HCE*, it is the Secant of the given ∠ of 30°, and confequently the Radius of the required Circle; therefore with the Radius *CH*, and Center *P*, crofs the Circle *HIK* in *K*. With the Radius *KP*, and Center *K*, defcribe the Circle *FPL* required.

By the Sector.

With the Tangent of 30°, and Center *E*, defcribe the Circle *HIK*, with the Secant thereof, and Center *P*, crofs the Circle *HIK* in *K*. On the Center *K*, and Radius *KP*, defcribe the *FPL* as before. (Fig. 26)

Prop. XIII. Prob.

To draw a great Circle to make a proposed Angle of any Number of Degrees, &c. (suppose 25° 30') with a given oblique Circle EPK, at a given Point P, in that Circle. (FIG. 27.)

Rule.

Through the given Point *P* and Center *S* draw the right Line *BD*, also through *S* draw *AC* ⊥ to *BD*, and from *A* draw *APF* to cut the primitive Circle in *F*, make *CI* = 2 *BF*, from *I* draw *IA* to cut *BD* in *M*, and through *M* draw *OQ* parallel to *AC*, in which Line *OQ* will be found the Centers of all great oblique Circles passing through the Point *P*. Find *H* the Center of the given oblique Circle *EPK*, and make an ∠ *HPN* = 25° 30', and draw *PN*; on the Center *N*, with the Radius *NP* describe the Circle *GPL*, which will intersect *EPK* in *P*, and make an Angle therewith of 20° 30', as was required.

By the Sector.

Through *SP* draw the Diameter *BD*, and through *S* draw *AC* ⊥ *BD*, measure *SP* on the Semitangents, set the Tangent of its Complement from *S* to *M*, and through *M* draw *OQ* ⊥ *BD*, find the Center *H*, measure *MH* (=41° 00') on the Tangents, then 41° 00" — 25° 30' = 15° 30', the Tangent of which set from *M* to *N*, the Center of the required Circle. *Note*, If one Circle is to be drawn perpendicular to another, it

muſt

muſt paſs through its Poles, as the right Circle *AC* is ⊥ to the right Circle *BD*, paſſing through its Poles *A*, *C*; it is alſo perpendicular to the Primitive *ABCD*.

Prop. XIV. Prob.

Through a given Point P *to draw a great Circle, to make a given Angle* (= 70° 00′) *with a given great Circle* BD. (Fig. 28.)

Rule.

Draw the great Circle *EF* about the given Point *P* conſidered as a Pole, by Prop. 8, and find *p* the Pole of the given great Circle *BD*, by Prop. 3, round the Pole *p* draw the leſſer Circle *IKL* (by Prop 6) at 70° Diſtance from it, to cut the great Circle *EF* in *I*, around the Pole *I* draw another great Circle *EPF* (by Prop 8) which will not only paſs through the given Point *P*, but will alſo cut the given great Circle *BD*, and make an Angle with it of 70°, as was required. For as *p* is the Pole of the given great Circle *BD*, and *I* is the Pole of the required Circle *EPF*, thoſe two Poles are diſtant from each other, the Space of the leſſer Circle *IKL* from its Pole, viz 70° (the Quantity of the given Angle), and conſequently the two great Circles muſt interſect each other in an Angle of 70°.

By the Sector.

Through the Center *C* and the given Point *P* draw the right Line *CP*, find *p* the Pole of the given great Circle

Circle BD, measure CP on the Semitangents, set the Tangent thereof from C to x, with the Radius Ex, or the Secant of the Degrees in CP, and Center x, describe the great Circle EF. Then Cp measured on the Semitangents is 34°, and 70 − 34 = 36°, therefore make Cr = Tangent of 18°, also 70 + 34 = 104°, the Tangent of whose Half 52 set from C to s, around the Diameter rs describe the small Circle IKL, to cut EF in I, again, find the Degrees in CI, the Tangent of which set from C to v, on the Center v with the Radius Ev, or the Secant of the Degrees in CI, describe the great Circle EPF, which will pass through the Point P, and cut the given great Circle BD in an Angle of 70 Degrees, as was required.

Prop XV. Prob.

Given two great Circles BE, FD, *through which a great Circle is to be drawn, to make an Angle of* 72° *with* BE, *and of* 56° *with* FD. (Fig. 29)

Rule.

Find x, v the Poles of the given great Circles BE, FD, about these Poles draw two small Circles prn, pon (by Prop 6.) at the Distance of 72° from the Pole x, and of 56° from the Pole v, about their Point of Intersection p describe the great Circle AG, by Prop. 8, which will cut BE and FD at the required Angles.

Prop XVI. Prob.

To measure any Part FH *of a great oblique Circle* BFE, *or to lay any Number of Degrees thereon.* (F. 30)

Rule.

Sect. IV.   *Of the* Sphere.   209

Rule.

Find the internal Pole *P* of the given Circle *BFE*, through the Extremities of the Arch *FH* draw *PG, PA*, to cut the primitive Circle in *G* and *A*, then the Arch *AG* is the Measure of $FH = 51°$. Or lay the Chord of 51° from *A* to *G*, and draw *AP, GP* to cut *BFE* in *F, H*, so is the Arch $FH = 51°$, Or, if you use the external Pole *p*, set the given Degrees (51°) from *D* to *I*, and draw *pHI, pFD*, cutting off an Arch *FH* = Measure of the Arch $DI = 51°$. Or the Pole *p* being found, if from *p* you draw *pFD, pHI*, it will cut off an Arch *FH* as before. (Fig. 30)

Prop. XVII Prob.

To measure any Part FE *of a right Circle* AC, *or to set any Number of Degrees thereon.* (Fig. 25)

Rule.

From the Pole *D* draw the Line *DEK*, to cut the Primitive in *K*, then *BK* measured on the Chords, is 36° = the Measure of *FE*, as also is $AK = 54°$ = the Measure of *AE*.

By the Sector.

Take *FE* in your Compasses, and apply it to the Tangents, and it will give 18°, whose Double 36° is the Measure of *FE*.

Ee 2   Or

Or the Tangent of Half the given Degrees set from *F* towards *A*, will give *FE* = the said Quantity. If the Part *AE* is to be measured, apply it to the Tangents from 45° backwards; or if the Degrees are to be set from *A* towards *F*, take off the Degrees from 45° towards the Beginning of the Tangents, and set from *A* towards *F*.

Prop XVII. Prob.

To measure any Part NO *of a lesser Circle* NRS, *or to lay any Number of Degrees on it.* (Fig. 31)

Rule.

Find *P*, *p* the internal and external Poles of the given Circle *NRS*, also let *ABCD* be the primitive Circle, whose Pole is *E*. *PN* measured is 64° = Distance of the given Circle *NRS* from its internal Pole *P*, also 180° − 64° = 116° its Distance from its external Pole *p*, then with the Tangent of 58° (= 116° ÷ 2) describe the Circle *IGH* parallel to the Primitive; through the Extremities of the Arch *NO*, from the internal Pole *P* draw the right Lines *POF*, *PNp*, to cut the parallel Circle *IGH* in *I* and *F*, then is *IF* the Measure of the Arch *NO* = 57°. Or 57° being set from *I* to *F*, and the Lines *INP*, *FOP* being drawn, will cut off the Arch *NO*.

Or thus, draw a Circle *KLQ* parallel to the Primitive, at 64° Distance from it (viz. the given Circle's Distance from its external Pole *p*), from *p* draw the Lines *pNH*, *pOG*, which will cut off an Arch *TQ* = 57°

Sect. IV.   *Of the* Sphere.   211

$57°$ = the Measure of the Arch *NO*. Or if $57°$ be set from *T* to *Q*, and the Lines *pNH*, *pOG* being drawn, will cut off an Arch *NO* as before. (Fig. 31.)

Prop. XIX. Prob.

To measure any Angle FEB.

Rule.

Find the Poles *M*, *N* of the adjoining Sides *FE*, *BE*, by Prop 3, (the nearest if the Angle be acute, but the furthest if it be obtuse), through the angular Point and these Poles, draw Lines to cut the Primitive in *K* and *L*; the Chord of the Arch *KL* is $35°$ = the Measure of the given Angle *FEB* (Fig. 32)

Or thus, about the angular Point *E*, as a Pole, describe the great Circle *FMG* to cut the containing Sides *FE*, *BE* in *F* and *O*, thro' these Points *F*, *O*, from the angular Point *E* draw Lines to cut the Primitive in *I* and *A*, then the Arch *IH* is the Measure of the Angle *FEB* = $35°$, as before.

GENERAL PROBLEM.

To project the Sphere on any Plane.

Before the Circles of the Sphere be projected upon the Plane of any of its Circles, it is requisite that you be acquainted with the Position of several of the principal Circles of the Globe, their Names and other astronomical Terms made use of in a Work of that Sort.

The

The Names of the principal Points, Circles great and small, Angles and circular Arches are as follows.

1. Points.

1 The Zenith Z is the vertical Point, or that Point in the Heavens which is directly over our Heads (Fig 33, 34, 35, 36.)

2. The Nadir is that Point which is opposite to the Zenith and is directly under our Feet, as N, these Points are the Poles of the Horizon.

3. The Poles of the World P, p are those Points, upon which the Earth turns in its diurnal Motion round the Sun

4. Equinoctial Points are the Points of Intersection of the Equinoctial and Ecliptic, as ♈ ♎.

5. Solstitial Points ♋ ♑ are 90° distant from the Equinoctial Points.

2. Great Circles.

1. The Equinoctial FG is distant from the Poles of the World 90 Degrees

2. Meridians, are Circles passing through the Poles of the World, and cutting the Equinoctial at right Angles, as PFp, $P\odot p$, &c

3 The Equinoctial Colure, is a Meridian cutting the Ecliptic in the Equinoctial Points ♈ and ♎, as PEp

4 The Solstitial Colure, is a Meridian passing through the Solstitial Points, P ♋ p.

5 Elliptic, is that Circle through which the Sun seems to move in the Space of a Year; it is divided into

to 12 equal Parts called Signs, whose Characters are ♈, ♉, ♊, ♋, ♌, ♍, ♎, ♏, ♐, ♑, ♒, ♓, and read thus, Aries, Taurus, Gemini, Cancer, Leo, Virgo, Libra, Scorpio, Sagitary, Capricorn, Aquaries, Pisces.

6. Horizon, is a Circle 90° distant from the Zenith and Nadir, as *AC*

7 Azimuths, are vertical Circles passing through the Zenith and Nadir, as *Z ⊙ N*.

8. Circles of Longitude, pass through the Poles of the Ecliptic.

3. LESSER CIRCLES

1. Tropics, are two Circles parallel to the Equinoctial, and distant from it 23° 30', the one is called the Tropic of Cancer, being on the Northern Side of the Equinoctial, and the other the Tropic of Capricorn, being on the South Side of the Equinoctial.

2 Polar Circles, are distant from each Pole 34° 30'; that towards the North Pole is called the Arctic Circle, and that towards the South, the Antarctic Circle

3. Parallels of Latitude, with Respect to the Earth, are parallel to the Equator

4 Parallels of Latitude, with Regard to the Heavens, are parallel to the Ecliptic

5 Parallels of Declination, are parallel to the Equinoctial, as *HMI*.

6. Parallels of Altitude, are small Circles parallel to the Horizon, as *K ⊙ L*.

4. Ar-

4. ANGLES and CIRCULAR ARCHES

1. Azimuth, is an Arch of the Horizon, between a vertical Circle and the North or South Points of the Horizon, as *AB* is the Sun's Azimuth from the South, whose Supplement *BC* is the Azimuth from the North.

2. Amplitude, is an Arch of the Horizon, between the Sun at his rising, or setting, and the East or West Points of the Horizon as *EN*.

3. Altitude, is an Arch of an azimuth Circle between the Sun or Star and the Horizon, as ☉ *B*.

4. Right Ascension, is an Arch of the Equinoctial, between the first Point of Aries and that Meridian which passes through the Body of the Sun or Star, as ♈ *o*.

5. Ascensional Difference, is an Arch of the Equinoctial intercepted between the Sun's Meridian at his Rising, and the Hour-circle of six, or it is the Angle at the Pole between those two Hour-circles.

6. Oblique Ascension, is the Sum or Difference of the right Ascension and ascensional Difference.

7. Sun's Place or Longitude, is an Arch of the Ecliptic, between the first Point of Aries and the Sun, as ♈ ☉.

EXAMPLE I.

To project the Sphere on the Plane of the Meridian, for Lat. $54°\frac{1}{2}$, at Half an Hour past 9 o'Clock before Noon, *May* 15, 1769.

1. Orthographically.

With a Chord of 60° describe the primitive Circle *ZANC*,

Pl V.

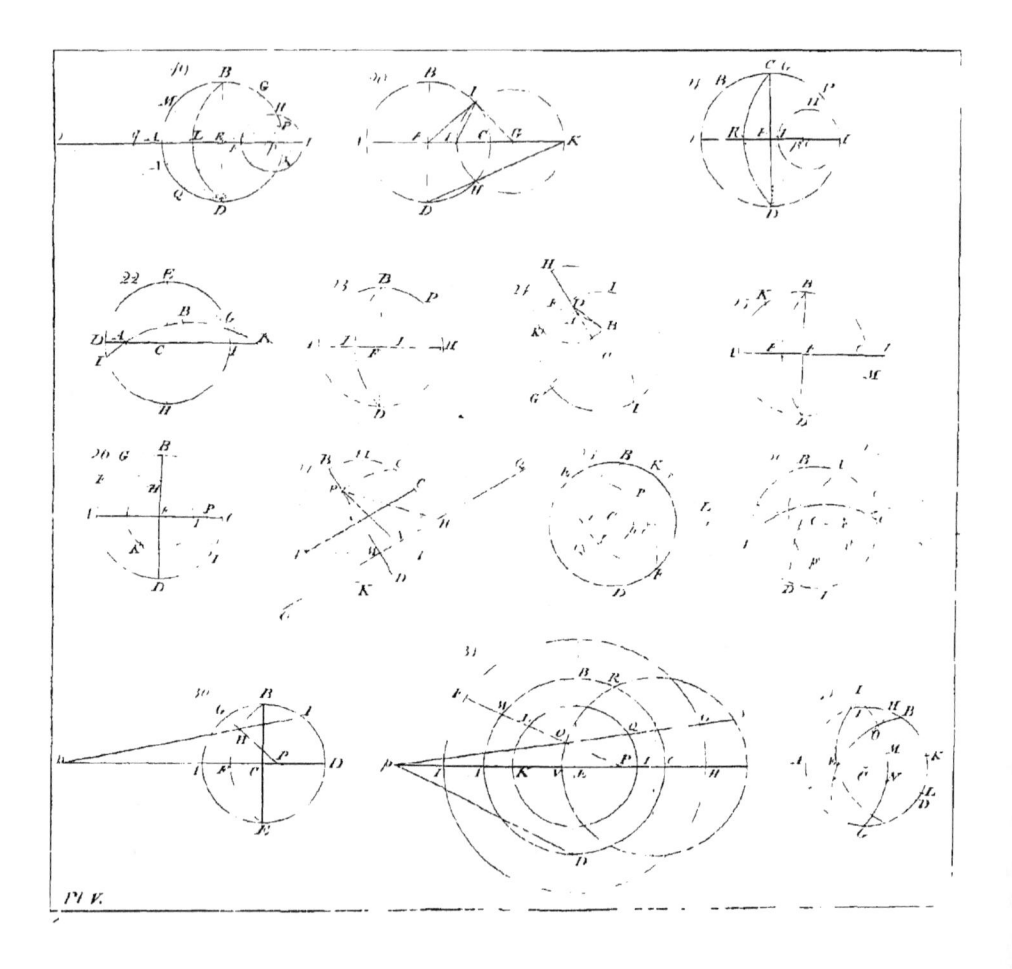

Sect. IV.   *Of the* SPHERE.   215

$ZANC$, representing the Meridian, set the Chord of the Lat (54°½) from C to P, and from Z to F, and draw FEG the Equinoctial, and PEp the Earth's Axis, or Hour-circle of Six   By Prop. 8, draw the Meridian $P\odot p$, at 3½ Hours (or 52° 30′) from Six, set the Sun's Declination for the given Time (19°) from G to I, and from F to H, and draw the Parallel of Declination HI, to cut the Hour-circle $P\odot p$ in $\odot$ the Place of the Sun at Half an Hour past 9 o'clock before Noon. Through $\odot$ draw the Parallel of Altitude $K\odot L$; also draw the Parallel of Twilight 18° below the Horizon, Ss. Through $\odot$ describe the Azimuth Circle $Z\odot N$ by Prop. 8. Then MN measured by Prop. 11, and converted into Time, is what the Sun rises before Six; CD is his Altitude at Six, CL ($= AK$) his Altitude at Half an Hour past Nine, AB his Azimuth from the South at the same Time, BC his Azimuth from the North, and EQ his Altitude when due East. EN is the Sun's Amplitude at rising or setting As the Parallel of Twilight is not cut by the Parallel of the Sun's Declination, therefore there is no real Night in that Latitude, but Twilight (FIG. 33.)

2. *Stereographically.*

With a Chord of 60° describe the Circle $ZANC$ for the Plane of the Meridian, draw AC the Horizon, at right Angles to which draw the prime Vertical ZN. Set the Latitude 54°½ from C to P, and from Z to F, and draw the Axis PEp, at right Angles to which, through the Center E, draw the Equinoctial FEG, so is P the North Pole of the Globe, and p the South

Pole Set $3\frac{1}{2}$ Hours (or 52° 30′) from E to O upon the Equinoctial, and draw the Hour-circle POp by Prop. 11 By Prop. 5, draw the Parallel of the Sun's Declination 19° for May 15, HOI, which will interfect the Hour-circle POp in ☉ the Sun's Place Th1o' ☉ draw the Parallel of Altitude K☉L, by Prop 5, and the Azimuth Circle ZON, by Prop 11, alfo draw Ss parallel to the Horizon, at the Diftance of 18° below it; this is the Parallel of Twilight. Through ☉, by Prop. 14, draw a great Circle ♈☉♎, to cut the Equinoctial FEG in an Angle of $23°\frac{1}{2}$, this Circle is called the Ecliptic. (Fig 37.)

Now it is evident by the Projection, that at 12 o'Clock at Night the Sun is at I, rifes at N, is upon the Axis (or Hour-circle of Six) at M, full Eaft at Q, at O at Half an Hour paft Nine in the Morning, and at H at 12 at Noon The Arch MN meafured, and converted into Time, is what the Sun rifes and fets before and after Six o'Clock, AB meafured by Prop 18, is the Sun's Azimuth from the South, and BC his Azimuth from the North, or the $\angle AZB$ meafured by Prop. 19, is the Azimuth from the South, and the $\angle BZC$ (= Supplement of the $\angle AZB$) the Azimuth from the North ☉B meafured by Prop 16, is the Sun's Altitude at Half an Hour paft Nine, QE his Altitude when Eaft, and CD his Altitude at Six in the Morning and Evening. EN meafured by Prop. 17, is the Amplitude North, at the Sun's rifing or fetting. ♈☉ is the Sun's Longitude, and ♈O his right Afcenfion at the given Time. (Fig. 34)

Ex-

Example II.

To project the Sphere on the Plane of the Meridian of the solstitial Colure, for May 22, 1769, at 10 o'Clock in the Morning, Latitude $54°\frac{1}{2}$.

Stereographically.

Let $PFpG$ be the Plane of the solstitial Colure; draw PEp the Axis, and FG perpendicular to it for the Equinoctial. Make $F♋ = 23°\frac{1}{2}$, and draw $♋E♑$ the Ecliptic. Set the Sun's Longitude $61°\ 57'$ from $♈$ to $☉$, by Prop. 17, and through $☉$ draw the 10 o'Clock Meridian $P☉p$. Make $KI = 30°$ or two Hours, and draw PKp the Meridian of the Place. Set the Latitude $54°\frac{1}{2}$ upon the Meridian from K to Z the Zenith of the Place, by Prop. 16, also about the Pole Z describe, by Prop 8, the great Circle AHC the Horizon, through Z, $☉$ draw the vertical Circle $Z☉B$, by Prop 7. Then $☉B$ measured by Prop. 16, is the Sun's Altitude at 10 o'Clock, $Z☉$ his Zenith Distance, $I☉$ his Declination North, $♈I$ his right Ascension, the $\angle LZ☉$ his Azimuth from the South, the $\angle PZ☉$ his Azimuth from the North, L is the culminating Point, or Point of the Ecliptic in the Meridian at the given Time, and M is the Point of the Ecliptic setting in the West, or the Point of Intersection of the Ecliptic and Horizon. (Fig. 35.)

Example III.

To project the Sphere on the Plane of the Horizon, Lat. $54°\frac{1}{2}$, at the last-mentioned Time, viz. May 22, 1769.

Stereographically.

With a Chord of 60° defcribe the primitive Circle $CEDQ$, reprefenting the Horizon. Draw CD for the Meridian, and EQ perpendicular to it, for the prime Vertical, or Eaſt and Weſt Azimuth Circle. Make $ZP = 35°\frac{1}{2}$ the Complement of the Latitude, fo is P the North Pole of the Globe, about which, by Prop 8, defcribe the Equinoctial EAQ, make $AG = 30°$ (or 2 Hours), and draw the 10 o'Clock Meridian BPF, fet the Sun's Declination 19°, from G to $\odot$ the Place of the Sun at 10 o'Clock, and through $\odot$ draw the Ecliptic $\Upsilon \odot \libra$, by Prop. 14, to cut the Equinoctial in Υ and $\libra$, in an Angle of $23°\frac{1}{2}$, alfo from Z through $\odot$ draw the vertical Circle ZOR. About A as a Pole, draw the Six o'Clock Hour-circle EPQ. Then $G\odot$ is the Sun's Declination, $\odot R$ his Altitude at 10 o'Clock, DR his Azimuth from the South, CR his Azimuth from the North, $\Upsilon \odot$ is his Longitude or Place in the Ecliptic, ΥG his right Afcenfion, S the Point of the Ecliptic that is in the Meridian, T the Point of the Ecliptic that is rifing in the Eaſt, H is the Point of the Ecliptic fetting in the Weſt; the $\angle CTS$ or STD is the Cufp of the Afcendant, and the $\angle CHS$ or SHD is the Cufp of the Defcendant. (Fig 36)

BOOK V.

Spheric Trigonometry, *or the* Doctrine *of* Spheric Triangles.

Definitions

1. Spheric Trigonometry teacheth us to meafure the Sides and Angles of fpheric Triangles

2. A great Circle of the Globe or Sphere is fuch, as divideth it into two equal Parts or Hemifpheres; thefe Circles are infinite in Number, but the fix following are accounted the chief, viz. the Equinoctial, Ecliptic, Meridian, Horizon, and the Equinoctial and Solftitial Colures, which Colures are Meridians, the one cutting the Ecliptic in two oppofite Points ♈ and ♎, and is called the Equinoctial Colure, the other interfecting the Ecliptic in two oppofite Points ♋ and ♑, and thence called the Solftitial Colure.

3. All fpheric Triangles are made by the Interfection of three great Circles of the Sphere

4. The neareft Diftance between any two Places on the Surface of the Globe, is an Arch of a great Circle paffing over or through the faid two Places

5. A fpheric Angle is conftructed by the Interfection of two great Circles of the Sphere, their Point of Interfection being the Angle, and hence the oppofite Angles at the Interfection are equal, as $ACB = ICH$. (Fig. 37.)

6. The greateft Angle is ever oppofite to the greateft Side,

Side, and the least Angle to the least Side, also equal Angles have equal Sides

7. The greatest Side always subtends the greatest Angle, the least Side the least Angle, and equal Sides equal Angles

8. Every spheric Angle is measured upon the Arch of a great Circle, at the Distance of a Quadrant or 90 Degrees from it, as ED is the Measure of the Angle A in the Triangle ABC, the Arch AE being a Quadrant

9. As in Plain Trigonometry, so in Spherical, the Radius is a mean Proportional between the Tangent of an Arch, and the Tangent Complement of the same Arch

10. Any great Circle passing through the Poles of another great Circle, these Circles intersect each other at right Angles.

11. The Sides of any spheric Triangle ABC may be turned into Angles, and the Angles into Sides, ever observing that the Complement of the greatest Side, or the Complement of the greatest Angle to a Semicircle (or 180°) must be used in the Conversion, for in the Triangle ABC, the Arch DE is the Measure of the Angle A, because AD and AE are Quadrants, also FG is the Measure of the Angle FBG (it being the Complement of the obtuse Angle B), and HI is the Measure of the Angle C, because CH and CI are Quadrants. Then it is evident in the Diagram, that KL is equal to the Arch DE, because KD and LE are Quadrants, and LD is a Complement common to both. ML is = the Arch FG, because MF and FG are Quadrants, and LF is their common Complement
MK

MK is = Arch HI, becaufe MH and KI are Quadrants, and their common Complement is KH, and therefore the Sides of the Triangle MKL are equal to the Angles of the Triangle ABC, taking the Complement of the greateft Angle B (viz the $\angle DBL$) Alfo it is in like manner demonftrable, that the Sides of the Triangle ABC, are equal to the Angles of the Triangle MKL, the greateft Side being equal to the Complement of the greateft Angle to a Semicircle, for AB is equal to the Arch EG = the Meafure of the Angle MLK, and BC is = the Arch FH = the Meafure of the Angle KML, alfo AC is = the Arch DI = the Meafure of the Angle HKP = the Complement of the obtufe Angle MKL. And therefore the Sides of any fpheric Triangle may be changed into Angles, and the Angles into Sides. (Fig 37.)

12. The three Sides of any fpherical Triangle, are lefs than two Semicircles.

13. The three Angles of any fpherical Triangle added together, are greater than two right Angles; and hence it is, that the Quantity of any two Angles being known, the third is not of courfe known, as it is in plain Triangles.

14. If any fpherical Triangle hath one or more of its Sides Quadrants, it is called a quadrantal Triangle.

15. If any fpherical Triangle hath one or more right Angles, it is called a right-angled fpherical Triangle.

16. Thofe Triangles having neither a right Angle, nor any Side a Quadrant, are called oblique fpherical Triangles.

17. If a fpherical Triangle be both right-angled and

qua

quadrantal, the Sides are equal to their opposite Angles, as *HMC*.

SECT I.

The SOLUTION *of the several* CASES *of* RIGHT-ANGLED SPHERICAL TRIANGLES

THERE are in every right-angled spherical Triangle five Parts, besides the right Angle, as in the right-angled spherical Triangle *ABC*, the two Legs *AB*, *BC*, the two oblique Angles *A*, *C*, and the Hypothenuse *AC* are the five Parts, of which five Parts, those three farthest from the right Angle are never used in any Operation, but only their Complements, for it is plain by the Triangle *ABC*, that if the Hypothenuse *AC* be continued to a Quadrant, the Arch *CD* is the Complement of *AD* to a Quadrant or 90°, also *ED* is the Measure of the Angle *A*, and being continued to a Quadrant, is the Complement of *EI*, the Arch *FG* is = the Measure of the Angle *C*, and is the Complement of the Quadrant *FH*, and therefore the Hypothenuse *AC*, and the two oblique Angles *A* and *C* are never used in trigonometrical Calculations, but their Complements (according to Lord Neper), but the Complements of the Legs *AB* and *BC* are *AH*, and *CI*, which are never used, but the Sines themselves, or the Tangents themselves.

In

Sect. I.   SPHERICAL TRIANGLES.   223

In the Solution of any right-angled fpherical Triangle, two Things (befides the right Angle) muſt be given, to find a fourth (the right Angle being always rejected, and the two Legs ſuppoſed to ſtand together. Of which three Things concerned in the Queſtion, one is always termed the middle Part, and the other two are always Extreams either conjunct (lying together), or disjunct (being ſeparated by ſome other Part). And therefore to know which of the three Things concerned in any Queſtion, is the middle Part, always obſerve if the three Parts ſtand together, the Middlemoſt of the three is the middle Part, as ſuppoſe AC and AB be given, and the Angle A required, here the three Parts ſtand together, and the Angle A is in the Middle, and is therefore the middle Part. But when the three Things concerned in the Queſtion do not ſtand together, that which ſtands by itſelf is the middle Part. As ſuppoſe AC and AB were given, and BC required, here the Parts AB and BC ſtand together (the right Angle B making no Separation) and AC ſtands by itſelf, ſeparated from the others by the Angles A, C, which are unconcerned in the Queſtion, and therefore AC is the middle Part. (FIG 38.)

There are 16 Caſes of right-angled ſpherical Triangles, all of which take their Solution from this one univerſal Propoſition, viz

The Sine of a middle Part and Radius, are reciprocally proportional with the Tangents of the Extreams conjunct, and Co-ſines of the Extreams disjunct. That is,

As Radius : Tangent of one Extream conjunct :: Tangent of the other Extream conjunct : Sine of the middle Part. Alſo,

As Radius · Co-sine of one Extream disjunct ∷ Co-sine of the other Extream disjunct ∷ Sine of the middle Part.

When the middle Part is required, Radius must come first in the Analogy, but if one of the Extreams be required, the other Extream must be first in the Analogy, and then the Radius either the second or third, it matters not which.

When at any Time a Complement in the Analogy falls upon a Complement in any of the circular Parts, you must take the Sine itself, or the Tangent itself; for Co-sine of Co-sine is = Sine, and Co-tangent of Co-tangent is = Tangent.

Secants may any Time be introduced into any Analogy consisting of Sines and Tangents, by observing these Proportions, viz.

1. As the Tangent ∶ Radius ∷ Radius ∶ the Co-tangent
2. As the Sine ∶ Radius ∷ Radius ∶ Co-secant
3. As the Tangent of an Arch ∶ Tangent of an Arch ∷ Co-tangent of the latter Arch ∶ Co-tangent of the former
4. As the Sine of an Arch ∶ the Sine of an Arch ∷ Co-secant of the latter Arch ∶ the Co-secant of the former. See *Martin*'s Trigon vol 2 pa 103

The several Cases of right-angled spherical Triangles are resolved by stereographic Projection, and also logarithmically.

Right-angled spherical Triangles.

CASE I

Given the Hypothenuse CB = 42° 36′, and the Angle C = 54° 40, to find the adjacent Side CA. (FIG 39)

1. By

Sect. IV.   SPHERICAL TRIANGLES.   225

1 By ftereographic Projection.

With a Chord of 60° fweep the Circle $DEFG$, make $FI =$ the Chord of 54° 40′ (the given Angle), and draw the Diameter HI, make $CB =$ the Half-tangent of 42° 36′, and through B, at right Angles to DF, draw the oblique Circle EBG, fo fhall ABC be the Triangle in which the Quefitum fhall be found. Then CA meafured on the Half-tangents is 28 00′.

2 Logarithmically.

As Radius	——	90° 00′	—— 10 000000
To Tan Hyp CB	——	42 36	—— 9 963574
So Col $\angle C$	——	54 40	—— 9 762177
To Tan. CA	——	28 00	—— 9 725751

CASE II.

Given the Hypothenufe $CB = 42°\ 36′$, *and the Angle* $C = 54°\ 40′$, *to find the oppofite Side* AB. (FIG. 39.)

1. By ftereographic Projection

Project the Triangle ABC by Cafe 1; then AB meafured by Prob. 16, is 33° 31′.

2. Logarithmically.

As Radius $S\,CB = 42°\ 36′$ $S.\angle C = 54°\ 40′$
$S.\,AB = 33°\ 31′$.

G g 2   CASE

CASE III.

Given the Hypothenuse CB = 42° 36', *and the Angle* C = 54° 40, *to find the other Angle* B (FIG. 39)

1. By stereographic Projection.

Construct the Triangle *ABC* by Case 1, then the Angle *B* measured by Prob 19, is 43° 55'.

2 Logarithmically.

As Radius Tan ∠ C 54° 40' Cof CB 42° 36' : Cot ∠ B 43° 55'.

CASE IV.

Given the Hypothenuse CB = 42° 36', *and the Leg* CA = 28° 00', *to find the adjacent Angle* C. (FIG. 39)

1. By stereographic Projection.

Make *CA* = the Half-tangent of 28° 00', through *A* draw *EAG* ⊥ to *DF*, also with the Half-tangent of 42° 36' draw the parallel Circle *KBA*, which will cut the great oblique Circle *EAG* in *B*; through *B* draw the right Circle *HBI*, compleating the Triangle *ABC* Then the ∠ C measured by Prob 19, is 54° 40'.

2 Logarithmically.

As Radius . Cotan. Hyp *CB* 42° 36' .. Tan. Leg *CA* 28° 00' Cof. ∠ *C* 54° 40'.

Sect. I.   SPHERICAL TRIANGLES.   227

CASE V

Given the Hypothenuse CB = 42° 36′, *and the Leg* CA = 28° 00′, *to find the opposite Angle* B   (FIG. 39.)

1. By stereographic Projection.

Project the Triangle *ABC* by Case 4. Then measure the ∠ B by Prob 19, which will be found 43° 55′.

2. Logarithmically.

As *S.*CB 42° 36′ : Radius ∷ *S* CA 28° 00′ : *S*∠B 54° 40′

CASE VI.

Given the Hypothenuse CB = 42° 36′, *and the Leg* CA = 28° 00′, *to find the other Leg* AB.   (FIG 39)

1. By stereographic Projection

Project the Triangle *ABC*, as in the last Case: Then *AB* measured by Prob. 16, is 33° 31′.

2. Logarithmically.

As Cof Leg. CA 28° 00′ : Radius ∷ Cof. Hyp. CB 42° 36′ : Cof. Leg *AB* 33° 31′.

CASE VII.

Given the Side CA = 28° 00′, *and the adjacent Angle* C = 54° 40′, *to find the opposite Side* AB.   (FIG 39.)

1 By

1. By ſtereographic Projection.

Make $CA = 28°\ 00'$ by Prob 17, and the $\angle C = 54°\ 40'$ by Prob 10. Through A draw EAG perpendicular to DF, to cut HI in B, then AB meaſured by Prob. 16, is $33°\ 31'$

2. Logarithmically

As Radius · S Side CA 28° 00′ :: Tan $\angle C$ 54° 40′ Tan Side AB 33° 31′

CASE VIII.

Given the Side $CA = 28°\ 00'$, and the adjacent Angle $C = 54°\ 40'$, to find the oppoſite Angle B (FIG. 39)

1. By ſtereographic Projection

Project the Triangle ABC by the laſt Caſe, then is the Angle B meaſured by Prob. 19, $= 43°\ 55'$

2 Logarithmically

As Radius S adjacent Angle C 54° 40′ .: Coſ Side CA 28° Coſ opp. Angle B 43° 55′.

CASE IX

Given the Side $CA = 28°\ 00'$, and the adjacent Angle $C = 54°\ 40'$, to find the Hypothenuſe CB. (FIG. 39)

1 By ſtereographic Projection

Project the Triangle ABC by Caſe 7, then the Hypothenuſe CB meaſured by Prob. 17, is 42° 36′

2. Lo-

2. Logarithmically

As Radius . Cof ∠ C 54° 40'   Cotan. Side CA 28° 00' . Cotan Hyp. CB 42° 36'.

CASE X.

Given the Side AB = 33° 31', *and the opposite Angle* C = 54° 40', *to find the adjacent Side* CA   (FIG 39.)

1 By stereographic Projection.

Project the ∠ C = 54° 40', by Prob 10, draw LM parallel to DF, at 33° 31' Distance from it, to cut HI in B, through B draw EBG perpendicular to DF, and the Triangle is constructed. Then CA measured, is 28° 00'.

2 Logarithmically.

As Radius Cotan opp ∠ C 54° 40'   Tan Side AB 33° 31' S. Side CA 28° 00'.

CASE XI.

Given the Side AB = 33° 31', *and the opposite Angle* C = 54° 40', *to find the adjacent Angle* B   (Fig 39.)

1 By stereographic Projection

Project the Triangle ABC by the last Case. Then the Angle B measured, is 43° 55'.

2. Logarithmically.

As Cof. AB 33° 31' Radius   Cof ∠ C 54° 40' S. adjacent ∠ B 43° 55'

CASE XII.

Given the Side AB = 33° 31′, *and the opposite Angle* C = 54° 40′, *to find the Hypothenuse* CB (FIG. 39)

1. By ſtereographic Projection.

The Triangle being projected by Caſe 10, CB meaſured is 42° 36′.

2. Logarithmically

As S. opp. ∠ C 54° 40′ : Radius . S Side AB 33° 31′ . S Hyp CB 42° 36′.

CASE XIII.

Given the Side CA = 28° 00′, *and the Side* AB = 33° 31′; *to find the Angle* C. (FIG. 39.)

1. By ſtereographic Projection

Make CA = 28° 00′, and through A draw EAG perpendicular to DF, alſo make AB = 33° 31′, and draw the right Circle HI through the Point B Then the ∠ C meaſured by Prob 19, is 54° 40′.

2 Logarithmically.

As Radius Cotan Side AB 33° 31′ S Side CA 28° 00′ Cotan ∠ C 54° 40′.

CASE XIV

Given the Side CA = 28° 00′, *and the Side* AB = 33° 31′, *to find the Hypothenuſe* CB. (FIG. 39)

1. By

1. By ſtereographic Projection.

Project the Triangle ABC, by the laſt Caſe: Then CB meaſured, is 42° 36'.

2. Logarithmically.

As Radius : Coſ. Side CA 28° 00' :: Coſ. Side AB 33° 31' Coſ. Hypothenuſe CB 42° 36'.

CASE XV.

Given the Angle $C = 54° 40'$, *and the Angle* $B = 43° 55'$; *to find the Side* AB. (Fig 39)

1 By ſtereographic Projection.

Make the Angle $C = 54°\ 40'$, alſo through the Poles E, G of the right Circle DF, draw the great oblique Circle EAG, by Prob. 14, to cut the right Circle HI, and make therewith an Angle of 43° 55', which will project the Triangle ABC Then AB meaſured, is 33° 31'.

2. Logarithmically.

As S. Angle B 43° 55' Radius : Coſ. Angle C 54° 40' : Coſ. Side AB 33° 31'.

CASE XVI.

Given the Angles B *and* C *as before, to find the Hyp.* CB. (Fig. 39.)

H h   1. By

1. By ftereographic Projection.

Conftruct the Triangle *ABC* by the laft Cafe, then the Hypothenufe *CB* meafured, is = 42° 36'.

2. Logarithmically.

As Radius : Cotan. Angle *C* 54° 40' ∶ Cotan Angle *B* 43° 55' ∶ Cof. Hyp. *CB* 42° 36'.

SECT. II.

The SOLUTION *of the feveral Cafes of* OBLIQUE-ANGLED SPHERICAL TRIANGLES.

THERE are feveral Ways of folving oblique fpherical Triangles, either by letting fall a Perpendicular, or without it. The Method given in the laft Section for refolving the Cafes of right-angled Triangles, will equally ferve for oblique; letting fall a Perpendicular from one of the Angles, which will either divide the given oblique Triangle into two right-angled ones, or otherwife will make two right-angled Triangles, by adding a right-angled Triangle to it, and this will do in every Cafe, except the 1ft, 4th, and two laft. In the firft Triangle, there are two Things given to find a third, which muft be either a vertical Angle or Bafe. In the fecond Triangle there is one Thing given, or at leaft may be eafily known, by Means of the firft Operation in the firft Triangle, and in the fe-

cond

cond Triangle is always the Answer to the Question. In these two Triangles you have either both the Bases, or both the vertical Angles, and by Help of these to find the Answer or Thing sought, compare these three Things in the second Triangle together, viz the Perpendicular, the Thing known, and the Thing required, and see which of the three is the middle Part, and which are the Extreams either conjunct or disjunct Proceed thus with the first Triangle, so will the middle Part and Extreams in one Triangle, be proportional to the middle Part and Extreams in the other Triangle (letting aside the Perpendicular in both Triangles)

As for Example. In the Triangle ABC, given the Side BC, and the Angles B and C, to find the Side AC. The Perpendicular CD being let fall, divides the oblique Triangle ABC into two right-angled Triangles DBC, DAC; then in the Triangle DBC, as Radius. Cos. BC Tan. DBC Cotan. DCB. Then the $\angle C$ being given, from thence the $\angle DCA$ becomes known; so in the Triangle DAC, the $\angle DCA$ is the middle Part, and CD and CA are Extreams conjunct, also in the Triangle DBC, the $\angle DCB$ is the middle Part, and CD and CB are conjunct Extreams; then rejecting the Perpendicular CD, it will be, as Cos. $\angle DCB$ Cos $\angle DCA$ Cotan. BC : Cotan. AC ——Note, In letting fall a Perpendicular, always observe to let it fall from the End of a given Side, and opposite to a given or known Angle, and if the three Things given stand together, let it fall from the End of a required Side, or opposite to a required Angle. (Fig. 40, 41.)

There are four Axioms, by which the twelve Cafes of oblique fpherical Triangles may be refolved without a Perpendicular.

AXIOM I.

As the Sine of a Side AB :
The Sine of its oppofite Angle C ∶:
The Sine of any other Side AC
The Sine of its oppofite Angle B.

Alfo;

As the Sine of an Angle C :
The Sine of its oppofite Side AB ∷
The Sine of any other Angle B :
The Sine of its oppofite Side AC.

AXIOM II.

As the Sine of ½ Sum 2 Sides containing an Angle, $\frac{AB+AC}{2}$:
The Sine of Half their Difference $\frac{AB-AC}{2}$ ∷
The Cotan. Half the included Angle, $\frac{1}{2} A$ ·
The Tangent Half Differ 2 unknown Angles, $\frac{C \backsim B}{2}$

Alfo;

As Cof. ½ Sum 2 Sides including an Angle, $\frac{AB+AC}{2}$;
The Cof Half their Difference $\frac{AB-AC}{2}$ ∷
The Cotan. Half the included Angle, $\frac{1}{2} A$.
The Tan. ½ Sum of the other two Angles, $\frac{C+B}{2}$.

Then

Then $\frac{C+B}{2} + \frac{C\infty B}{2}$ = greater Angle C, and $\frac{C+B}{2} - \frac{C\infty B}{2}$ = lesser Angle B.

Axiom III.

As Sine ½ Sum 2 Angles, $\frac{A+C}{2}$:

The Sine ½ their Differ. $\frac{C-A}{2}$.

The Tan. ½ contained Side, $\frac{AC}{2}$.

The Tan. ½ Differ. other 2 Sides, $\frac{AB \infty BC}{2}$.

Also;

As Cos. ½ Sum of 2 Angles, $\frac{A+C}{2}$:

The Cos. ½ their Difference $\frac{C-A}{2}$..

The Tan ½ contained Side, $\frac{AC}{2}$:

The Tan ½ Sum of the other 2 Sides, $\frac{AB+BC}{2}$.

Then $\frac{AB+BC}{2} + \frac{AB \infty BC}{2}$ = greater Side AB, and $\frac{AB+BC}{2} - \frac{AB \infty BC}{2}$ = lesser Side BC.

Axiom IV.

As Rectangle Sines of the 2 containing Sides.
The Square of Radius ∷
The Rectangle Sines of ½ Sum 3 Sides, and of Differ.
    Side opposite thereto
The Square of the Cosine of ½ contained Angle.

But

But if a Perpendicular CD be let fall from the obtuse Angle C, upon the longest Side or Base AB, then the Solution may be obtained thus. As Tan Half the Base or longest Side AB Tan. $\frac{1}{2}$ Sum of the other 2 Sides, $\frac{AC+BC}{2}$: Tan. $\frac{1}{2}$ Differ. of these 2 Sides, $\frac{AC-BC}{2}$: Tan. $\frac{1}{2}$ Differ. Segments of the Base. Then the Half Difference added to the Half Base, gives the greater Segment AD, but subtracted from the Half Base, gives the lesser Segment BD.

Or, in Case a Perpendicular is not let fall, you may find an Angle thus

Take Half the Difference of the two Sides containing the required Angle, which add to and subtract from Half the Side opposite thereto; this Sum and Difference keep. Then to the Complement arithmetical of the logarithmic Sines of the two containing Sides, add the logarithmic Sines of the Half Sum and Difference, Half the Sum of these four Logarithms, is the logarithmic Sine of Half the required Angle.

Or the first Part of the Work, viz. the finding the Sum and Difference, may be performed more easily thus, from the Half Sum of the three Sides subtract the two Sides (separately) containing the required Angle, these Differences will be the same with the Sum and Difference found by the former Part of the Rule; with which work as before directed, and you will have the Answer.

Oblique

Sect. II.   SPHERICAL TRIANGLES.   237

Oblique spherical Triangles.

CASE I

Given the Side AC = 41° 00', the Side BC = 39° 30', and an opposite Angle A = 29° 31', to find the other opposite Angle B. (FIG. 40, 41.)

1. By stereographic Projection.

Make $AC = 41°$, draw ABH (by Prop. 11) to make an Angle at $A = 29°\ 31'$, also about C, as a Pole, draw the parallel Circle KBL, at the Distance of 39° 30' from it, which will cut ABH in B, through the Points C, B draw (by Prop. 7) the great Circle CBI. Then the Angle B measured (by Prop. 19) is 30° 33'.

2. Logarithmically.

As S Side BC 39° 30'   S its opp $\angle A$ 29° 31'
S. Side AC 41° 00' : S its opp $\angle B$ 30° 33'.

Now $\frac{AC + BC}{2}$ is of the same Affection as $\frac{A+B}{2}$, and if $\frac{A+B}{2}$ be of the same Affection with $\frac{A + \text{Sup } B}{2}$, then the $\angle B$ is ambiguous.

CASE II.

Given the Sides AC and BC, and the Angle A the same as before; to find the included Angle C. (FIG. 40, 41.)

1. By

1 By stereographic Projection.

Project the Triangle ABC, as in the last Case, then the $\angle C$ measured, is $132°\ 22'$.

2 Logarithmically.

By Case 3 of right-angled Triangles, Radius Cof $AC\ 41°$ Tan $A\ 29°\ 31'$ Cotan $DCA\ 66°\ 51'$.

Then Cotan $AC\ 41°\ 00'$ Cof $DCA\ 66°\ 51'$: Cotan $BC\ 39°\ 30'$ Cof. $DCB\ 65°\ 31$; then $DCA + DCB = 66°\ 51' + 65°\ 31' = 132°\ 22' = \angle C$.

Then, because BC and the $\angle A$ are of the same Affection, DCB is acute, otherwise obtuse

Then because in the present Case, the Sides AC, BC are of the same Affection, the Perpendicular falls within the Triangle, and the Angles A and B are of the same Affection.

Therefore to the lesser Arch of $DCB = 65°\ 31'$, add $DCA = 66°\ 51$, and the Sum is $132°\ 22'$, also to the greater Arch of $DCB = 114°\ 29'$, add $DCA = 66°\ 51'$, the Sum is $181°\ 20'$. Then because the greater Arch of DCB, with DCA added to it, exceeds $180°$, the lesser Arch of DCB can only be admitted. But had both these Sums been less than $180°$, then either the greater or less Arch of DCB might have been added to DCA, for the Angle C, which would have been ambiguous.

But when the Angles A and B at the Base, are of a different Affection, the Perpendicular will then fall out of the Triangle. And if the greater Arch DCB is

less

less than the Angle DCA, the Angle C will be had by subtracting either Arch of DCB from DCA, and the Angle C will be ambiguous; but when the greater Arch of DCB is greater than the Angle DCA, the lesser Arch of DCB subtracted from DCA, will only give the Quantity of the Angle C, which then is not ambiguous.

CASE III.

Given the Sides AC *and* BC, *and the Angle* A *the same as before, to find the third Side* AB. (Fig. 40, 41)

1 By stereographic Projection.

Project the Triangle ABC, by Case 1, then AB measured, is 72° 28'.

2. Logarithmically.

By Case 1 of right-angled Triangles, Rad Cos. A 29° 31' Tan. AC 41° 00' Tan AD 37° 6'.

Then Cos. AC 41° 00' Cos. AD 37° 6' . Cos. BC 39° 30' Cos. BD 35° 22'.

Then $AD + BD = 37° 6' + 35° 22' = 72° 28' = AB$.

If AD be greater than BD, then $AD - BD = AB$, also if $AD + BD$ be less than 180°, $AD + BD = AB$, if both be less than 180°, AB is ambiguous.

CASE IV.

Given the Angle A = 29° 31', *the Angle* B = 30° 33', *and an opposite Side* AC = 41°, *to find the other opp. Side* BC. (Fig. 40, 41)

1 By

1. By stereographic Projection.

Draw ABH to make an Angle with the Primitive at $A = 29° 31'$, also make $AC = 41°$, by Prop. 14, draw a great Circle CBI to cut ABH in an Angle of $30° 33'$, as in B. Then BC measured, is $39° 30'$.

2. Logarithmically.

As S $\angle B$ $30° 33'$ S. opp Side AC $41°$. S. $\angle A$ $29° 31'$ S its opp. Side BC $29° 30$.

$\frac{AC + BC}{2}$ is of the same Affection as $\frac{A \perp B}{2}$.

If $\frac{BC + AC}{2}$ be of the same Affection as $\frac{AC + \text{Supp } BC}{2}$, then BC is ambiguous.

That is $\frac{29° 30' + 41° 00'}{2} = \frac{70° 30'}{2} = 35° 15'$.

Also $\frac{41° 0' + 150° 30'}{2} = \frac{191° 30'}{2} = 95° 45'$, by which the required Side BC is proved to be not ambiguous.

CASE V.

Given the Angles A *and* B, *with the opposite Side* AC *the same as before in the last Case, to find the included Side* AB. (FIG. 40, 41)

1. By stereographic Projection.

Project the Triangle by Case 4, so will AB measured, $= 72° 28'$.

2. Lo-

2 Logarithmically.

By Cafe 1 of right-angled Triangles,
Radius Cof. ∠ A 29° 31′   Tan. AC 41° ∶ Tan. AD = 37° 6′.

Then Cotan. ∠ A 29° 31′ ∶ S. AD 37° 6′   Cotan. ∠ B 30° 33′ S. BD 35° 22′.

As the ∠s A, B are of the fame Affection, AD + BD = AB. If BD + AD, and BD + Supp. AD, be each lefs than 180°, AD (and confequently AB) is ambiguous.

If the Angles A, B are of different Affection, AD − BD = AB. Alfo if AD and Supp AD be greater than BD, then AD and AB are ambiguous.

CASE VI.

Given the Angles and Side as above; to find the Angle C. (FIG 40, 41.)

1. By ftereographic Projection.

Project the Triangle ABC by Cafe 4; then the ∠ C meafured, is 132° 22′.

2. Logarithmically.

By Cafe 3, right-angled Triangles, Radius Cof AC 41°   Tan. ∠ A 29° 31′ Cotan ∠ DCA 66° 51′.

Then Cof. ∠ A 29° 31′   Cof ∠ B 30° 33′ ∶ S. ∠ DCA 66° 51 S ∠ DCB 65° 31′.

Then DCA + DCB = 66° 51′ + 65° 31′ = 132° 22′ = ∠ C.

When the $\angle$s A and B are of the same Affection, $DCA + DCB$ are $= \angle C$. If $DCB + DCA$, and $DCB +$ Sup DCA be less than 180°, then DCA and C are ambiguous

If A and B are of different Affection, then $DCA - DCB = \angle C$, but if both DCA and its Sup be greater than the $\angle DCB$, then the $\angle DCA$, and C are ambiguous.

Note, Those who desire to see more into the Nature of Ambiguities, may consult Mr *Emerson*'s Trigonometry, which I have closely kept to, in compiling this Compendium.

CASE VII.

Given the Side AC = 41°, *the Side* AB = 72° 28′, *and the included Angle* A = 29° 31′, *to find an opposite Angle* B. (FIG 40, 41)

1 By stereographic Projection.

Make $AC =$ the Chord of 41°, draw ABH to make an Angle at A of 29° 31′, and make $AB = $ 72° 28′, through C, B draw the great oblique Circle CBI, so is ABC the Triangle, in which the $\angle B$ measured, is 30° 33′.

2. Logarithmically.

(By Case 1, right $\angle$s) Radius Cos $\angle A$ 29° 31′ ·
Tan AC 41° Tan AD 37° 6′ Then $AB - AD$
$= 72° 28′ - 37° 6′ = 35° 22′ = BD$.

Then

Then S. AD 37° 6′ : Cotan. $\angle A$ 29° 31′ :: S. BD 35° 22′ Cotan $\angle B$ 30° 33′.

Now according as AD is lesser or greater than AB, the Angles A and B are of the same or different Affection.

CASE VIII

Given the Sides and Angle the same as before, to find the third Side BC. (FIG. 40, 41.)

2. By stereographic Projection.

Project the Triangle by the last Case; then BC measured, is $= 39°\ 30'$.

2. Logarithmically.

(By Case 1, right $\angle$ s) Radius Cos $\angle A$ 29° 31′ : Tan AC 41° : Tan AD 37° 6′, from whence BD is found $= 35°\ 22'$.

Then Cos. AD 37° 6′ : Cos AC 41° 00 :: Cos. BD 35° 22′ : Cos BC 39° 30′.

Then as BD and $\angle A$ are of the same or different Affection, BC is accordingly less or greater than a Quadrant.

CASE IX.

Given the Angle A $= 29°\ 31'$, *the Angle* C $= 132°\ 22'$, *and the intended Side* AC $= 41°$, *to find an opp Side* BC (FIG. 40, 41.)

1. By

1. By stereographic Projection.

Make $AC = 41°$; draw ABH to make an Angle at A of $29° 31'$, and CBI to make an Angle at C of $132° 22'$, then the Side BC measured, $= 39° 30'$.

2. Logarithmically

By Case 3, right $\angle$s, Radius · Cos AC 41 · Tan. $\angle A$ 29° 31' : Cotan $\angle DCA$ 66° 51'; and hence the $\angle DCB = 65° 31'$.

Then Cos. $\angle DCA$ 66° 51' · Cotan. AC 41° 00' . Cos. $\angle DCB$ 65° 31' . Cotan BC 39° 30'.

According as DCB and A are of the same or different Affection, the Side BC is less or greater than a Quadrant.

CASE X.

Given the Angles and Side the same as before; to find the third Angle B (FIG. 40, 41.)

1. By stereographic Projection.

Project the Triangle ABC, as before in the last Case, then the $\angle B$ measured, $= 30° 33'$.

2. Logarithmically.

By Case 3, right $\angle$s, Radius Cos AC 41° 00' Tan A 29° 31' Cotan DCA 66° 51', from whence DCB is found $= 65° 31'$.

Then S DCA 66° 51' S. DCB 65° 31' . Cos. A 29° 31' Cos. B 30° 33'.

Then

Sect. II. SPHERICAL TRIANGLES. 245

Then as the Angle DCA is less or greater than the Angle ACB, the ∠s A and B are of the same or different Affection

CASE XI.

Given all the three Sides $AC = 41°$, $BC = 39° 30'$, *and* $AB\ 72° 28'$, *to find an Angle* A. (FIG. 40, 41)

1. By stereographic Projection.

Make $AC = 41°$; about the Point A draw the Parallel MN, at $72° 28'$ Distance from it, also round C draw another Parallel KL, at the Distance of $39° 30'$, to cut the former in B, through their Point of Intersection B, from C draw the great Circle CBI, and compleat the Triangle ABC. Then the ∠ A measured, is $= 29° 31'$.

2. Logarithmically.

As Tan $\frac{1}{2} AB = 36° 14'$ Tan. $\frac{AC + BC}{2} = 40° 15'$: Tan $\frac{AC \sim BC}{2} = 0° 45'$ · Tan. Arch $= 0° 52'$. Then as $\frac{1}{2} AB = 36° 14'$, is greater than the Arch $0° 52'$, the Perp falls within the Triangle, otherwise not

Then $\frac{1}{2} AB + $ Arch, $= 36° 14' + 0° 52' = $ greater Segment $AD = 37° 6'$, and $\frac{1}{2} AB \sim $ Arch, $= 36° 14' \sim 0° 52' = $ lesser Segment $BD = 35° 22'$.

Then by Case 4, right ∠s, Radius Cotan AC $41°$ Tan. AD $37° 6'$ Cos. ∠ A $29° 31'$.

CASE

CASE XII.

Given all the 3 Angles, viz. $A = 29° 31'$, $B = 30° 33'$, *and* $C = 132° 22'$, *to find a Side* AC. (FIG 40, 41)

1. By stereographic Projection.

The Angles being converted into Sides, project the Triangle, as by the last Case, so will AC measured, give $41°$.

2. Logarithmically.

As A, B are of the same Affection, the Perp. falls within the Triangle, otherwise without.

As Cotan. $\frac{A+B}{2} = 30° 2'$ · Tan. $\frac{A \backsim B}{2} = 0° 31'$
Tan. $\frac{1}{2} C = 66° 11'$ Tan Arch $= 0° 40'$

Then $\frac{1}{2} C +$ Arch $= 66° 11 + 0° 40' =$ greater $\angle DCA$ $66° 51'$, at the Vertex   And $\frac{1}{2} C \backsim$ Arch $= 66° 11' \backsim 0° 40' =$ lesser $\angle DCB$ $65° 31'$, at the Vertex.

Then by Case 16, right $\angle$s, Radius · Cotan A $29° 31'$ · Cotan. DCA $66° 51'$ · Cof. AC $41° 00'$

BOOK VI.
ASTRONOMY.

1. AStronomy hath its Derivation from the two Greek Words Aster, a Star, and Nomos, a Law, for by it we are taught the Motions of the Sun, Moon, and Stars, and whatever in any wife pertains to them.

2. Before we proceed to perform Conclusions in Astronomy, it is requisite to know the Sun's Place in the Ecliptic, the Latitude of the Place, and the Sun's greatest Declination, that is, the Angle that the Sun's Orbit (the Ecliptic) makes with the Equinoctial.

3. The Sun's Place in the Ecliptic is to be obtained from astronomical Tables, which I have here inserted, whose Uses are evident from the Examples in Prob 1.

4. The Reader must not expect, that this shall be a full and complete Course of Astronomy, but only a Collection of the most useful astronomical Problems, necessary to be known by every Person, who would deservedly acquire the Name and Character of an able Surveyor.

SECT. I.

ASTRONOMICAL PROBLEMS, *requisite to be known in the Practice of* SURVEYING.

PROB. I

To calculate the Sun's true Place in the Ecliptic.

TAKE out of the Tables of the Sun's mean Motion, the Longitude and Anomaly answering to the given Year, Month, Day, Hour, Minute, Second, &c. which being severally added together, will give the Sun's mean Motion for the proposed Time; observing in Leap Year, to find the Day of the Month in the Column on the right Hand Side of the monthly Pages after February, noted on the Top with Bissex.

Enter the Table of the Sun's Elliptic Equation, with the mean Anomaly thus collected; which find on the Top of the Table, if the Anomaly be less than 6 Signs, but on the Bottom if more; that is, if the mean Anomaly is less than 6 Signs, look out the Sign on the Head of the Table, and the Degrees in the left Hand Column descending; but if the Anomaly exceeds 6 Signs, look out the Sign in the Bottom of the Table, and the Degrees in the right Hand Column ascending, and in the Angle, or Place of meeting is the Sun's Elliptic Equation, which added to, or subtracted from (according to the Title in the Table) the Sun's mean Longitude before found, will give his true Ecliptic Place.

But

Sect. I.   Astronomical Problems.   249

But as the Table of Equation is only calculated to even Degrees, when the Anomaly confists of Signs, Degrees, Minutes, and Seconds, find the proportional Part for the Minutes and Seconds, by the Rule of Three, which added to, or subtracted from the Degrees, &c. which were first taken out of the Table, the Sum or Difference will be the mean Anomaly truly found.

EXAMPLE I.

Let the Sun's true Place be found for June 16, 1769, at Noon.

OPERATION.

	Long ☉ S ° ′ ″	Anom ☉ S ° ′ ″		L.L
The Radix 1761	9 8 41 20	6 0 33 50	As 60′ 0″	0
Current Years 8	0 0 3 37	11 29 55 13	To 1 55	14956
			So 4 46	10999
M Mot for 1769	9 8 44 57	6 0 29 3	To 0 9	25955
June the 16th	5 14 36 11	5 14 35 43	This propor. Part	
Mean Motion	2 23 21 8	11 15 4 46	subt. from 0° 29′ 30″	
Equation add	0 29 21		(Equa. of 11 s 15°)	
			Remaind. 0° 29′ 21″	
Sun's Place	2 23 50 29		is the true Equat.	

EXAMPLE II.

Let the Sun's Place be fought for June 28, at 43 Min. past 10 o'Clock in the Forenoon, 1769.

Note, Astronomical Time begins and ends at Noon; and each Day begins at its own Noon, and ends at the Noon of the next succeeding Day. Therefore, the

K k 2   above-

250   ASTRONOMICAL PROBLEMS. Book VI.

above-mentioned Time expres'd in aftronomical Terms, will be 1769, June 27 d. 22 hrs. 43 min. Alfo the following folar Tables are accommodated to the Meridian of London (the Metropolis of England).

OPERATION

	Longit ☉ S ° ′ ″	Anom ☉ S ° ′ ″	
			L L
The Radix 1761	9 8 41 20	6 0 33 50	As 60′ 00″ 0
Current Years 8	0 0 3 37	11 29 55 13	To 1 59 14808
			So 51 16 683
M Mot for 1769	9 8 44 57	6 0 29 3	To 1 42 15491
June 27	5 25 26 43	5 25 26 14	
Hours 22	0 54 13	0 54 13	Then 0° 7′ 57″ —
Min 43	1 46	1 46	1′ 42″ = 0° 6′ 15″
Mean Motion	3 5 7 39	11 26 51 16	= Ellip Equat
Equat. add	0 6 15		
Sun's Place	3 5 13 54		

But if you have the Sun's Place to calculate under any other Meridian, Eaft or Weft of the Meridian of London, by the following Tables, then you muft reduce the Time at the propofed Place, to the Time at London

As fuppofe you be at Leverpool, and want to calculate the Sun's true Place at 8 h 40 m. in the Morning

As the Meridian of Leverpool is 10′ in Time, Weft of the Meridian of London, therefore add 10′ to 8 h. 40 m. (the Time at Leverpool) and the Sum 8h. 50 m. is the Time at London, to which calculate the Sun's Place as before,

But

Sect. I.　Astronomical Problems.　　251

But if the Place you are to calculate for, or at, be East of the Meridian of London, the Difference of Meridians in Time, must be subtracted from the given Time, the Remainder is the Time at London. This is so very easy, Examples are needless.

Prob II.

To find the Latitude of any Place.

There are several Methods of doing this, but the easiest and best, is by taking the Sun's Meridian Altitude with a very good Quadrant or Theodolite, which is done thus: If it be a Theodolite of the best Sort; level the Limb, and a little before the Sun comes to the Meridian, elevate the Telescope, till you observe the horizontal Hair therein, touch the Sun's lower or upper Limb; and as the Sun rises, elevate the Telescope to it, till you observe the Sun begins to descend, then will the Index give on the vertical Arch, the Meridian Altitude of the Sun's lower or upper Limb; to or from which Altitude, add or subtract 16 Min. (the Sun's apparent Semidiameter) and the Sum or Difference (according as you use the lower or upper Limb) is the apparent central Altitude, or the apparent Altitude of the Sun's Center, which being corrected by Refraction and Parallax, will give the Sun's true central Altitude.

Or thus;

Level your Theodolite, and about 2 or 3 Hours before Noon direct the Telescope till the horizontal Hair

touch

touch the Sun's lower or upper Limb as before, then faften the Inftrument in this Pofition, and note upon Paper the Degrees, &c. of Altitude, as alfo the Degrees, &c. cut off by the Index on the Limb. Let the Inftrument remain in this Pofition till the Afternoon, (or if it be altered, fix the Index to the fame Degree, &c. upon the vertical Arch,) and then obferve when the horizontal Hair juft touches the fame Edge of the Sun, as before in the Morning Obfervation, the Index will cut the Limb of the Inftrument at fome particular Degree, &c. which note

Now from the Evening Obfervation fubtract the Morning Obfervation, and to Half the Remainder add the Morning Obfervation; to the Degree, &c. of this Sum, fix the Index on the Limb of the Theodolite, fo will the Telefcope and Arch exactly ftand in the Plane of the Meridian But if the Obfervation on the Limb, which was made in the Morning, exceed that of the Afternoon, then increafe the latter by 360°, after which work as before, and if the Remainder exceed 360°, fubtract 360° therefrom.

The Inftrument, that is, the Telefcope and vertical Arch being thus fixed in the Plane of the Meridian, muft remain in the fame Place and Direction, till the next Day, or till the firft Opportunity offers, of the Sun paffing vifibly over the Meridian; by which his apparent Meridian Altitude (and from thence his true Altitude) may be obtained

Note, In the Morning it is neceffary to take 3 or 4 Obfervations, at any convenient Diftance of Time from

one

one another; becaufe whatever Elevation the Telefcope ftands at in the Morning Obfervation, the Sun will exactly fall in with the fame, in the Evening Obfervation; and if Clouds happen to interpofe at that Inftant, your Labour is loft But by having feveral Morning Obfervations, if you fail in one, you may fucceed in another.

The Sun's Meridian Altitude being determined by either of the foregoing Methods, (the former is the better and the moft practical) the Latitude of the Place is eafily found by the two following Rules.

Rule I.

If the Sun's Zenith Diftance and Declination be of the fame Name, that is, both North or both South, then the Difference of the Zenith Diftance and Declination, is the required Latitude, which is always of the fame, or contrary Name with the Declination, according as the Declination is greater or lefs than the Zenith Diftance.

Rule II.

When the Sun's zenith Diftance and Declination are of a contrary Name, that is, the one North, the other South, then the Sum of the Zenith Diftance and Declination, is the Latitude, which is ever of the fame Name with the Sun's Declination

Note, The Zenith Diftance is equal to the Complement of the Altitude.

Example I.

Suppose the Sun's Meridian Altitude South (when corrected by Refraction and Parallax) = 54° 48′ 32″; required the Latitude of the Place of Observation; the Sun's Declination North being 18° 20′.

90° − 54° 48′ 32″ + 18° 20′ = 53° 51′ 28″ = Latitude North.

Example II.

Let the Sun's corrected Meridian Altitude South, be 54° 48′ 32″, and his Declination South, at the same Time, 18° 20′; required the Latitude of the Place of Observation.

90° − 54° 48′ 32″ − 18° 20′ = 16° 51′ 28″ = Latit. North, because the Altitude and Declination are of the same Name (both South) and because the Declination is less than the Zenith Distance.

The Truth of the two foregoing Rules, is proved and demonstrated by Projection thus.

First, let us suppose the Sun's true Meridian Altitude = 41° 11′ 47″, his true Place in the Ecliptic = 0s 14° 12′ 31″, and his Declination North = 5° 36′ 47″, all taken and found for the same Time. (Fig 42.)

Then with a Chord of 60° describe the primitive Circle *HZON*, representing the Plane of the Meridian of the solstitial Colure, draw *HO* the Horizon, and *ZN* perpendicular thereto, for the prime Vertical; so is *Z* the Zenith of the Place whose Latitude is required.

Set

Sect. I.   ASTRONOMICAL PROBLEMS.   255

Set $48° \ 48' \ 13''$ (= the Comp. ☽ Altitude) from Z to ☉, also set $5° \ 36' \ 47''$ (= ☉ Declin.) from ☉ Southwards to E, because the Declination is North, had it been South, it must have been set the contrary Way, viz. North from a to E. so will E be the Point of Intersection of the Meridian and Equinoctial. Draw EAQ the Equinoctial, and PS perp. thereto for the Earth's Axis, and draw the Parallels of Declination ☉c, ab. Then it is evident from the Diagram, that ZE = Latitude of the Place; and that $Z☉ + ☉E = 48° \ 48' \ 13'' + 5° \ 36' \ 47'' = 54° \ 25'$ = ZE = the Latitude of the Place of Observation. But if the Declination had been South, then it would have been $Za - aE = ZE$ the Latitude required. For the Latitude of any Place, is the Distance upon the Meridian, between the Zenith of that Place and the Equinoctial.

Prob. III.

To find the Obliquity of the Ecliptic, or the Angle that the Ecliptic makes with the Equinoctial; which is equal to the Sun's greatest Declination.

With an exquisite astronomical Quadrant take the Sun's Meridian Altitude very accurately, on the Days of the Summer and Winter Solstice, that is, on the Days the Sun touches the first Scruple of the tropical Signs Cancer and Capricorn.

Then subtract those two Meridian Altitudes one from the other, Half the Remainder is the Angle of Obliquity.

Ex-

EXAMPLE.

At Winton, on the Days of the Summer and Winter Solstice, the two Meridian Altitudes of the Sun taken by me, were, viz. at the Summer Solstice $59° 4'$, and at the Winter Solstice $12° 6'$, from whence the Angle of Obliquity is required.

PROJECTION.

Make the Arch $ZB = 30° 56' =$ the Sun's zenith Distance at the Summer Solstice, and $ZD = 77° 54' =$ the Sun's zenith Distance at the Winter Solstice. Bisect BD in E, so will $EB (= ED)$ be the Arch of the Sun's greatest Declination, which in Numbers is found thus, (Fig. 42.)

From $ZD = 77° 54' = \odot$ zenith Dist. at Winter Solst.
Take $ZB = 30\ 56 = \odot$ zenith Dist. at Summer Sol.

Rem. $BD = 46\ 58 =$ Breadth of the Zodiac.

Half of which $= 23\ 29 =$ Obliquity of the Ecliptic.

PROB. IV.

Given the Sun's Place in ♉ $29° 50' 3''$, and his greatest Declination $23° 29'$, to find his present Declination.

In the right-angled spherical Triangle ♈$B\odot$, right-angled at B, there are given the Hypothenuse ♈$\odot = 59° 50' 3'' =$ Distance of the Sun from the nearest Equinoctial Point ♈, and the $\angle$ of Obliquity B♈$\odot = 23° 29'$, to find $B\odot$ his present Declination. (FIG. 43.)

Analogy

Sect. I. Astronomical Problems.

Analogy, by Case 2, right ∠s.

As Radius : S. ♈☉ = 59° 50′ 3″ : S. ∠ B♈☉ = 23° 29′ S. B☉ = 20° 9′ 8″ = Sun's Declination North.

Note, If the Sun be in any of the southern Signs, his Declination is then South; and the Quæsita may be obtained in the right-angled spherical Triangle ♎Dc, the Equinoctial Point ♎ being the nearest.

Prob V

Given the Sun's present Declination = 20° 9′ 8″, and the Obliquity of the Ecliptic = 23° 29′; to find his Longitude, or Place in the Ecliptic.

This Prob. is just the Reverse of the last, and is solved in the right-angled Triangle B♈☉ (Fig. 43.)

Analogy, by Case 12, right ∠s.

As S. ∠ B♈☉ = 23° 29′ : Radius :: S B☉ = 20° 9′ 8″ S. ♈☉ = 59° 50′ 3″ = Sun's Longitude.

That is, the Sun's true Place is ♉ 29° 50′ 3″, because his Declination is North, had it been South, it would have been ♏ 29° 50′ 3″, because then ♎ would have been the nearest Equinoctial Point.

Prob. VI.

Given the Sun's Longitude ♈☉ = 59° 50′ 3″, and his greatest Declination B♈☉ 23° 29′, to find his right Ascension ♈B. (Fig. 43.)

Analogy, by Cafe 1, *right* ∠ s.

As Radius : Tan ♈O = 59° 50′ 3″ :: Cof ∠ B♈☉ = 23° 29′ : Tan. ♈B = 57° 38′ 15″ = Sun's right Afcenfion.

Note, If the Sun be in the firft Quadrant of the Ecliptic (as it is in the prefent Cafe) viz. in ♈, ♉, ♊; then the fourth Arch (as found above, is the Sun's right Afcenfion from Aries But if the Sun be in the fecond Quadrant of the Ecliptic, viz in ♋, ♌, ♍, then the fourth Arch muft be taken from 180°; and the Remainder is the right Afcenfion from Aries. When the Sun is in the third Quadrant, viz. in ♎, ♏, ♐, the fourth Arch muft be added to 180°, and the Sum is the right Afcenfion from Aries. Laftly, when the Sun is in the fourth Quadrant, viz. in ♑, ♒, ♓; the fourth proportional Arch muft be fubtracted from 360°; and the Remainder is the Sun's right Afcenfion from Aries.

Prob. VII.

Given the Latitude of the Place = 54° 25′, *and the Sun's Declination* = 20° 9′ 8″, *to find his Amplitude.*

In the right-angled fpherical Triangle *POC*, there are given the Leg *PO* = 54° 25′ = the Latitude, and the Hypothenufe *PC* = 69° 50′ 52″ = Comp Decl or the Diftance of the Sun from the North Pole of the Globe; to find the Leg *CO* = the Compl. Amplitude. (Fig. 43.)

Analogy

Sect. I.   ASTRONOMICAL PROBLEMS.   259

Analogy, by Cafe 6, right ∠s.

As Cof $PO = 54° 25'$ Radius ·· Cof. $PC = 69° 50' 52''$ Cof $CO = 53° 41' 46''$, whofe Complement $\Upsilon C = 36° 18' 14''$ is the Sun's true Amplitude.

PROB. VIII.

Given the Latitude of the Place $= 54° 25'$, and the Sun's Declination $= 23° 29'$; to find the afcenfional Difference, and confequently the true Time of the Sun's Rifing and Setting, with the Length of the Day and Night.

In the right-angled fpherical Triangle POF, there are given $PO = 54° 25'$, and $PF = 66° 31'$, to find the Angle $FPO = $ the Complement of the afcenfional Difference.

Analogy, by Cafe 4, right ∠s.

Radius Tan. $PO = 54° 25'$. Cotan. $PF = 66° 31'$: Cof $∠ FPO = 52° 36' 58'$, whofe Complement $37° 23' 22''$ is the Sun's afcenfional Difference, which converted into Time ($15°$ of the Equinoctial being $=$ to 1 Hour of Time) is 2 h. 29 m. 33 fec. 28 th. which taken from, and added to 6 Hours, the former $=$ 3 h. 30 m. 26 fec. 32 th is the true Time of the Sun's Rifing, and the latter $=$ 8 h. 29 m. 33 fec. 28 th. is the true Time of the Sun's Setting in the Latitude of $54° 25'$ North.

But fuppofing the Sun's Declination South, then this afcenfional Difference in Time muft have been added to, to, and subtracted from 6 Hours, and the former = 8h. 29′ 33″ 28‴ is the true Time of the Sun's Rising; and the latter 3 h 30′ 26″ 32‴ is the true Time of the Setting.

Note, Double the Time of the Sun-rising gives the Length of the Night, and double the Time of the Sun-setting the Length of the Day.

Prob IX.

Given the right Ascension and ascensional Difference; to find the oblique Ascension and oblique Descension.

In North Latitudes

Rule

If the Declination be North, the ascensional Difference added to, and subtracted from the right Ascension, the latter is the oblique Ascension, and the former the oblique Descension. But if the Declination be South; the former is the oblique Ascension, and the latter the oblique Descension.

In South Latitudes just the contrary.

Example.

Suppose the Sun's right Ascension = 90° 00′ (as in the Beginning of ♋) and the ascensional Difference = 37° 23′ 22″, in the Latitude of 54° 25′ North; required the oblique Ascension and oblique Descension.

Oper

Sect. I. **Astronomical Problems.**

OPERATION.

Right Ascension — —	90° 00′ 00′
Ascens. Differ. subtr. and add —	37 23 22
Remainder is the oblique Ascension	52 36 38
Sum is the oblique Descension —	127 23 22

In such-like Cases as these, we always suppose the Sun's Declination unalterable for one whole Day (which in Reality is not so), therefore whenever we mean to be accurate in our Calculations, we take Care to get the true Declination, as near the precise Time in the Question, as possibly we can.

P R O B. X.

Given the Latitude = 54° 25′ *North, and the Declination of the Sun, Moon, or Star* = 20° 9′ 8″ *North; to find their oblique Ascension and oblique Descension, and consequently their Time of Rising and Setting.*

In the right-angled spherical Triangle PCO, given $PO = 54° 25′ =$ the Latitude, and $PC = 69° 50′ 52″$, $=$ Complement of the Declination, to find the ∠ at P $=$ the Time from Midnight (Fig. 43)

Analogy, by Case 4, *right* ∠ *s.*

As Radius · Tan. $PO = 54° 25′$ Cotan. $PC = 69° 50′ 52″$ Cos. ∠ $P = 59° 8′ 32″$.

This 59° 8′ 32″ is the semi-nocturnal Arch, which in Time is $= 3$ h. 56′ 34″ 8‴ $=$ the true Time of their Rising.

Prob XI.

Given the Latitude $= 54° 25'$ *North, and the Sun's Declination* $= 23° 29'$ *North, to find the Time he will be due East and West.*

In the right-angled spherical Triangle ZAP, given $ZP = 35° 35' =$ Co-latitude, and $AP = 66° 31' =$ Distance of the Sun from the North Pole; to find the $\angle P =$ the Hour from Noon, when the Sun is upon the prime Vertical, or East and West Line ZN. (Fig. 44)

Analogy, by Case 4, *right* $\angle s$.

Radius · Tan. $ZP = 35° 35'$ · Cotan. $PA = 66° 31'$: Cos. $\angle P = 71° 54'$.

Then $71° 54'$ converted into Time is $= 4$ h $47' 0'' 36'''$ = the true Time of the Sun's Westing; whose Compl. to 12 Hours, is 7 h. $12' 59'' 24'''$ the true Time of his Easting. But had the Declination been South, then the former Easting ($= 7$ h. $12' 59'' 24'''$) is the then Westing, as also is the former Westing ($= 4$ h. $47' 0'' 36'''$) the present Easting, as is evident from the other Triangle SaN in the same Diagram.

Prob. XII.

Given the Latitude of the Place $= 54° 25'$ *North, and the Sun's Declination* $= 23° 29'$ *North; to find its Altitude when East or West.*

Sect. I.   ASTRONOMICAL PROBLEMS.   263

In the right-angled spherical Triangle ZAP, there are given $ZP = 35° 35' = $ Comp. Latitude, and $PA = 66° 31' =$ Compl. Sun's Declination, to find $ZA =$ the Compl. his Altitude when East or West. (FIG. 44.)

Analogy, by Case 6, *right* ∠*s.*

Cof $ZP = 35° 35'$: Radius ∴ Cof $AP = 66° 31'$: Cof. $ZA = 60° 40'$, whose Complement $29° 20'$ is the Sun's Altitude required; but if the Declination had been South, then $29° 20'$ would have been the Depression below the Horizon.

PROB. XIII.

Given the Latitude of the Place $= 54° 25'$ *North, and the Declination of the Sun* $= 23° 29'$ *North; to find his Azimuth at the Hour of Six.*

In the right-angled spherical Triangle ZPA, there are given $ZP = 35° 35' = $ Compl. Latit. and $PA = 66° 31' =$ Sun's Declin. N. to find the ∠ Z his Azimuth from the North, which is $=$ Arch BO of the Horizon. (FIG. 45.)

Analogy, by Case 13, *right* ∠*s.*

Tan. $PA = 66° 31'$ Radius.   S $ZP = 35° 35'$: Cotan. ∠ Z $75° 49' =$ Sun's Azimuth from the North. But if the Declination had been South, it would have been his Azimuth from the South; whose Comp to $90°$, is the Azimuth from East or West.   Also the

M m   Sup-

Supplement of the Azimuth from the North or South, will be the Azimuth from the South or North.

P r o b. XIV.

Given the Latitude of the Place = 54° 25′, *and the Sun's Declination North* = 23° 29′; *to find his Altitude at the Hour of Six.*

In the right-angled spherical Triangle ZAP, there are given $ZP = 35°\ 35′ =$ Comp. Lat and $PA = 66°\ 31′ =$ Dist. Sun from the elevated Pole, to find ZA the Comp. Altit. at Six o'Clock. (Fig. 45.)

Analogy, by Case 14, *right* ∠s.

Radius Cos. $ZP = 35°\ 35′$ ∷ Cos $PA = 66°\ 31′$ Cos. $ZA = 71°\ 6′$, whose Compl. 18° 54″ is the Sun's Altitude at the Hour of Six, but if the Declination had been South, it would have been the Depression.

P r o b. XV.

Given the Latitude of the Place = 54° 25′ *North, and the Sun in the Equinoctial, to find the Altitude at* 10 *o'Clock in the Morning, or at Two in the Afternoon.*

In the right-angled spherical Triangle ♈MN, are given ♈M 60° = the Time from Six, and M♈N = 35° 35′ = Compl Latitude, to find MN the Sun's Altitude at that Time. (Fig. 45.)

Analogy

Sect I.   Astronomical Problems.   265

Analogy, by Case 2, right ∠s.

Radius S ♈M = 60° · S ∠ M♈N = 35° 35′ :
S MN = 30° 15′ = Sun's Altitude at Ten in the Morning, or Two in the Afternoon.

Prob XVI

Given the Latitude of the Place = 54° 25′ North, and the Sun's Azimuth from the East or West = 16° 13′ North, to find his Altitude at that Time, the Sun then being in 0 Degr ♋.

In the right-angled spherical Triangle ♈BA, given ♈B = 16° 13′ = Sun's Azimuth from the East or West towards the North, and the Angle A♈B = 54° 25′ = Latitude, to find AB the Altitude at that Time (Fig. 45.)

Analogy, by Case 7, right ∠s.

Radius · Tan. ∠ AZB = 54° 25′ S. ♈B = 16° 13′ : Tan AB = 21° 19′ = Sun's Altitude.

Prob. XVII.

Given the Latitude of the Place = 54° 25′ North, the Sun's Declination North = 23° 29′, and the Time of the Day = 10 o'Clock in the Morning, to find the Sun's Altitude.

In the oblique-angled spherical Triangle ZPR, given the Side ZP = 35° 35′ = Compl. Latitude, RP = 66° 31′

M m 2

66° 31′ = Sun's Distance from the North Pole of the Globe, and the ∠ ZPR = 30°; to find RZ the Complement of the Sun's Altitude. (Fig. 45.)

First, for the Segment dP, *by Case* 1, *right ∠s*

Cotan. ZP = 35° 35′   Radius . Cos ∠ ZPR = 30′ 00″ : Tan dP = 31° 47′

Then RP — dP = 66° 31′ — 31° 47′ = 34° 44′ = Rd.

Then Cos. dP = 31° 47′   Cos. ZP = 35° 35′ :· Cos. Rd = 34° 44′   Cos. RZ = 38° 11′, whose Complement 51° 49′ is the Sun's Altitude.

A General Rule *to be observed.*

If the given Time be between Six in the Morning and Six at Night, the fourth Arch found as above, must be subtracted from the Sun's Distance from the North Pole, but if the given Time be before Six in the Morning, and after Six at Night, the fourth Arch must be added to the Sun's Distance from the North Pole, the Sum or Difference is the fifth Arch.

Prob. XVIII.

Given the Latitude of the Place = 54° 25′, *the Sun's Declination* = 23° 29′ *North, and his Altitude* = 48° 30′, *to find the Hour of the Day.*

In the oblique-angled spherical Triangle AZP, given all the three Sides, viz. ZP = 35° 35′, AP = 66° 31′, and ZA = 41° 30′; to find the Angle P the Hour from Noon. (Fig. 46.)

Op L-

Sect. I. ASTRONOMICAL PROBLEMS. 267

OPERATION.

	°	′
ZP = Complement of the Latitude	35	35
AP = Complement of the Sun's Declination	66	31
AZ = Complement of the Sun's Altitude	41	30
Sum of the three Sides	143	36
Half Sum	71	48
Complement of the Latitude subtr.	35	35
Difference	36	13
Half Sum	71	48
Complement of the Declination subtr.	66	31
Difference	5	17

The Requisites being obtained, proceed thus:

Side ZP Comp. Latitude S. Co Ar. 35° 35′	0·235162
Side AP Comp Declinat. S Co. Ar. 66 31	0·037547
Differ. Co-latitude and ½ Sum S. 36 13	9·771470
Differ. Co-declinat. and ½ Sum S. 5 17	8·964170
Sum of the Logarithms	19·008349
Half is the Sine of — 18° 37′ 10″	9·504174

Doubled is — — 37 14 20 which converted into Time, is 2 h. 28′ 57″ 20‴, that is 9 h. 31′ 2″ 40‴ in the Morning, the Time of this Observation.

PROB.

Prob XIX.

Given the Latitude of the Place = 54° 25′, *the Sun's Declination* N = 23° 29′, *and the Altitude* = 48°; *to find his Azimuth from the North.*

In the oblique spherical Triangle AZP, given all the Sides, viz. ZP = 35° 35′ = Co-latitude, AP = 66° 31′ = Comp Sun's Declinat. North, and AZ = 42° = Compl Altitude, to find the $\angle Z$ = the Sun's Azimuth from the North. (Fig. 47.)

Operation.

ZP = Complement of the Latitude	—	35° 35′
AP = Complement of the ☉ Declination		66 31
AZ = Compl ☉ Altitude —	—	42 00
Sum of the three Sides —	—	144 6
Half Sum — —	—	72 3
Compl. Latitude subtract —	—	35 35
Difference — —	—	36 28
Half Sum — —	—	72 3
Complement Altitude subtract —	—	42 0
Difference — —	—	30 3

Then

Sect. I.   ASTRONOMICAL PROBLEMS.   269

Then proceed thus;

Side ZP = Comp Latit S Co. Ar 35° 35′   0·235162
Side AZ = Comp Altit S Co Ar. 42 00   0·174489
Differ Comp. Lat and ½ Sum S 36 28   9·774046
Differ. Comp. Altit. and ½ Sum S 30   3   9·699626

Sum of the Logarithms ———   19·883323

Half is the Sine of — — 60 58   9·941661

Then 60° 58′ doubled is 121° 56′ = $\angle Z$ = Sun's true Azimuth from the North, whose Complement to a Semi-circle is 58° 4′ = the Azimuth from the South.

Prob. XX

Given the Latitude of the Place = 54° 25′ *North, the Sun's Altitude* = 46° 28′, *and the Time of the Day* = 10 *o'Clock*, 43 *Min. before Noon, to find the Sun's Azimuth from the North*

In the oblique spheric Triangle AZP, there are given ZP = 35° 35′ = Compl Latit AZ = 43° 32′ = Compl. ☉ Altitude, with the $\angle P$ = 19° 15′, to find the $\angle Z$, the Sun's Azimuth from the North (Fig. 48)

The Perpendicular being let fall from Z upon AP, we have two right angled spherical Triangles PBZ, ABZ; in the Triangle PBZ, we have given ZP = 35° 35′, and the $\angle$ at P = 19° 15′; to find the $\angle PZB$.

Analogy

Analogy, by Cafe 3, right ∠s.

Radius Tan. ∠ $P = 19° 15'$: Cof. $ZP = 35° 35'$: Cotan. ∠ $PZB = 74° 9'$.

Then Cotan. $ZP = 35° 35'$ Cof. ∠ $PZB = 74° 9'$ ∴ Cotan. $AZ = 43° 32$ Cof ∠ $AZB = 78° 8'$

Then $AZB + PZB = 78° 8' + 74° 9' = 152° 17' = AZP =$ Sun's true Azimuth from the North; whofe Supplement $27° 43'$ is the Azimuth from the South.

Prob. XXI.

Given the Latitude of the Place $= 54° 25'$ North, the Sun's Declination North $= 6° 45'$, and his Diftance from the Zenith (always) $= 108°$; to find the true Time of Day-break in the Morning, and the End of the Evening Twilight.

Note, Day-break in the Morning, and the End of the Evening Twilight, is when the Sun is $18°$ below the Horizon.

In the oblique-angled fpherical Triangle ZPA, there are given $ZP = 35° 35' =$ Compl Latitude, $AP = 83° 15' =$ Compl Declination, and $AZ = 108° =$ Sun's Diftance from the Zenith; to find the ∠ $P =$ the Hour from Noon of the End of the Evening Twilight. (Fig. 49.)

Sect. I.   ASTRONOMICAL PROBLEMS.   271

OPERATION.

ZP the Complement of the Latitude	35° 35'
AP Complement of the ☉'s Declinat.	83 15
AZ ☉'s Zenith Distance	108 00
Sum of the three Sides	226 50
Half Sum	113 25
Compl Latit subtr.	35 35
Difference	77 50
Half Sum	113 25
Compl Declination subtr.	83 15
Difference	30 10

Then,

Side ZP Compl. Latit. S. Co. Ar. 35° 35' = 0·235162
Side AP Compl Declin S Co Ar. 83 15 = 0·003021
Diff. Compl. Latit and ½ Sum S. 77 50 = 9·990134
Diff. Compl. Decl and ½ Sum S 30 10 = 9·701151

Sum of the Logarithms   19·929468

Half is the Sine of — — 67 13 = 9·964734
Doubled is — — 134 26 = ∠ at the
Pole, which converted into Time is 8h 57m 44s the
End of the Evening Twilight, whose Complement to
12 Hours, is 3h. 2m. 16s. the true Time of Day-break.

N n   SECT

272　*The* SUN's MEAN MOTION　Book VI.

SECT II.

TABLES *of the* SUN's MEAN MOTION.

Years complete	Sun's Longitude S ° ′ ″	Sun's Anomaly S ° ′ ″
1	11 29 45 40	11 29 44 37
2	11 29 31 20	11 29 9 14
3	11 29 17 0	11 29 13 51
B 4	0 0 1 49	11 29 57 37
5	11 29 47 29	11 29 52 14
6	11 29 33 9	11 29 26 51
7	11 29 18 49	11 29 11 28
B 8	0 0 3 37	11 29 55 13
9	11 29 49 18	11 29 39 51
10	11 29 34 58	11 29 4 28
11	11 29 20 38	11 29 9 5
B 12	0 0 5 26	11 29 52 50
13	11 29 51 6	11 29 37 27
14	11 29 36 47	11 29 2 5
15	11 29 22 27	11 29 6 42
B 16	0 0 7 15	11 29 50 27
17	11 29 52 55	11 29 35 4
18	11 29 38 35	11 29 19 41
19	11 29 24 15	11 29 4 18
B 20	0 0 9 03	11 29 48 4

Years current	Sun's Longitude S ° ′ ″	Sun's Anomaly S. ° ′ ″
1701	9 8 14 8	6 1 9 38
1721	9 8 23 12	6 0 57 42
1741	9 8 32 16	6 0 45 46
1761	9 8 41 20	6 0 33 50
1781	9 8 50 24	6 0 21 54
1801	9 8 0 19	5 29 10 49
1821	9 8 9 23	5 28 58 53
1841	9 8 18 27	5 28 46 57
1861	9 8 27 31	5 28 35 1
1881	9 8 36 35	5 28 23 5
1901	9 7 46 30	5 27 12 0
1921	9 7 55 34	5 27 0 4
1941	9 8 04 38	5 26 48 8
1961	9 8 13 42	5 26 36 12
1981	9 8 22 46	5 26 24 16
1991	9 8 31 50	5 26 12 20

Sect II. *in* MONTHS *and* DAYS. 273

Com. Year	JANUARY Sun's Long S ° ′ ″	Sun's Anom S ° ′ ″	Com Year	FEBRUARY Sun's Long S ° ′ ″	Sun's Anom S ° ′ ″
1	0 0 59 8	0 0 59 8	1	1 1 32 26	1 1 32 21
2	0 1 58 17	0 1 58 17	2	1 2 31 35	1 2 31 30
3	0 2 57 25	0 2 57 25	3	1 3 30 43	1 3 30 38
4	0 3 56 33	0 3 56 33	4	1 4 29 51	1 4 29 46
5	0 4 55 42	0 4 55 42	5	1 5 29 0	1 5 28 55
6	0 5 54 50	0 5 54 50	6	1 6 28 8	1 6 28 3
7	0 6 53 58	0 6 53 57	7	1 7 27 16	1 7 27 11
8	0 7 53 7	0 7 53 6	8	1 8 26 25	1 8 26 20
9	0 8 52 15	0 8 52 14	9	1 9 25 33	1 9 25 27
10	0 9 51 23	0 9 51 22	10	1 10 24 41	1 10 24 35
11	0 10 50 31	0 10 50 30	11	1 11 23 49	1 11 23 43
12	0 11 49 40	0 11 49 39	12	1 12 22 58	1 12 22 52
13	0 12 48 48	0 12 48 47	13	1 13 22 6	1 13 22 0
14	0 13 47 57	0 13 47 55	14	1 14 21 15	1 14 21 9
15	0 14 47 5	0 14 43 3	15	1 15 20 23	1 15 20 17
16	0 15 46 13	0 15 46 10	16	1 16 19 31	1 16 19 24
17	0 16 45 22	0 16 45 19	17	1 17 18 40	1 17 18 32
18	0 17 44 30	0 17 44 27	18	1 18 17 48	1 18 17 40
19	0 18 43 38	0 18 43 35	19	1 19 16 56	1 19 16 48
20	0 19 42 47	0 19 42 43	20	1 20 16 05	1 20 15 57
21	0 20 41 55	0 20 41 52	21	1 21 15 13	1 21 15 5
22	0 21 41 3	0 21 41 0	22	1 22 14 21	1 22 14 12
23	0 22 40 12	0 22 40 8	23	1 23 13 30	1 23 13 21
24	0 23 39 20	0 23 39 16	24	1 24 12 38	1 24 12 29
25	0 24 38 28	0 24 38 24	25	1 25 11 46	1 25 11 37
26	0 25 37 37	0 25 37 33	26	1 26 10 55	1 26 10 46
27	0 26 36 45	0 26 36 41	27	1 27 10 3	1 27 9 54
28	0 27 35 53	0 27 35 48	28	1 28 9 11	1 28 9 1
29	0 28 35 2	0 28 34 56	29	1 29 8 20	1 29 8 10
30	0 29 34 10	0 29 34 5			
31	1 0 33 18	1 0 33 14			

The Sun's Mean Motion — Book VI.

Com Year	MARCH Sun's Lon S ° ′ ″	Sun's Ano S ° ′ ″	Bissextile	Com Year	APRIL Sun's Lon S ° ′ ″	Sun's Ano S ° ′ ″	Bissextile
1	1 29 8 20	1 29 8 10	0	1	2 29 41 36	2 29 41 22	0
2	2 0 7 28	2 0 7 18	1	2	3 0 40 40	3 0 40 32	1
3	2 1 6 36	2 1 6 26	2	3	3 1 39 55	3 1 39 40	2
4	2 2 5 44	2 2 5 33	3	4	3 2 39 3	3 2 38 46	3
5	2 3 4 53	2 3 4 42	4	5	3 3 38 12	3 3 37 56	4
6	2 4 4 1	2 4 3 50	5	6	3 4 37 20	3 4 37 4	5
7	2 5 3 9	2 5 2 58	6	7	3 5 36 28	3 5 36 12	6
8	2 6 2 18	2 6 2 7	7	8	3 6 35 37	3 6 35 20	7
9	2 7 1 26	2 7 1 15	8	9	3 7 34 45	3 7 34 28	8
10	2 8 0 34	2 8 0 22	9	10	3 8 33 53	3 8 33 36	9
11	2 8 59 42	2 8 59 30	10	11	3 9 33 1	3 9 32 44	10
12	2 9 58 51	2 9 56 39	11	12	3 10 32 10	3 10 31 53	11
13	2 10 57 59	2 10 57 47	12	13	3 11 31 18	3 11 31 1	12
14	2 11 57 8	2 11 56 56	13	14	3 12 30 27	3 12 30 10	13
15	2 12 56 16	2 12 56 4	14	15	3 13 29 35	3 13 29 18	14
16	2 13 55 24	2 13 55 1	15	16	3 14 28 43	3 14 28 26	15
17	2 14 54 33	2 14 54 20	16	17	3 15 27 52	3 15 27 34	16
18	2 15 53 41	2 15 53 28	17	18	3 16 27 0	3 16 26 42	17
19	2 16 52 49	2 16 52 36	18	19	3 17 26 8	3 17 25 50	18
20	2 17 51 58	2 17 51 54	19	20	3 18 25 17	3 18 24 58	19
21	2 18 51 6	2 18 50 53	20	21	3 19 24 25	3 19 24 7	20
22	2 19 50 14	2 19 50 0	21	22	3 20 23 33	3 20 23 15	21
23	2 20 49 23	2 20 49 9	22	23	3 21 22 42	3 21 22 23	22
24	2 21 48 31	2 21 48 17	23	24	3 22 21 50	3 22 21 31	23
25	2 22 47 39	2 22 47 25	24	25	3 23 20 58	3 23 20 39	24
26	2 23 46 48	2 23 46 31	25	26	3 24 20 7	3 24 19 48	25
27	2 24 45 56	2 24 45 42	26	27	3 25 19 15	3 25 18 56	26
28	2 25 15 4	2 25 14 49	27	28	3 26 18 23	3 26 18 4	27
29	2 26 44 13	2 26 43 58	28	29	3 27 17 32	3 27 17 12	28
30	2 27 43 21	2 27 43 6	29	30	3 28 16 40	3 28 16 20	29
31	2 28 42 29	2 28 42 15	30		3 29 15 48	3 29 15 28	30
	2 29 41 38	2 29 41 43	31				

MAY

Sect II. *in* MONTHS *and* DAYS.

MAY

Com. Year	Sun's Lon S ° ′ ″	Sun's Ano S. ° ′ ″	Differ
1	3 29 15 48	3 29 15 28	0
2	3 0 14 56	3 0 14 36	1
3	4 1 14 4	4 1 13 44	2
4	4 2 13 12	4 2 12 51	3
5	4 3 12 21	4 3 12 0	4
6	4 4 11 29	4 4 11 8	5
7	4 5 10 37	4 5 10 16	6
8	4 6 9 46	4 6 9 25	7
9	4 7 8 54	4 7 8 33	8
10	4 8 8 2	4 8 7 40	9
11	4 9 7 10	4 9 6 48	10
12	4 10 6 19	4 10 5 57	11
13	4 11 5 27	4 11 5 5	12
14	4 12 4 36	4 12 4 14	13
15	4 13 3 44	4 13 3 22	14
16	4 14 2 52	4 14 2 29	15
17	4 15 2 1	4 15 1 38	16
18	4 16 1 9	4 16 0 46	17
19	4 17 0 17	4 16 59 54	18
20	4 17 59 26	4 17 59 3	19
21	4 18 58 3	4 18 53 11	20
22	4 19 57 42	4 19 57 18	21
23	4 20 56 21	4 20 56 27	22
24	4 21 55 35	4 21 55 35	23
25	4 22 55 7	4 22 54 43	24
26	4 23 54 16	4 23 53 52	25
27	4 24 53 24	4 24 53 0	26
28	4 25 52 32	4 25 52 8	27
29	4 26 51 41	4 26 51 16	28
30	4 27 50 49	4 27 50 24	29
31	4 28 49 57	4 28 49 32	30
	4 29 49 6	4 29 41 41	31

JUNE

Com. Year	Sun's Lon S ° ′ ″	Sun's Ano S. ° ′ ″	Differ
1	5 29 49 6	4 29 48 41	0
2	5 0 48 14	5 0 47 50	1
3	5 1 47 23	5 1 46 58	2
4	5 2 46 31	5 2 46 6	3
5	5 3 45 40	5 3 45 14	4
6	5 4 44 48	5 4 44 22	5
7	5 5 43 56	5 5 43 30	6
8	5 6 43 5	5 6 42 39	7
9	5 7 42 13	5 7 41 47	8
10	5 8 41 21	5 8 40 55	9
11	5 9 40 29	5 9 40 3	10
12	5 10 39 38	5 10 39 11	11
13	5 11 38 46	5 11 38 19	12
14	5 12 37 55	5 12 37 27	13
15	5 13 37 3	5 13 36 35	14
16	5 14 36 11	5 14 35 43	15
17	5 15 35 20	5 15 34 51	16
18	5 16 34 28	5 16 34 0	17
19	5 17 33 36	5 17 33 8	18
20	5 18 32 45	5 18 32 17	19
21	5 19 21 53	5 19 31 25	20
22	5 20 31 1	5 20 30 33	21
23	5 21 30 10	5 21 29 40	22
24	5 22 29 18	5 22 28 40	23
25	5 23 28 26	5 23 27 57	24
26	5 24 27 35	5 24 27 6	25
27	5 25 26 43	5 25 26 11	26
28	5 26 25 51	5 26 25 22	27
29	5 27 25 0	5 27 24 30	28
30	5 28 24 8	5 28 23 3	29
	5 29 23 16	5 29 22 46	30

JULY

The Sun's Mean Motion — Book VI.

Com Year	JULY Sun's Lon S ° ′ ″	JULY Sun's Ano S ° ′ ″	Bissex	Com Year	AUGUST Sun's Lon S ° ′ ″	AUGUST Sun's Ano S ° ′ ″	Bissex
1	5 29 23 16	5 29 23 16	0	1	6 29 56 33	6 29 55 57	0
2	6 0 22 24	6 0 21 53	1	2	7 0 55 42	7 0 55 6	1
3	6 1 21 32	6 1 21 1	2	3	7 1 54 50	7 1 54 14	2
4	6 2 20 40	6 2 20 9	3	4	7 2 53 58	7 2 53 22	3
5	6 3 19 49	6 3 19 17	4	5	7 3 53 7	7 3 52 30	4
6	6 4 18 57	6 4 18 25	5	6	7 4 52 15	7 4 51 37	5
7	6 5 18 5	6 5 17 33	6	7	7 5 51 23	7 5 50 45	6
8	6 6 17 14	6 6 16 42	7	8	7 6 50 32	7 6 49 53	7
9	6 7 16 22	6 7 15 50	8	9	7 7 49 40	7 7 49 2	8
10	6 8 15 30	6 8 14 58	9	10	7 8 48 48	7 8 48 10	9
11	6 9 14 38	6 9 14 6	10	11	7 9 47 56	7 9 47 18	10
12	6 10 13 47	6 10 13 14	11	12	7 10 47 5	7 10 46 26	11
13	6 11 12 55	6 11 12 22	12	13	7 11 46 13	7 11 45 34	12
14	6 12 12 4	6 12 11 31	13	14	7 12 45 22	7 12 44 43	13
15	6 13 11 12	6 13 10 39	14	15	7 13 44 30	7 13 43 51	14
16	6 14 10 20	6 14 9 47	15	16	7 14 43 38	7 14 42 58	15
17	6 15 9 29	6 15 8 55	16	17	7 15 42 47	7 15 42 7	16
18	6 16 8 37	6 16 8 3	17	18	7 16 41 55	7 16 41 15	17
19	6 17 7 45	6 17 7 11	18	19	7 17 41 3	7 17 40 23	18
20	6 18 6 54	6 18 6 20	19	20	7 18 40 12	7 18 39 32	19
21	6 19 6 2	6 19 5 28	20	21	7 19 39 20	7 19 38 40	20
22	6 20 5 10	6 20 4 36	21	22	7 20 38 28	7 20 37 48	21
23	6 21 4 19	6 21 3 44	22	23	7 21 37 36	7 21 36 56	22
24	6 22 3 27	6 22 2 52	23	24	7 22 36 45	7 22 36 4	23
25	6 23 2 35	6 23 2 0	24	25	7 23 34 53	7 23 35 12	24
26	6 24 1 44	6 24 1 9	25	26	7 24 35 2	7 24 34 21	25
27	6 25 0 52	6 25 0 17	26	27	7 25 34 10	7 25 33 29	26
28	6 26 0 0	6 25 59 25	27	28	7 26 33 18	7 26 32 37	27
29	6 26 59 9	6 26 58 33	28	29	7 27 32 27	7 27 31 45	28
30	6 27 58 17	6 27 57 41	29	30	7 28 31 35	7 28 30 53	29
31	6 28 57 25	6 28 56 49	30	31	7 29 30 43	7 29 30 1	30
	6 29 56 33	6 29 55 57	31		8 0 29 52	7 0 29 10	31

SEP-

Sect II.   *in* MONTHS *and* DAYS.   277

Com Year	SEPTEMBER Sun's Lon S ° ′ ″	Sun's Ano S ° ′ ″	Bissex	Com Year	OCTOBER Sun's Lon. S ° ′ ″	Sun's Ano S ° ′ ″	Bissex
1	8 0 29 52	8 0 29 10	0	1	9 0 4 2	9 0 3 17	0
2	8 1 29 0	8 1 28 18	1	2	9 1 3 11	9 1 2 25	1
3	8 2 28 9	8 2 27 26	2	3	9 2 2 19	9 2 1 33	2
4	8 3 27 17	8 3 26 35	3	4	9 3 1 27	9 3 0 41	3
5	8 4 26 56	8 4 25 44	4	5	9 4 0 36	9 3 59 49	4
6	8 5 25 31	8 5 24 52	5	6	9 4 59 44	9 4 58 57	5
7	8 6 24 42	8 6 24 0	6	7	9 5 58 52	9 5 58 5	6
8	8 7 23 51	8 7 23 8	7	8	9 6 58 1	9 6 57 13	7
9	8 8 22 59	8 8 22 16	8	9	9 7 57 9	9 7 56 21	8
10	8 9 22 7	8 9 21 24	9	10	9 8 56 17	9 8 55 29	9
11	8 10 21 15	8 10 20 32	10	11	9 9 55 25	9 9 54 37	10
12	8 11 20 24	8 11 19 41	11	12	9 10 54 34	9 10 53 45	11
13	8 12 19 32	8 12 18 50	12	13	9 11 53 42	9 11 52 53	12
14	8 13 18 40	8 13 17 57	13	14	9 12 52 49	9 12 52 2	13
15	8 14 17 48	8 14 17 5	14	15	9 13 51 58	9 13 51 11	14
16	8 15 16 57	8 15 16 13	15	16	9 14 51 7	9 14 50 19	15
17	8 16 16 6	8 16 15 22	16	17	9 15 50 16	9 15 49 28	16
18	8 17 15 14	8 17 14 30	17	18	9 16 49 24	9 16 48 36	17
19	8 18 14 22	8 18 13 38	18	19	9 17 48 32	9 17 47 44	18
20	8 19 13 31	8 19 12 47	19	20	9 18 47 41	9 18 46 52	19
21	8 20 12 39	8 20 11 55	20	21	9 19 46 49	9 19 46 1	20
22	8 21 11 47	8 21 11 3	21	22	9 20 45 57	9 20 45 9	21
23	8 22 10 56	8 22 10 11	22	23	9 21 45 6	9 21 44 17	22
24	8 23 10 4	8 23 9 19	23	24	9 22 44 14	9 22 43 25	23
25	8 24 9 12	8 24 8 27	24	25	9 23 43 22	9 23 42 33	24
26	8 25 8 21	8 25 7 35	25	26	9 24 42 31	9 24 41 41	25
27	8 26 7 29	8 26 6 44	26	27	9 25 41 39	9 25 40 49	26
28	8 27 6 37	8 27 5 52	27	28	9 26 40 47	9 26 39 57	27
29	8 28 5 46	8 28 5 1	28	29	9 27 39 56	9 27 39 5	28
30	8 29 4 54	8 29 4 9	29	30	9 28 39 4	9 28 38 13	29
	9 0 4 2	9 0 3 17	30	31	9 29 38 12	9 29 37 20	30
					10 0 37 20	10 0 36 28	31

N O-

NOVEMBER

Con. Year	Sun's Lon S ° ′ ″	Sun's Ano S ° ′ ″	Bissex
1	10 0 37 20	10 0 36 28	0
2	10 1 36 29	10 1 35 36	1
3	10 2 35 37	10 2 34 44	2
4	10 3 34 45	10 3 33 52	3
5	10 4 33 54	10 4 33 0	4
6	10 5 33 2	10 5 32 8	5
7	10 6 32 10	10 6 31 16	6
8	10 7 31 19	10 7 30 25	7
9	10 8 30 27	10 8 29 33	8
10	10 9 29 35	10 9 28 40	9
11	10 10 28 43	10 10 27 48	10
12	10 11 27 52	10 11 26 57	11
13	10 12 27 0	10 12 26 5	12
14	10 13 26 9	10 13 25 14	13
15	10 14 25 17	10 14 24 22	14
16	10 15 24 25	10 15 23 29	15
17	10 16 23 34	10 16 22 38	16
18	10 17 22 42	10 17 21 46	17
19	10 18 21 50	10 18 20 54	18
20	10 19 20 59	10 19 20 3	19
21	10 20 20 7	10 20 19 11	20
22	10 21 19 15	10 21 18 18	21
23	10 22 18 24	10 22 17 27	22
24	10 23 17 32	10 23 16 35	23
25	10 24 16 40	10 24 15 43	24
26	10 25 15 49	10 25 14 52	25
27	10 26 14 57	10 26 14 0	26
28	10 27 14 5	10 27 13 8	27
29	10 28 13 14	10 28 12 16	28
30	10 29 12 22	10 29 11 24	29
	11 0 11 30	11 0 10 32	30

DECEMBER

Con. Year	Sun's Lon S ° ′ ″	Sun's Ano S ° ′ ″	Bissex
1	11 0 11 30	11 0 10 32	0
2	11 1 10 39	11 1 9 40	1
3	11 2 9 47	11 2 8 48	2
4	11 3 8 55	11 3 7 56	3
5	11 4 8 4	11 4 7 4	4
6	11 5 7 12	11 5 6 12	5
7	11 6 6 20	11 6 5 20	6
8	11 7 5 29	11 7 4 28	7
9	11 8 4 37	11 8 3 36	8
10	11 9 3 45	11 9 2 44	9
11	11 10 2 53	11 10 1 52	10
12	11 11 2 2	11 11 1 0	11
13	11 12 1 10	11 12 0 8	12
14	11 13 0 19	11 12 59 17	13
15	11 13 59 27	11 13 58 25	14
16	11 14 58 35	11 14 57 33	15
17	11 15 57 44	11 15 56 42	16
18	11 16 56 52	11 16 55 50	17
19	11 17 56 0	11 17 54 48	18
20	11 18 55 9	11 18 54 6	19
21	11 19 54 17	11 19 53 14	20
22	11 20 53 25	11 20 52 22	21
23	11 21 52 34	11 21 51 30	22
24	11 22 51 42	11 22 50 39	23
25	11 23 50 50	11 23 49 47	24
26	11 24 49 59	11 24 48 55	25
27	11 25 49 7	11 25 48 3	26
28	11 26 48 15	11 26 47 11	27
29	11 27 47 24	11 27 46 19	28
30	11 28 46 32	11 28 45 28	29
31	11 29 45 40	11 29 44 37	30
	0 0 44 48	0 0 43 45	31

Sect. II. *in* Hours, Min. Sec. 279

H , ″ ‴ ‷	Sun's Long. ° ′ ″ ′ ″ ‴ ″ ‴ ⁗ ‴ ⁗ v	Sun's Anom. ° ′ ″ ′ ″ ‴ ″ ‴ ⁗ ‴ ⁗ v	H , ″ ‴ ‷	Sun's Long. ° ′ ″ ′ ″ ‴ ″ ‴ ⁗ ‴ ⁗ v	Sun's Anom ° ′ ″ ′ ″ ‴ ″ ‴ ⁗ ‴ ⁗ v.
1	0 2 28	0 2 28	31	1 16 23	1 16 23
2	0 4 56	0 4 56	32	1 18 51	1 18 51
3	0 7 24	0 7 24	33	1 21 19	1 21 19
4	0 9 51	0 9 51	34	1 23 47	1 23 47
5	0 12 19	0 12 19	35	1 26 15	1 26 15
6	0 14 47	0 14 47	36	1 28 43	1 28 43
7	0 17 15	0 17 15	37	1 31 11	1 31 11
8	0 19 43	0 19 43	38	1 33 39	1 33 39
9	0 22 11	0 22 11	39	1 36 6	1 36 6
10	0 24 38	0 24 38	40	1 38 44	1 38 44
11	0 27 6	0 27 6	41	1 41 2	1 41 2
12	0 29 34	0 29 34	42	1 43 30	1 43 30
13	0 32 2	0 32 2	43	1 45 58	1 45 58
14	0 34 30	0 34 30	44	1 48 25	1 48 25
15	0 36 58	0 36 58	45	1 50 53	1 50 53
16	0 39 25	0 39 25	46	1 53 21	1 53 21
17	0 41 53	0 41 53	47	1 55 49	1 55 49
18	0 44 21	0 44 21	48	1 58 17	1 58 17
19	0 46 49	0 46 49	49	2 0 44	2 0 44
20	0 49 17	0 49 17	50	2 3 12	2 3 12
21	0 51 45	0 51 45	51	2 5 40	2 5 40
22	0 54 13	0 54 13	52	2 8 8	2 8 8
23	0 56 40	0 56 40	53	2 10 36	2 10 36
24	0 59 8	0 59 8	54	2 13 3	2 13 3
25	1 1 36	1 1 36	55	2 15 31	2 15 31
26	1 4 4	1 4 4	56	2 17 59	2 17 59
27	1 6 32	1 6 32	57	2 20 27	2 20 27
28	1 9 0	1 9 0	58	2 22 55	2 22 55
29	1 11 27	1 11 27	59	2 25 23	2 25 23
30	1 13 55	1 13 55	60	2 27 51	2 27 51

O o A

A Table of the Sun's Equation — Book VI.

Me in Anom	Sign 0 sub Equation ° ′ ″	Sign 1 sub Equation ° ′ ″	Sign 2 sub Equation ° ′ ″	Sign 3 sub Equation ° ′ ″	Sign 4 sub Equation ° ′ ″	Sign 5 sub Equation ° ′ ″	Mean Anom.
0	0 0 0	0 57 7	1 39 41	1 56 19	1 41 48	0 59 15	30
1	0 1 59	0 58 51	1 40 42	1 56 20	1 40 48	0 57 26	29
2	0 3 59	1 0 33	1 41 41	1 56 19	1 39 46	0 55 37	28
3	0 5 58	1 2 15	1 42 39	1 56 16	1 38 41	0 53 48	27
4	0 7 57	1 3 55	1 43 35	1 56 12	1 37 35	0 51 57	26
5	0 9 56	1 5 35	1 44 29	1 56 5	1 36 27	0 50 5	25
6	0 11 55	1 7 14	1 45 21	1 55 56	1 35 17	0 48 13	24
7	0 13 53	1 8 51	1 46 11	1 55 45	1 34 5	0 46 19	23
8	0 15 51	1 10 27	1 47 0	1 55 31	1 32 52	0 44 25	22
9	0 17 49	1 12 1	1 47 46	1 55 15	1 31 37	0 42 30	21
10	0 19 47	1 13 35	1 48 31	1 54 58	1 30 20	0 40 34	20
11	0 21 45	1 15 7	1 49 13	1 54 38	1 29 1	0 38 37	19
12	0 23 42	1 16 38	1 49 53	1 54 16	1 27 41	0 36 40	18
13	0 25 38	1 18 7	1 50 32	1 53 52	1 26 19	0 34 41	17
14	0 27 35	1 19 36	1 51 9	1 53 26	1 24 55	0 32 42	16
15	0 29 30	1 21 3	1 51 44	1 52 58	1 23 30	0 30 43	15
16	0 31 25	1 22 28	1 52 17	1 52 27	1 22 3	0 28 43	14
17	0 33 20	1 23 51	1 52 20	1 51 55	1 20 35	0 26 42	13
18	0 35 14	1 25 14	1 53 16	1 51 0	1 19 5	0 24 41	12
19	0 37 8	1 26 35	1 53 43	1 50 44	1 17 33	0 22 39	11
20	0 39 1	1 27 55	1 54 7	1 50 5	1 16 0	0 20 37	10
21	0 40 53	1 29 13	1 54 30	1 49 24	1 14 26	0 18 34	9
22	0 42 44	1 30 29	1 54 50	1 48 42	1 12 50	0 16 31	8
23	0 44 35	1 31 13	1 55 9	1 47 57	1 11 13	0 14 28	7
24	0 46 25	1 32 56	1 55 25	1 47 11	1 9 34	0 12 24	6
25	0 48 14	1 34 8	1 55 39	1 46 22	1 7 54	0 10 21	5
26	0 50 2	1 35 18	1 55 51	1 45 31	1 6 13	0 8 17	4
27	0 51 50	1 36 26	1 56 1	1 44 38	1 4 31	0 6 13	3
28	0 53 36	1 37 32	1 56 9	1 43 43	1 2 47	0 4 9	2
29	0 55 22	1 38 38	1 56 15	1 42 47	1 1 2	0 2 4	1
30	0 57 7	1 39 41	1 56 19	1 41 48	0 59 15	0 0 0	0
	Sign 11 add	Sign 10 add	Sign 9 add	Sign 8 add	Sign 7 add	Sign 6 add	

Mr

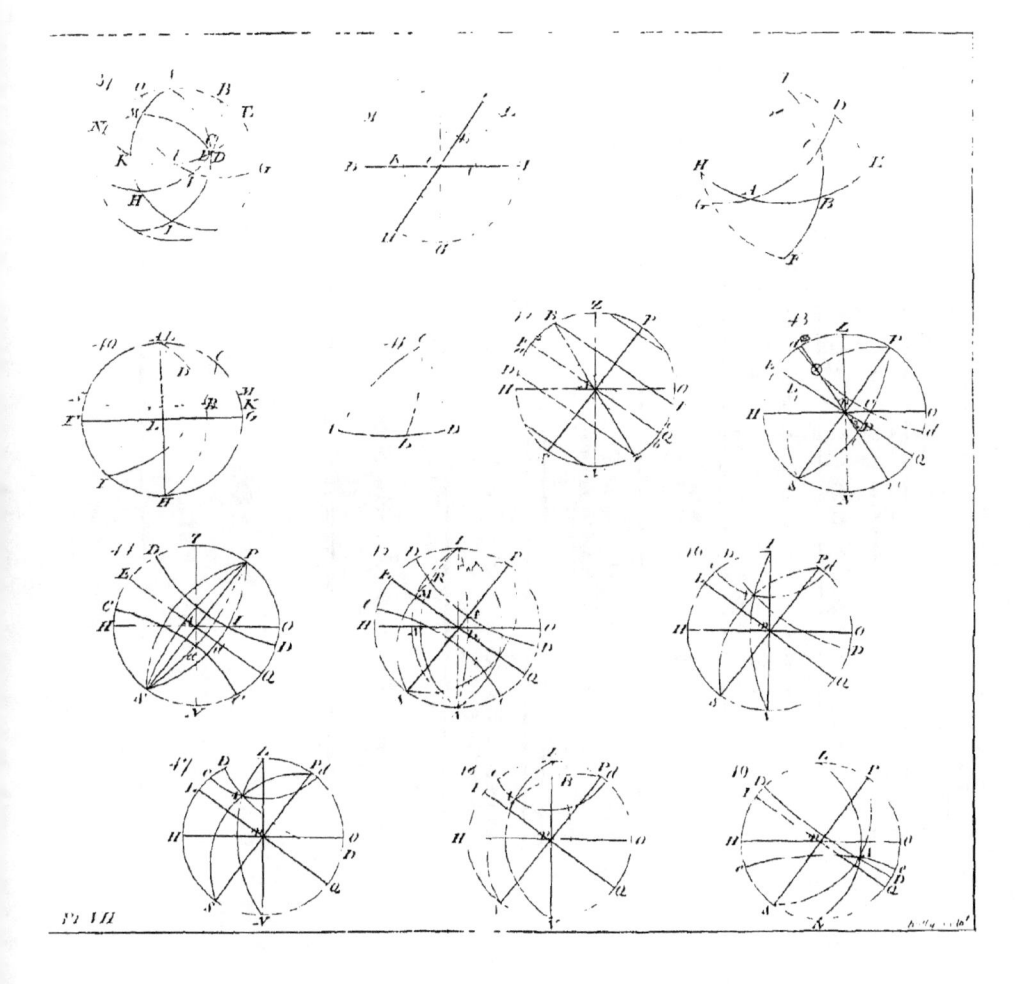

Sect II. *Mr* Flamstead's *Table of Refractions,* &c.

Altit		Refrac		Altit	Refrac		Altit	Par Sun	Altit	Par. Sun
°	′	′	″	°	′	″	°	″	°	″
0	0	33	00	25	1	45	0	10	90	0
0	30	26	38	26	1	40	3	10		
1	0	23	22	27	1	36	6	10		
1	30	20	17	28	1	31	9	10		
2	0	17	26	29	1	27	12	9		
2	30	15	15	30	1	23	15	9		
3	0	13	23	31	1	20	18	9		
3	30	11	53	32	1	17	21	9		
4	0	10	39	33	1	14	24	8		
4	30	9	38	34	1	11	27	8		
5	0	8	48	35	1	9	30	8		
6	0	7	26	36	1	7	33	7		
7	0	6	25	37	1	5	36	7		
8	0	5	27	38	1	2	39	7		
9	0	5	2	39	1	0	42	6		
10	0	4	33	40	0	58	45	6		
11	0	4	6	41	0	56	48	6		
12	0	3	45	42	0	54	51	5		
13	0	3	29	43	0	52	54	5		
14	0	3	13	44	0	50	57	5		
15	0	3	0	45	0	48	60	4		
16	0	2	48	46	0	46	63	4		
17	0	2	38	47	0	45	66	4		
18	0	2	29	48	0	44	69	3		
19	0	2	21	49	0	42	72	3		
20	0	2	14	50	0	40	75	2		
21	0	2	7	55	0	34	78	2		
22	0	2	1	60	0	29	81	1		
23	0	1	55	70	0	19	84	1		
24	0	1	50	80	0	9	87	0		
				90	0	0				

BOOK VII.

The DESCRIPTION *and* USE *of the several* INSTRUMENTS *required in making an actual* SURVEY.

THE whole Practice of making an actual Survey, can only be said to consist of two Parts, *viz.* 1. The Measuring of Distances, 2. The taking of Angles. The Instruments mostly in Use for Measuring of Distances, are the Chain, and the Perambulator (or surveying Wheel) the latter being chiefly used in Surveying of Roads.

But for the ascertaining the true Quantity of any Angle, there are several Instruments, as the Theodolite, the plain Table, the Semi-circle, and the Circumferentor; but the two latter are out of Use at this Day, the Preference being (deservedly) given to the two former.

Lastly, there are other Instruments used in plotting a Survey, as a Scale decimally divided the whole Length, commonly called a Feather-edged Scale, a Protractor, a Parallel Ruler, &c. of which in their Order.

SECT

SECT. I.

The Description and Use of GUNTER's 4 POLE CHAIN.

THERE have been various Sorts of Chains made and contrived, according to the particular Notions of different Surveyors, but that called and known by the Name of *Gunter*'s Chain, is preferable to all others as yet contrived, both for its Exactness, and easy Application, in the Practice of making an actual Survey. Its Length is just 22 Yards, or 66 Feet, or 4 Poles, at 5½ Yards to the Pole, decimally divided the whole Length, into 100 equal Divisions, by Means of as many Links, the Length of each of which is 7 92 Inches.

This Chain is marked at the End of every 10 Links, with Pieces of Brass, which Number from each End thereof to the Middle and no further, where is hung a circular Piece of Brass, denoting 50 Links or the Middle of the Chain, and so may any Number of Links be readily discerned, during the Time of measuring a Distance.

The Manner of working or measuring with the Chain, is thus

First provide a Staff exactly 6 Feet, 7 Inches, and 2 tenth Parts long, which must be divided into 10 equal Parts, and is in Length exactly equal to 10 Links of the Chain, with this you must measure your Offsets,

Offsets, as shall be shewn hereafter, and is thence named an Offset-staff

You must also be provided with 10 short Sticks like Arrows, about two Feet in Length, pik'd with Iron at one End, and of a convenient Thickness, so as easily to be grasped in one Hand.

Being thus accommodated, let the Man who carries the fore End of the Chain, (commonly called the Leader of the Chain), take the ten Sticks or Arrows in his Hand, and going forward with the Chain, let the Person who carries the hinder End thereof, stand at the Station, and hold the End exactly to it, and then he must direct the Leader of the Chain, by making a proper Signal, 'till he fix him in a direct Line with the next Station; there let him put down a Stick. Then going forward towards the Station, measure the Distance, and make the Offsets, but the Manner of doing these shall be more fully described when we come to lay down the Method of making an actual Survey by the Chain only. It is only further to be remarked, that the Person who carries the hinder End of the Chain, must be careful to take up every Stick as he comes to it, for losing a Stick is losing a Chain's Length; and to guard against that, the Man who carries the hinder End of the Chain, must frequently enquire of the Leader of the Chain, how many Sticks or Arrows he hath; and if the Number each Man hath, when put together, make ten, there can be no Error in that Measurement, if otherwise, there is a Mistake, which only can be remedied by a second Measuring, which by no Means must be omitted

ted, as the Truth of the whole Survey is greatly dependent thereon.

SECT. II.

The Description and Use of the PERAMBULATOR, *or* SURVEYING-WHEEL.

THIS Instrument consists of a Wheel neatly laid round with Iron, to prevent its wearing, whose outside Circumference is 99 Inches, or Half a Statute Pole, it has a wooden Frame three Feet long (including the Handle and Cheeks), within which the Wheel turns in Time of Practice. It has likewise a Box of about ten Inches Diameter, containing a Motion-work of Brass, on the Face of which are three concentric Circles, to each of which belongs an Index or Hand.

One of these Circles is divided into 100 equal Parts, shewing the Links, one Revolution of which is equal to one *Gunter's* Chain. Another is divided into 80 equal Parts, denoting the Chains, one Revolution of which answers to one Mile. And the other Circle is divided into 50 equal Divisions, noting the Miles; one Revolution of which is equal to 50 Miles. So the Distance passed over by the Wheel at any Time, will be expressed in Miles, Chains, and Links.

The Motion-work in the Box being acted upon by the Rotation of the Wheel, gives Motion to the three Hands or Indices before described. The Length of the whole Instrument, from the Extremity of the Wheel

Wheel to the Handle, is little more than four Feet; but as to its Size, it may be greater or less, and so contrived, as to take in Pieces, (the Wood-work being of Mahogany) and put together again, for the Convenience and Ease of Carriage.

This Instrument having a Theodolite adapted to it, is very expeditious in practical Surveying, where too great Exactness is not required, seeing by it any Surveyor will measure a Parcel of Ground in Half the Time that it can be done by any other Instrument. And though it be objected, that in passing over Ant-hills and Plow-ridges, the Distance given by the Wheel is longer than that given by the Chain, occasioned by its passing over the Tops and Bottoms of such Hills and Ridges; this I say cannot be denied to be Truth, for there will be some little Difference between the Distance given by this Instrument, and that given by the Chain, but then of these two Measures, give me Leave to ask the Question, which of them is nearest the Truth? For I esteem it a Matter of Difficulty, to gain the true and exact horizontal Distance between any two Places, by measuring upon the Surface of the Earth, let the same be performed with the utmost Care, for though the Chain be free from some Objections, which the other Instrument is liable to, yet what Person can pretend to lead a Chain in that horizontal Position, which is required to make a true Distance For the swaying of the Chain, the Uncertainty of pricking down the Arrows, and withal the Variableness of its being stretched so tight as it should be, all these seem to denote as much Uncer-

tainty

Sect. II. *The* INSTRUMENTS *described*

tainty, and make it subject to the same Censure of Fallibility.

Having sufficiently described all the Parts of the Perambulator, I shall in the next Place shew its Use in practical Surveying, which is as follows:

Being well assured of the Truth of your Instrument before you begin to measure your Distance observe to set the three Hands or Indices to o, or the Beginning of the Divisions of their respective Circles, and then driving the Wheel right before you, towards a destined Station, you (for Example) looking upon the Indices, observe the Mile Index to stand between o and the first Mark, the Chain Index at its 30th Division, and the Link Index at o, the Distance then gone over by the Wheel is 30 Chains.

Again, suppose upon a View the Mile Index stands between the 1st and 2d Divisions, the Chain Index between the 40th and 41st Divisions, and the Link Index at its 64th Division; the Distance gone over by the Wheel is one Mile, 40 Chains, and 64 Links.

Thus you may measure any Distance without Trouble or Disturbance to the Mind, and may measure the Length of a whole Day's Run, letting the Indices revolve, and need not have the Trouble of regulating them at every new Station, though I account it very safe to regulate the Indices at every Station, neither does it take up much Time.

SECT.

SECT III.

The Description and Use of the common or plain THEODOLITE.

THIS Instrument consisteth of a Brass Plate, of 13 or 14 Inches Diameter, but may be made greater or less at Pleasure. The Limb is divided into 360 Degrees, each of these Degrees is subdivided by other smaller Divisions, which, by the Help of Diagonals projected between the outermost and innermost concentric Circles drawn upon the Plate, Angles may be taken in Degrees and Minutes. There are two plain Sights fixed perpendicular to the Plate; and some Theodolites have a Box and Needle fixed to the Plate, and some to the Index; so there can but be said to be two Sorts of plain Theodolites, viz. one whose Box is fixed to the Plate, and the other having its Box fixed to the Index.

There are likewise two plain Sights fixed to the Index. On the under Side of the Plate is a Brass Ball, made and fitted to a Socket upon the Top of a three-legg'd Staff, by Means of which and a Spirit Level, the Instrument is to be reduced to an horizontal Position.

All plain Theodolites that are most useful, have either the Box fixed to the Index, and the Numbers on the Plate contrary to those in the Box (the Eye being conceived in the Center,) or the Box fixed to the Plate, and the Numbers in the Box increase the same Way

Way with those on the Plate (the Eye being supposed in the Center,) then a Protractor whose Numbers increase the same Way with those on the Plate, will be fit to lay down both the Angles and Bearings.

If you have a Theodolite whose Box is fixed to the Index, and the Numbers on the Plate contrary to those in the Box, then the fixed Sights must always be directed back to the last Station, and the Index to the next, but if it be a Theodolite with its Box fixed to the Plate and the Numbers in the Box increase the same Way with those on the Plate, then the fixed Sights must always be directed to the next Station and the Index to the last.

Also further observe, that if the Beginning of the Degrees are kept towards you when the fixed Sights are directed, and the Flower-de-luce towards you when the Index is directed, then the End of the Index next you, will note on the Limb the Angle, and the South End of the Needle in the Box, will point out the Bearing.

The further Uses of this Instrument shall be hereafter shewn, in practical Surveying.

SECT. IV.

The Description and Use of the new improved (or best) THEODOLITE.

THIS is the most complete, commodious, and universally useful Instrument now in being, for sur-

surveying and plotting of Ground, seeing by it all Sorts of Ground in whatever Situation the same shall be, and though it be ever so hilly or uneven, may be truly and accurately delineated or plann'd

This Instrument hath a vertical Arch of the same Radius with the Limb, and fixed perpendicular to it; being accurately divided into 180 Degrees, by two Nineties, from the Vertex downwards either Way.

On this Arch is mounted a Telescope, with a Spirit Level fixed thereto at right Angles, to which is another Spirit Level in the Box; by Means of which perpendicular Levels, and four Screws playing between two Brass Plates on the Head of the Staff, the Instrument is readily brought to an horizontal Level, that is, the Plate of the Instrument lies parallel to the Plane of the Horizon.

There is an Index belonging to the vertical Arch, which by Help of Tooth and Pinion, is accurately moved round the same, and carries the Telescope along with it, so that the Elevation or Depression of any Object above or below the Horizon is readily known. This Index has a Vernier or Nonius to three Minutes, so that Angles of Elevation or Depression may be taken to three Minutes of a Degree.

Within the Degrees on the vertical Arch, are two Lines numbered downwards with 10, 20, 30, &c. to 100, and are cut by the Edge of the Index, these shew the Altitude or Depression of any Object, in the 100th Parts of the Distance the Instrument is placed at in Time of Observation, on the Right-hand Side is engraved Elevation, and on the Left Depression. By

these

these we estimate the Height of any standing Tree, &c. Below these are other Divisions cut by the lower Edge of the Index, and shew the Difference between the Hypothenuse and Base of a right Angle Triangle, always supposing the Hypothenuse to consist of 100 equal Parts; and consequently is given by Inspection, the Number of Links to be deducted from each Chain's Length, in measuring up or down any Ascent or Descent, in order to reduce it to a true horizontal Distance.

Upon the Telescope are fixed two plain Sights, which may be used in short Distances, they are also useful in continuing the same straight Line both Ways from any Station.

The Plate of the Instrument is accurately divided into 360 Degrees, and cut by three Indices with *Nonius*'s Divisions on each and distant from each other 120°, therefore whatever Division on the Limb, is cut by the Index under the Eye glass of the Telescope, the very same will always be found to be cut by the other two.

There is in some Theodolites another small Index, which is made to cut other particular Divisions on the Limb, useful in taking of Breadths, when the perspective View of any House or Building is to be taken.

The whole Index with the Box fixed thereon, turns round on a conical Center, by Means of Tooth and Pinion without stirring the Needle, there is also a Spring and Screw adapted to the Index, by which it may be readily fixed to any Part of the Limb, and will thereby be so secured, that there is not the least

Danger

Danger of its being joſtled out of its Place, while the Inſtrument is carrying to another Station. The further Uſes of this Inſtrument will be ſhewn hereafter.

SECT. V.

The Deſcription and Uſe of the PLAIN TABLE.

THE Plain Table is an Inſtrument made of Mahogany or very good Oak, being well dried and ſeaſoned, it is in Form, a Parallelogram about 15 Inches long, and 12 Inches broad; but may be made greater or leſs, keeping nearly the ſame Proportion

It has a Box-wood Frame fitted to it, which may be taken off and put on at Pleaſure, and by Means of Joints may be folded up and put in the Pocket, for Convenience of Carriage.

The Frame ſerves to hold on the Paper, when the Table is covered therewith, keeping down the Edges ſo tight and cloſe, that Schemes or Draughts may be drawn thereon.

On each Side of this Frame are Scales of Inches, each divided into 10 equal Parts, and properly numbred, whoſe Uſes are for the ready and quick drawing of parallel Lines upon the Paper, and for ſhifting the Paper when Occaſion requires it

One Side or Edge of this Frame is divided into 360 Degrees, from a Braſs Center in the Middle of the
Table

Table, and when put upwards, refembles the Limb of a Theodolite. The other Side or Edge is divided into 180°, each Degree being fubdivided into fmaller Divifions (like thofe on the other Side the Frame) according to the Magnitude of the Inftrument, and fupplies the Place of an Inftrument called a Semi-circle, the Center of this, is a fmall Hole exactly in the Middle between the two Ends of the Table, and about a fourth Part of the Breadth from one of its Sides or Edges.

There is a Box and Needle annexed to the Side of the Table, whofe Ufes are to take the Bearings from the Meridian, when it is ufed as a Theodolite, and to find a Meridian Line, when it is ufed as a Plain Table.

There is a Brafs Index belonging this Inftrument, whofe Length fomewhat exceeds the Diagonal of the Table, floped away on one of its Sides like a *Gunter*'s Scale, which is commonly called the Fiducial Edge. It has two Sights (one at each End) which ftand perpendicular to it, being both of the fame Height, and fo placed, that the vertical Hair fhall be parallel to, or in the fame Line with the Fiducial Edge. On the upper Side of the Index are Scales of equal Parts, Diagonal Scales, and a Scale of Chords.

This Inftrument moves upon a three-legg'd Staff, by Means of a Ball and Socket, by which it may be placed in any Pofition without removing the Legs. Its further Ufes will be fhewn hereafter, when we come to treat of Surveying by the Plain Table.

SECT.

SECT VI.

The Description and Use of PROTRACTORS.

THERE are several Sorts of Protractors used by Surveyors in laying down the Angles of a Survey, as

1. The Semi-circular Protractor, which is, according as its Name imports, a Semi circular Plate of Brass, of 6 or 8 Inches diameter (that being a suitable Size for protracting a Survey by,) whose Limb is divided into 180 Degrees, and numbered both Ways with 10, 20, 30, &c to 180, each of these Degrees is halved, or divided in two. In the Middle of its Diameter is a small Mark, which is the Center of the Protractor, and must always be laid to the Angle Point

2. The Circular Protractor is much more useful than the semi-circular One, in protracting of Angles. Its outside Edge or Limb is divided into 360 Degrees, like the Limb of a Theodolite, and numbered with 10, 20, 30, &c to 360, each Degree is subdivided into Halves, if the Size of the Instrument will admit of it. In the Middle of its Diameter is a small Mark, which must be laid to the Angle Point, when an Angle is to be protracted, and the Diameter (representing a Meridian) must be laid upon the Meridian Line of any Plan, when the Bearing of any Object is to be laid down.

All the Parts of this Instrument being so plain, and

Sect. IV.   *The* Instruments *described.*

its Application so simple and easy, 'tis needless to say more thereof.

3. The Round Protractor with open Center and a *Nonius*, is the best and most useful of all Protractors; it hath its Limb circular, and accurately divided into 360 Degrees, and made to number each Way, with 10, 20, 30, &c. to 360. It has an Index with a *Nonius* thereto to three Minutes of a Degree, which moves round the Limb of the Protractor upon an open conical Center; that Part of the Index beyond the Limb, has a Steel Point fixed at the End, whose Use is to prick off Angles, being in a direct Line with the Center of the Protractor and the Beginning of the Divisions of the *Nonius*. One of these Protractors I had from Mr *Ben. Cole*, Mathematical Instrument Maker, at the Orrery, No. 136, in *Fleet-street, London*; but perceiving that there might be some Improvement made therein, I returned the Instrument, and ordered him to open that Part of the Index beyond the Limb, and to make a fiducial Edge, exactly to answer the Center of the Protractor and the Steel protracting Point, which he performed very accurately. The Reason assigned for this Alteration is, that whereas it frequently happens in protracting of several Bearings from one Center, that there will be some Points falling so near each other upon the Paper, that it is difficult to distinguish which is which, when the Bearings are all prick'd down by the Steel Point above described, therefore to prevent Confusion, I would advise in such like Cases to point off the Bearings by the fiducial Edge of the In-

dex, which will give Room, and make it much less liable to commit an Error in protracting.

SECT. VII.

The Description and Use of SCALES.

IN Cases of drawing Instruments, commonly called portable Pocket Cases, besides Compasses, Drawing-pens, Dotting-wheel, &c Crayon (whose Uses are known at the first Glance) are a Semi-circular Protractor as before described, a Scale, and Sector; the two latter, together with a Feather-edged Scale used by Surveyors, shall be described in this and the next Section Also some very good Cases have in them a Parallel Ruler, which is an Instrument particularly requisite in practical Surveying.

The Scales commonly put in Cases of Instruments, have besides Scales of equal Parts of several Sizes, two Diagonal Scales; the Diagonal Scales, together with a Line of Inches, commonly possess one Side of the Scale. On the other Side are a Scale of Chords, Rhumbs, Sines, Tangents and Secants, all constructed from the same Radius of a Circle. Some of these Scales have only Scales of equal Parts, Diagonal Scales, and a Scale of Chords. The Lines of Chords, Rhumbs, Sines, Tangents

Sect. VII. *The* Instruments *described.*

Tangents and Secants are ufed in laying down Angles or Bearings from the Meridian, the Lines of equal Parts ferve to fet off Diftances.

But the Scale ufed by Surveyors (commonly called a Feather-edged Scale) is made of Brafs, Ivory or Wood, in Length about 10 or 12 Inches; but may be made longer or fhorter at Pleafure. It is decimally divided the whole Length, clofe by its Edges which are cut floping, to make it lie clofe to the Paper, and numbered 0, 1, 2, 3, 4, &c which are called Chains, and every one of the intermediate Divifions is 10 Links; the Numbers are fo placed, as to reckon backwards and forwards, and the Beginning of the Divifion is about 2 or 3 of the grand Divifions off the fore End of the Scale, thefe are numbered backwards from 0 towards the left Hand, with the Numbers or Figures 1, 2, 3, &c. The Application and Ufe of this Scale is both eafy and expeditious, for having any Number of Chains, &c. to lay down upon a given Line, apply 0 (or the Beginning of the Divifions) to the Beginning of the Line, and keeping its Edge clofe to the Line, with your protracting Pin, point off clofe by its Edge the given Diftance in Chains, or Chains and Links.

SECT. VIII.

The Description and Use of the SECTOR.

THE Sector is an Instrument of such extraordinary Use in the several Branches of the Mathematics, that to pass it over in Silence, without a Word or two in its Behalf, would be an Injury done to its Character

This Instrument has its Original from the 4. Euc. 6. *viz* that Equiangular Triangles are similar.

It consisteth of two Parts moving on a Joint like a Carpenter's Rule, and is made of Silver, Brass, Ivory, or Wood, being in Length 6, 9, or 12 Inches. The Lines used Sector-wise upon the Face of this Instrument, are the Line of Lines, or Line of equal Parts and is numbered 1, 2, 3, &c. to 10, and marked with *LL* the 1 may stand for 100, and if so, the 2 will be 200, the 3 will be 300, the 4 will be 400, &c. but if the 1 stand for 1000, the 2 will be 2000, the 3 will be 3000, &c. or if the 1 be 1 Tenth, the 2 will be 2 Tenths, the 3 will be 3 Tenths, &c Next to this Line is a Line of Chords flowing from the Center, and numbered with 10, 20, 30, &c. to 60, where is placed a Brass Point The Chord of 60° being

Sect. VIII.   *The* INSTRUMENTS *described.*   299

ing the Radius of every Circle, is equal to a Sine of 90°, or a Tangent of 45°, and is marked *C h o.*

On the other Face of the Sector is a Line of natural Sines issuing from the Center, numbered 10, 20, 30, &c. to 90, and marked at the End with *SS.* Next to this are two Lines of natural Tangents flowing from the Center, the one is numbered 10, 20, 30, &c to 45, and marked *TT* at the End between this and the Line of Sines, is a Line of lesser Tangents, issuing from two Brass Centers, which begin to number at 45, and so increases to 50, 60, and 75, where it is marked *tt*, and supplies the Place of the greater Tangents, when the Angle is above 45°.

On the same Face of the Sector with the Line of Chords, is the Line of natural Secants, flowing from two Brass Centers, between the Chords and the Line of Lines, and numbered 20, 30, 40, 50, 60, and 75, and marked with *ss* These Chords, Sines, Tangents, and Secants are all projected from the same Radius of a Circle There are several other Lines placed upon the Sector, which not being useful in Surveying, shall be passed over in Silence.

The Line of Lines is useful in reducing of Plans according to any Proportion, and hence any Plan may be enlarged or diminished at Pleasure. It also serveth to divide a Line into any proposed Number of equal Parts; to find the Proportion between two or more given Lines, two Lines being given to find a third in Proportion to them, to find a mean Proportion between any two given Lines, and lastly, to divide a Line in such Manner as any other given Line is divided.

The

The Lines of Chords, Sines, Tangents, and Secants are useful in laying down plain Angles, and also in projecting the Circles of the Sphere, as hath been heretofore shewn.

SECT. IX.

The Description and Use of the PARALLEL RULER.

THE Parallel Ruler is made of Brass, Ivory, or Wood, in Length from 4½ Inches to 36. It consisteth of two Rulers connected together by two metal Bars, which move round the Rivets that fasten their Ends; these Bars are placed in such a Manner, as to have the same Inclination to each Ruler, so will they be parallel to each other at every Distance, as also will the Rulers to whatever Extent they open.

But those Parallel Rulers are the best, whose Bars cross each other, and move on a Joint at their Intersection. One End of each Bar moves on a Center, and the other End slides on Grooves as the Rulers receed.

This Instrument is useful in resolving several geometrical Problems, as also in delineating the Lines of a Survey.

BOOK

BOOK VIII.

Surveying and Plotting of Ground, by the CHAIN *Plain Table, and* Theodolite.

Surveying of Land, is the Method of computing the true Content or Area of any Parcel of Ground: It also layeth down Rules and Precepts, for planning, or representing in Miniature, any Part or Portion of the terraqueous Globe.

SECT. I.

Surveying and plotting of Ground by the Chain.

Prop. I.

To find the Area of any Inclosure ABCDEFG, *whose Hedges are straight.* (Fig. 1)

Rule.

Set up Marks or Station-staves at every Corner of the Field, then the Field being divided into Triangles or Trapeziums, or both, begin at A, and measure the Base AC, as also the Perpendicular Ba: in like Manner measure the Diagonal AD, and two Perpendiculars Gb, Cc. Thus measure all the remaining Bases, Diagonals, and Perpendiculars, that is, take their Dimensions as above directed. Then find the Area of each Triangle, by Prob. 27. B. II. and of each Trapezium, by Prob. 28.

Note,

302   SURVEYING *by the* CHAIN.   Book VIII.

Note, To let fall Perpendiculars in the Field, use an Instrument called a Cross.

A Specimen of the Field-book belonging Surveys of this Kind, is as follows; in which, the first Column on the left Hand contains the Perpendiculars on the Left of the Bases or Diagonals, the second Column contains the Bases or Diagonals; the third the Perpendiculars on the Right of the Bases or Diagonals; the fourth the Multipliers, and the fifth the double Areas.

The FIELD BOOK.

Perpendiculars	Diagonals or Bases	Perpendiculars	Multipliers	Double Areas
B 102	1 (A) 0 405 790		790 × 102	80580
C 250	2 (A) 0 160 732 870	378 G	378 + 250 × 870	546360
F 220	3 (D) 0 250 820	.	820 × 220	180400
	4 (C) 0 290 615 close here	170 F	615 × 170	104550 911890 = double Area.

This 911890 being reduced by the latter Part of Rule 2, in Prob. 22, B. II. is = 4 *A.* 2 *r.* 9·5120 *p.* = Area of the given Field.   FIG. 1.   PROP.

Prop II.

To find the Number of Acres, &c. in any Inclosure ABCDEF, *whose Hedges contain several Bendings or Curves.* Fig 2.

Rule

Place a Station-staff a little distant from the several Corners A, B, C, &c of the Field. Then find the Area of the Part contained between the traverse Lines and the Hedges, by Prop 44 B II. also find by the last Prop. the Area of the Part contained within the traverse Lines, these two Areas added together, will give the Area of the whole Field. But you must observe, that at every Corner you have a small Square or Parallelogram, whose Area may be easily obtained, by multiplying the last and first Offsets together, all round the Field, as for Example, at the Corner B is a little Parallelogram, whose Breadth may be said to be $= 25$ $=$ Offset at 445 in ☉ 1, and its Length $30 =$ Offset at 0 in ☉ 2, these Dimensions insert in your Field Book, according to the Form hereafter prescribed, whose double Area being found, and added to the Rest, will give the double Area of the Whole.

Note, The Offsets are most commodiously measured with the Offset-staff before described, in the Description and Use of the Chain.

The FIELD BOOK.

	☉ L	☉ L	☉ R	M.	D A
		☉ 1 in	Riggs		
		0	30	60 × 25	1500
Corner {30 {25		275	42	275 × 72	19800
		415	25	170 × 67	11390
		☉ 2 in	Ditto		32690
		0	30	40 × 20	800
Cor. {20 {20		275	50	275 × 80	22000
		442	20	167 × 70	11690
		☉ 3 in	Ditto		67180
		0	20	64 × 28	1792
		20	35	20 × 55	1100
Cor {32 {28		180	30	160 × 65	10400
		362	32	182 × 62	11284
		☉ 4 in	Ditto		91756
		0	28		12600
		200	35	200 × 63	14300
		420	30	220 × 65	
		☉ 5 in	Ditto		118656
		0	30	90 × 30	2700
		155	60	155 × 90	13950
Cor {30 {45		300	30	145 × 90	13050
		☉ 6 in	Ditto		
		0	45	60 × 38	2280
Cor {38 {30		435	40	435 × 85	36975
		550	38	115 × 78	8970
		1o ☉ 1		carried over	196581

Sect. I. SURVEYING *by the* CHAIN. 305

The FIELD BOOK

	O L	⊙ L.	⊙ R	M	D A
To ⊙ 5	Ret. to 410	⊙ 2 in o 420 676 746 To ⊙ 4	Ditto 148 to ⊙ 3 746 × 558		brought over 196581 416268
To ⊙ 1	Ret to 320	⊙ 2 in o 318 740 755 To ⊙ 6	Ditto 755 × 614 To ⊙ 5 294		612849 463570 1076419 = 5 ac¹ 11 21 1352 p = the area

Note, On the Tops of the Columns in the Field Book, ⊙ L fignifieth Station-lines, O R — Offsets Right; O. L — Offsets Left, M — Multipliers, D. A — Double Areas. FIG. 2.

PROP. III.

To take the Quantity of any Angle BAC. FIG. 3, 4, 5.

RULE

Let *A, B, C* denote three Stations in a Field Hold one End of the Chain at *A,* and direct your Affiftant to place the other End at *D* and *E* fucceffively, where he muft ftick two very ftraight Staves, fo as to be in a direct Line with the Station-ftaves *A, B,* and *C,* meafure the Diftance between the Sticks *D, E,* which will be the Quantity of the Angle. But

R r 2

if the Angle be greater than a Sextant (or 60 Degrees,) take it at two, three, or more Times, as you find it most convenient. If the Angle exceed a Semi-circle, annex the Mark ⌐, to the Quantity found as above, but if it be less than a Semi-circle, prefix the Mark ∠ When the Angle to be taken is greater than a Semi-circle, it is best to take its Supplement, and prefix the Mark ∠ as above.

The Method of expressing the Quantity of an Angle, is thus,

Radius 100 } = The Measure of the Angle BAC
∠ Chord 80 } Fig. 3.

Radius 100 } = The Measure of the Angle
∠ Chord { 90 } BAC. Fig. 4
       { 75 }

Radius 100 }
       { 70 } = The Measure of the Angle
⌐ Chords { 85 } BAC. Fig. 5
       { 100 }

Prop IV.

To protract or lay down any Angle BAC, *having the Radius* AD, *and the Chords* DE, EF, *and* FG *given.* Fig 5

Rule

Draw *AB* at Pleasure. With the Radius *AD*, and one Foot of the Compasses on the Angle Point *A*, describe the Arch *DEG*, set the Chords *DE*, *EF*, and *FG* severally upon the Arch, from *D* to *E*, from
E

Sect I. SURVEYING *by the* CHAIN.   307

E to *F*, and from *F* to *G*. Through *G* draw a Line *AC*, so will *BAC* be the Angle required.

PROP. V.

To take the Plot of a Field ABCDEFG.

Take the Angles at the several Stations, by Prop 3, and measure the Distances and Offsets by Prop 2, which enter in a Field Book, according to the Form hereafter following

The FIELD BOOK

REMARKS	O	⊙ I	O	REMARKS
		⊙ 1 In	Hodge	Close
	R	00		
	C	00		
		0	28	
		160	30	
		240	20	
		375	30	
		⊙ 2 in	Ditto	
	R	100		
		70		
⟩	C	90		
		85		
		45		
		0		
		376	40	

The

308   SURVEYING *by the* CHAIN.   Book VIII.

The FIELD BOOK.

REMARKS	O	OL	O	REMARKS
		☉ 3 in	Ditto	
	R	100		
∠	C {	70		
		55		
		0	35	
		230	36	
		410	36	
		430		
		☉ 4 in	Ditto	
	R	100		
		80		
∠	C {	100		
		95		
		0		
		210	40	
		376	41	
		☉ 5 in	Ditto	
	R	100		
∠	C {	72		
		65		
		0	35	
		325	30	
		640	31	
		☉ 6 in	Ditto	
	R	100		
		80		
∠	C {	80		
		0	40	
		215	40	
		343	38	

The

Sect. I.   Surveying *by the* Chain.   309

The FIELD BOOK.

REMARKS	O	☉ L	O	REMARKS
		☉ 7 in	Ditto.	
	R	100		
⌐	6	95		
		100		
		88		
		0		Fig 6
		46	30	
		440	36	
		Close Hodge	Close at ☉ 1.	

To lay down the Plan

Draw a Line 1, 2, upon which set off the Distances 160, 240, and 375, as taken from the Field Book. At ☉ (or the Station set off an Offset = in Length to 28, at 160 lay down an Offset of 20, and because the Offsets stand in the right Hand Column of your Field Book, set them off on the right Hand Side of the traverse Line 1 2, at 375 prick down an Offset of 30 to the Right, for the Reason just now given. Through these Points draw a Line *AB*, for one Side or Hedge of the Field. At ☉ 2 lay down the Angle by Prop 3, and set off the Distances and Offsets as before, thus proceed at every Station, and you will have a true Plan.

Note, In laying down the Angles, I would recommend the Use of a larger Scale, than the other Part of the Work is perform'd by.

SECT.

SECT. II.

Surveying and Plotting of the GROUND *by the* PLAIN TABLE.

PROB. VI.

To take the Plot of a Field ABCDE, *from one Station* ⊙ *at or near the Middle thereof* FIG 7.

RULE FIG. 8.

LET *RSTV* represent the Plain Table covered with a Sheet of Paper, on which the Plan of the Field is to be drawn. Set up and level your Instrument at O. (7) and move the Table about, 'till the South Point of the Needle hang over the Flower-de-luce (or 360) in the Box. Fasten the Table in this Position, and draw a Line *Pp* (8) parallel to one of its Sides *SV* or *RT*, for a Meridian Line to the Plan. Then chuse some Point O upon the Paper, which must denote the Station ⊙, (7) where the Instrument is standing in the Field, upon ⊙ (8) as a Center, move the fiducial Edge of the Index, 'till through the Sights you observe the Marks or Corners *A*, *B*, *C*, *D*, *E*, (7) and close by its Edge draw the Lines ⊙ *A*, ⊙ *B*,

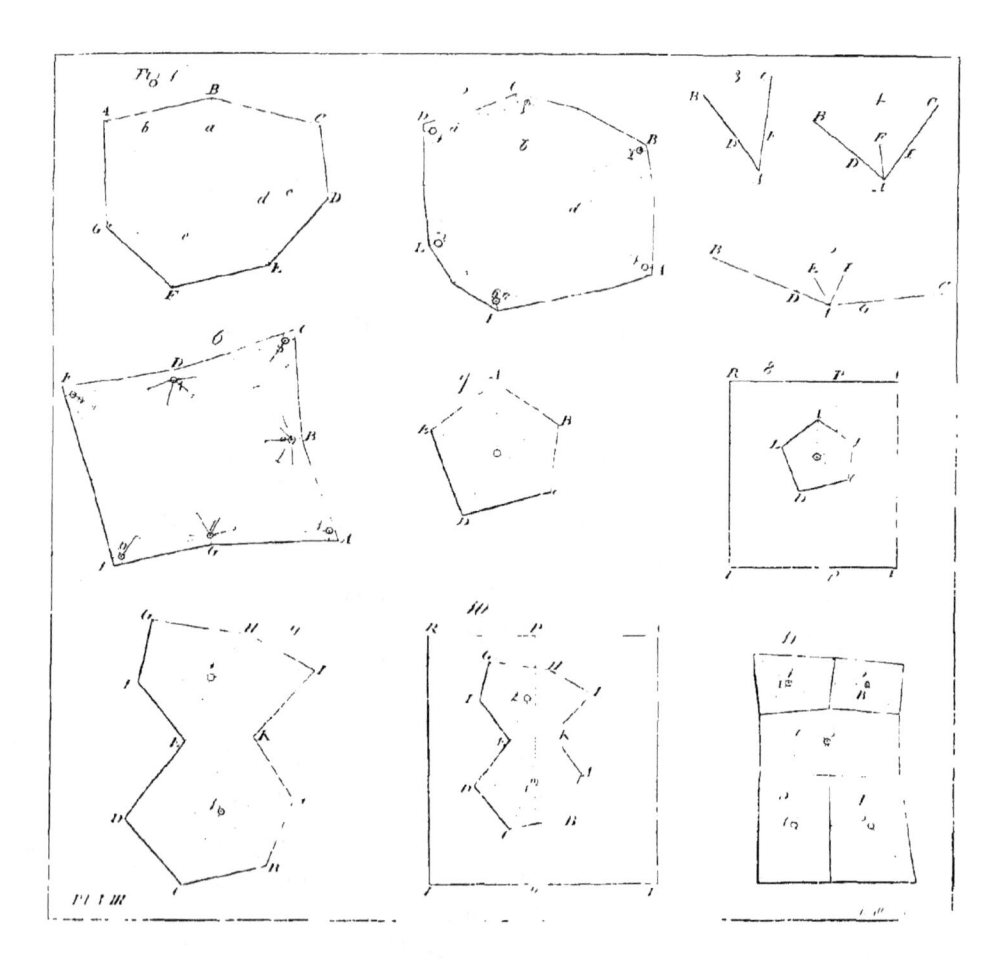

Sect. II. Surveying *by the* Plain Table. 311

⊙ *B*, ⊙ *C*, ⊙ *D*, ⊙ *E* (8) of any sufficient Length. Then measure the Distances from the Instrument at O, (7) to the several Marks, *A*, *B*, *C*, *D*, *E*, which set upon the Lines ⊙ *A*, ⊙ *B*, ⊙ *C*, ⊙ *D*, ⊙ *E*, (8) from ⊙ to *A*, *B*, *C*, *D*, *E*. Lastly, join these Points by drawing the Lines *AB*, *BC*, *CD*, *DE*, *EA*, which will compleat the Plan *ABCDE*, every Way proportional and similar to the given Field. Fig. 7, 8.

Prop VII.

To take the Plot of a Field GIBD, *from several Stations taken therein.* Fig 9, 10.

Rule.

Set up your Plain Table at ⊙ 1, (9) and project the Part *ABCD*, together with ⊙ 2, by Prop. 6. Then remove your Instrument to ⊙ 2, lay the Fiducial Edge of the Index along the Line 1 2 (10) and turn the Table this Way or that Way, 'till the vertical Hair cleave the Object at ⊙ 2, fasten the Instrument in that Direction, and on ⊙ 2 (10) as a Center, move the Index, and project as before, the remaining Part of the Field *HIKEFG*, (9).

Prop. VIII.

To take the Plot of several Fields lying together, from Stations taken therein. Fig. 11, 12.

Rule

Level your Plain Table at ⊙ 1, (11) and take the

S s   Plot

312 SURVEYING *by the* PLAIN TABLE. Book VIII.

Plot of the Field *A,* by Prop 6. Then take the Plot of the other Fields *B, C, D, E,* by Prop. 7, so will *A, B, C, D, E* (12) be the Plans of the Fields *A, B, C, D, E* (11)

PROP IX

To take the Plot of a large Field or Pasture ABCD. FIG 13

RULE.

Divide the Field or Pasture into the Parts *E, F, G, H, I, K, L, M,* these considered as so many different Fields, may be plotted as such by the last Prop

PROP. X.

To take the Plot of a Field ABCDEF, *by going round the same* FIG 14, 15

RULE

Set up Marks a little distant from the Hedges, which must be called Stations Then beginning the Survey at ⊙ 1, (14) adjust the Instrument, and draw the Meridian *Pp,* (15) by Prop 6 Chuse any Point ⊙ 1 for your first Station, and draw the traverse Line 1 2 Remove your Instrument to ⊙ 2 (14) in the Field, and lay down the Distances and Offsets as measured between the first and second Stations, and draw the Hedge *AB* (15). Then lay the Fiducial Edge of the Index on the Line 1 2, and turning the Table about, turn back the Sights to ⊙ 1, (14) and fasten

Sect II. SURVEYING *by the* PLAIN TABLE

ten it by Means of a Screw which plays in the Socket; then moving the Edge of the Index on ⊙ 2, (15) direct the Sights to ⊙ 3 (14) in the Field and draw the Line 2 3 (15) upon the Paper. Measure the Distances and Offsets between the second and third Stations in the Field, which being laid down upon the Line 2 3, (15) the Hedge *BC* may be drawn. Thus proceed at every Station in the Field, by which a true Plan will be obtained.

You must have a Field Book, in which to insert in a fair, regular, and formal Method, the several Distances and Offsets, with other remarkable Occurences which may happen during the Course of the Survey. A Specimen of which you have as follows.

Note, when the Instrument was standing at ⊙ 6, (14) and the Index directed forward to ⊙ 1 (where you begun the Survey) the Edge thereof would fall or lie upon ⊙ 1 (15) on the Paper, at the same Distance as measured in the Field, if the Work was right.

The FIELD BOOK.

REMARKS	0	⊙ L	0	REMARKS
		⊙ 1		In *ABCDEF*
		0	18	
		180	30	
		345	20	Corner
		⊙ 2		In Ditto
		0		
		170	28	
		330	15	

The FIELD BOOK.

REMARKS	O	L	O	REMARKS
	☉ 3			In Ditto
	0	20		
	250	10		
	520	22		
	☉ 4			In Ditto
	0	25		
	220	28		
	455	28		Corner
	☉ 5			In Ditto
	0	25		
	282	6		
	440	20		Corner
	☉ 6			In Ditto
	0	18		
	310	29		Corner. Clofe here
to	☉ 1			

Prop XI.

To take the Plot of feveral Fields A, B, C, D, E, F, *by Circulation* Fig. 16, 17.

Rule.

Take the Plot of the Field *A*, by Prop 10, then return to ☉ 2, (17) where fet up your Plain Table, lay the Fiducial Edge of the Index on the Station-line 1 2, (16) and take a Back-fight to ☉ 1, (17) that being the Station immediately preceding that you are at, (as I always make it cuftomary at my Return to any Station, to take a Back-fight to the next preceding Station)

Pl. IX

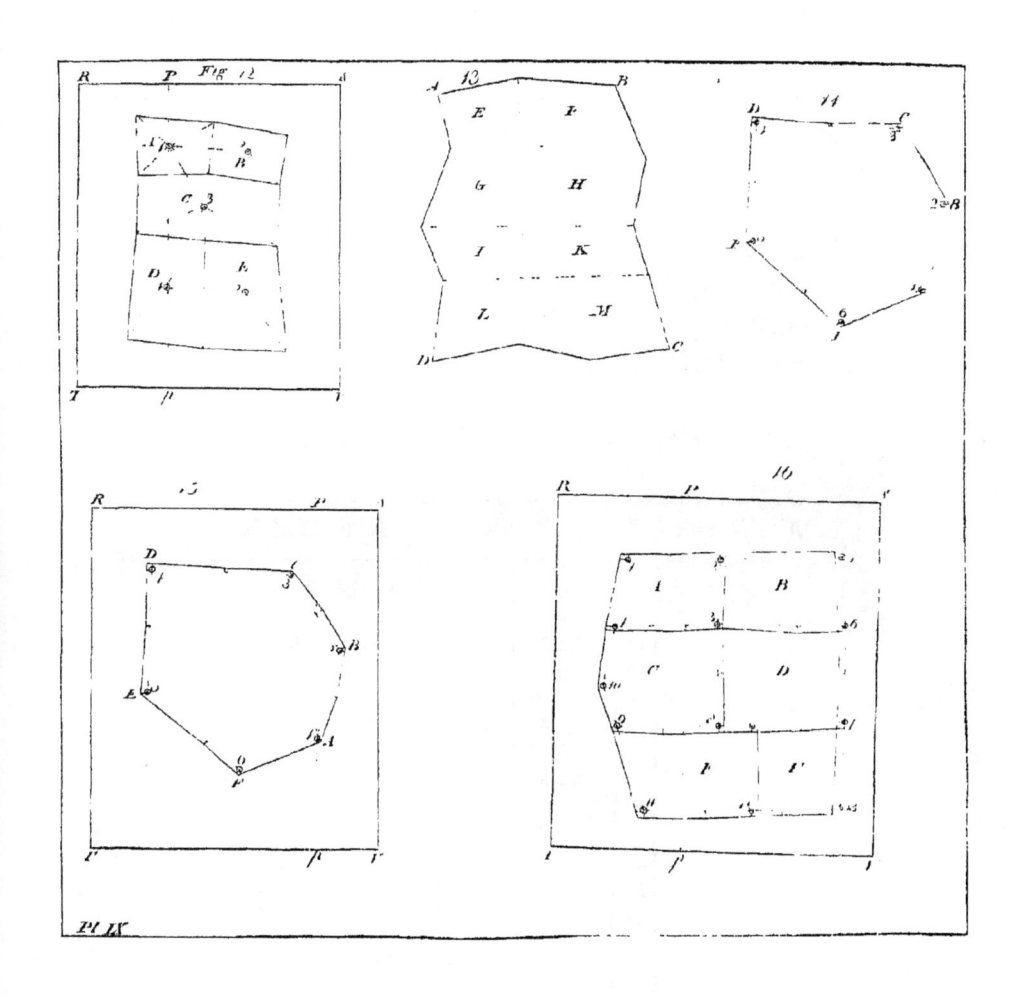

Sect II.   Surveying *by the* Plain Table.   315

tion) then the Table being secured in that Position, on ☉ 2 (16) as a Center, direct the Sights to ☉ 5, (17) and draw the traverse Line 2 5 (16) which make = Distance measured on the Ground. Thus proceed at ☉ 6, (17) which make = Distance measured on the Ground. Thus proceed at ☉ 6, (17) and if when the Index is directed to the closing ☉ 3, (17) its Edge just touch ☉ 3 (16) on the Table, your Work closes, and you are sure of being so far Right. The Distances and Offsets are to be measured and delineated, as in the foregoing Field *A*, after which take the Plot of the remaining Fields *C, D, E, F*, in the very same Manner as before. See the Field Book.

The FIELD BOOK.

REMARKS	☉	☉ L	☉	REMARKS
		☉ 1		In Field *A*
	20	0		
	10	140		
	18	290		
		☉ 2		In Ditto.
	18	0		
	20	220		
		☉ 3		In Ditto
	20	0		
	25	150		
	16	330		
		☉ 4		In Field *A*.
	28	0		
	24	220		To ☉ 1. Close here Field *A*

The

The FIELD BOOK.

REMARKS	⊙	L		REMARKS
Return to	⊙ 2			In Field *A*
	0			
Corner 20	20			
				Cross the Hedge into Field *B*
28	205			
Corner 16	380			
				Cross the Hedge into the open Field.
	400			
	⊙ 5			In the open Field.
	0	20		
	230	20		
	⊙ 6			In the open Field
	0			
Corner 20	20			
				Into Field *B*.
25	155			
15	315			
Close here 20	395			Cross the Hedge into Field *A*
	414			To ⊙ 3.
Return to	⊙ 6			In the open Field
	0			
	20	20		
	160	20		
	320	25		
	⊙ 7			In Ditto
	0			
12	25			
25	140			
25	280			
	300			By ⊙ for closing *E*.
Corner 20	390			Cross the Hedge into *D*
	414			

The

Sect II. Surveying *by the* Plain Table.   317

The FIELD BOOK.

REMARKS.	⊙	⊙L	⊙	REMARKS
		⊙ 8		In Field *D*
		0	24	
		180	20	
		328	20	Here *F* clofes
				Into Field *A*.
		345		To ⊙ 3 in *A*
Return to		⊙ 8		In Field *D*
	23	0		
	30	170		
	16	320		
		⊙ 9		In Ditto.
	20	0		
Corner	16	142		
		⊙ 10		In Ditto.
		0		
Here Field *D*	20	185		
clofes		200		To ⊙ 4
Return to		⊙ 9		In Field *D*.
		0		
		15	20	
				Into Field *E*.
		300	20	
		⊙ 11		In Field *E*.
		0	15	
		195	30	
		350	20	
		⊙ 12		In Ditto.
		0	20	
		265	16	Clofe here Field *E*
				Into Field *G*
		285		To bye ⊙ it 300 in Line 7, 8.

The

The FIELD BOOK.

REMARKS	O	C.L.	O	REMARKS
Return to		⊙ 12		In E
		0		
		25	15	
				Crofs the Hedge into F
		100	18	
		265	20	Corner
				into the open Field.
		290		
		⊙ 13		In the open Field.
	25	0		
	20	270		
Clofe F on Corner of L		290		To ⊙ 7 in the open Field

Of shifting the Papers.

In the Practice of Surveying it almost frequently happeneth, that the Whole of the Survey cannot be contained within the Compafs of one Sheet of Paper; when this is the Cafe, there is no other Remedy but taking off one Sheet, and putting on another, which is performed after the Method now to be explained in the following Example.

EXAMPLE.

Let *AFGL* be a Field to be plotted, the Plan of which cannot be contained on one Sheet of Paper. F. 18.

To illuftrate this, we will fuppofe *AB, BC, CE, EF, FG, GI, IK, KL, LA* to be all traverfe Lines. Then begin at the Station *A*, and by Prop. 10, work forwards to *B* and *C*, but in going further towards *E*, you

Sect. II.   Surveying *by the* Plain Table.   319

you find the traverse Line goes off the Table at *D*, where make a particular Mark. Then return to the Station *A* again, and work about the the contrary Way to *L*, *K*, and *I*, but in laying down the the next Distance *IG*, the Line is found to go off the Table as at *H*, where make a Mark as before upon the Paper, and also be sure to leave another in the Ground, which you must do at the other Place *D*. This done take off your Paper, and put a new Sheet on the Table, on which lay the taken-off Sheet towards the contrary End of the Table, by which you may easily project two Lines *DE*, *HG*, which will be in the same true Direction with *CD* and *IH* before laid down. Then fixing the Instrument at either of the Marks *D*, *H* in the Ground, perform the remaining Part of the Work as you have done in that which went before. Fig. 19.

The Plain Table may be used as a Theodolite or Semi-circle, by making Use of the Graduations on the Frame, and then the Angles are taken in Degrees and Minutes, which afterwards may be laid down upon Paper, by pricking off the Degrees, &c from the Limb of a good Protractor the Method of doing which will be fully shewn in the next Section, where the Use of the Theodolite will be displayed in every Part But indeed the Plain Table is not an Instrument at all fit to use as a Theodolite, for no Accuracy can be expected from it, therefore I would not by any Means recommend its Use, any otherwise than covered with a Sheet of Paper.

But all the Methods of Surveying by the Plain Table hitherto given, are at the best but tedious and
T t   trouble-

troublesome (especially in large Surveys where Numbers of Stations are concern'd, and where there is frequent Occasion for shifting of Papers) except the Surveyor be perfectly expert and skill'd in his Business, and even then he will find it a Difficulty, to close his Traverses so correctly as might be wished, after such piecing and patching of Papers. But a Method of Surveying by this Instrument, shall be hereafter shewn, which is free from all the Inconveniences above-mentioned, as the Trouble of shifting the Papers is entirely removed, and the Angles (though never so many) are all expeditiously taken and protracted at the same Time in the Field, within the Compass of a common Sheet of Paper, though you had Thousands of Acres to survey

SECT III.

Surveying and Plotting of GROUND *by the* THEODOLITE.

PROP XII.

To take the Bearings and Angles of ABCDEF.

RULE. FIG 20.

SET up your Theodolite at *A*, fix the Index to 360 on the Limb, level the Instrument, bring the South End of of the Needle to the Flower-de-luce (or 360) in the Box, and fasten the Limb, this is called adjusting the Instrument. Then moving the
Index

Sect III.　Surveying *by the* Theodolite　321

Index, 'till the vertical Hair cleave the Object *B*, the End thereof which is next you will cut on the Limb the Bearing as also will the South End of the Needle in the Box, if no Mistake has been committed. Remove your Theodolite to *B*, and take a Back-observation to the Object *A*, after which (the Limb being secured) direct the Index to the Mark *C*, and the End thereof which is towards you will give on the Limb the Angle, and the South End of the Needle in the Box will note the Bearing. *Note*, The Back-observation is always taken with the fixed Sights, if the Theodolite hath its Box fixed to the Index, and the Numbers in the Box increase the contrary Way with those in the Plate, otherwise the fixed Sights must be used for the Fore-observation. Then to prove the Truth of the Angle and Bearing, take the two following Rules.

I. To the present Angle add the last Bearing, from that Sum subtract 180°, and the Remainder is the present Bearing.

II. To the present Bearing add 180°, from that Sum deduct the preceding Bearing, the Remainder will be the present Angle.

But if the Number to be subtracted is the greater, add 360° (or a whole Circle) to the lesser, and perform Subtraction as before, and if the Remainder exceed 360°, abate 360° from it, and the Remainder will be the Bearing or Angle.

Having taken the Bearing at *A*, and the Bearing and Angle at *B*, and compared the one by the other, in like Manner must the Angles and Bearings at *C*, *D*,

T t 2　　　　　　　　　　　　　　　*E*,

E, F be found and compared, whose several Quantities are as below.

	BEARINGS		ANGLES	
A	206°	00'	104°	00'
B	173	45	147	45
C	84	30	90	45
D	32	00	127	30
E	347	45	135	45
F	282	00	174	15

To know whether the Plan will close or not : multiply 180 by a Number less by 2 than the Number of the internal Angles, the Product will be equal to the Sum of all the Angles in the Field, if there be outward Angles, use their Complements to 180°. So in the present Figure, the Number of internal Angles is 6, therefore $180 \times 4 (= 6 - 2) = 720 =$ the Sum of all the Angles both internal and the Complements of the external to 180°.

Prop XIII.

To take the Plot of a Field ABCDEF, *from one Station* ⊙, *at or about the Middle thereof.* Fig 21.

Rule.

Adjust your Theodolite at ⊙, by Prop 12, and direct the Index to A, B, C, D, E, F, and it will cut the Limb of the Instrument at the several Bearings Measure the Distance from the Instrument at ⊙, to the Corners A, B, C, D, E, F

Or

Sect. III Surveying *by the* Theodolite.   323

Or thus,

Direct the fixed Sights to *A*, fasten the Limb, and and direct the moveable Sights to the several Corners *B*, *C*, *D*, *E*, *F*, and the Index will cut on the Limb the Angles. The Bearings, Angles, and Distances are as below

	BEARINGS		ANGLES		DISTANCES
	D	M	D	M	L
A	15	30	0	00	345
B	76	45	61	15	450
C	128	00	112	30	468
D	187	30	172	00	320
E	242	00	226	30	440
F	305	00	289	30	420

To protract the Bearings and Angles

Draw the Meridian *NS*, in which assume any Point O for your Station, on which lay the Center of a Protractor, (its Diameter coinciding with *NS*) and prick off close by its Limb the several Bearings, as they stand in the foregoing Table. From O draw the Lines O *A*, O *B*, O *C*, O *D*, O *E*, O *F*, upon which lay the respective Distances in the Field Book, and join the Points *A*, *B*, *C*, &c. compleating the Plan. Or, if O *A* be drawn at Pleasure, you may round the Center O protract the Angles only, by laying the Diameter of the Protractor along the Line O *A*, after which close by its Limb prick off the several Angles, and then proceed as before.

Pror.

Prop XIV.

To take the Plot of a Field ABCDEFGHI, *from several Stations taken therein.* Fig. 22.

Rule.

Adjust the Theodolite at ☉ 1, and take the Bearings and Angles of *A, B,* ☉ 2, *G, H, I,* then remove your Instrument to ☉ 2, fix the Index to the Bearing thereof, and take a Back-observation to ☉ 1, and fasten the Limb, then by Prop. 13 take the Bearings and Angles of *C, D, E, F*. Measure the Distances from each Station to the Corners *A, B, C* &c as also the Distance between the two Stations, whose several Quantities are as expressed in the following Field Book.

Or thus,

After the Bearings and Angles are taken as above, instead of measuring from each Station into the several Corners *A, B, C,* &c you need only measure from ☉ 1 and ☉ 2, to the Corners *A, C,* as also the Distance between ☉ 1 and ☉ 2, after which take the Lengths of the Sides *AB, BC, CD,* &c

Sect III.   Surveying *by the* Theodolite.

The FIELD BOOK

	BEARINGS	ANGLES	DISTANCES
	☉ 1		LINKS
A	8° 20′	0° 00′	280
B	76 50	68 30	275
☉ 2	95 00	86 40	650
G	141 00	152 40	260
H	231 30	223 10	345
I	332 30	324 10	375
	☉ 2		
B			
C	348° 00′	337° 40′	220
D	75 30	67 10	276
E	152 15	143 55	307
F	247 15	238 55	215
G			

To draw the Plan.

Lay down the Part *AEGHI*, by Prop 13, and make the Line 1 2 equal the Diſtance between the Stations in the Field. Through ☉ 2 draw the Meridian *NS*, round which as a Center, lay down the remaining Bearings, by which the Reſt of the Plan *CDEF* may be drawn.

Prop. XV.

To take the Plot of ſeveral Fields, lying contiguous or adjoining one to another, from Stations taken towards the Middle of each Field   Fig. 23.

Rule.

Take the Plot of *A*, by Prop. 13, and the Plot of *B*, by

326 SURVEYING by the THEODOLITE. Book VIII.

by Prop. 14, in like Manner plot the other Fields C D The Bearings and Distances taken in the Field, are inserted in the Field Book, a Specimen of which immediately follows.

The FIELD BOOK.

REMARKS	O B	BEAR	DIS	REMARKS.
		⊙ 1		In *A*
The open	5	350° 15′	220	Field.
	6	62 15	250	B.
	⊙ 2	90 00	425	
	7	120 30	215	C
John Simpson's	8	240 45	225	Ground.
		O 2		In B.
The open	6	— — —		Field
William	9	65° 30′	240	Spencer's Ground
	10	118 55	244	D
B closes	7			it 7.
Return to		O 1		In *A*.
	⊙3	180° 00′	230	
		⊙ 3		In C.
	7			D
	O 4			
South	11	90° 10′	422	
John Wilson's	12	127 00	230	Field
C closes	8	234 15	237	Ground it 8
		O 4		In D
Henry Allison's	10	— — —		Ground,
South	13	126° 45′	260	Field
D closes	11			at

To draw the Plan.

This is wholly performed by Prop. 13 and 14.

PROP.

Sect III. Surveying *by the* Theodolite.

Prob. XVI.

To take the Plot of one or more Fields A, B, *lying together, by measuring round the same, which is the best practical Method.*

Rule.

Set up Marks a little distant from the Hedges, quite round the Fields, which Marks are named Stations. Then Beginning at ⊙ 1 in *A*, take the Bearing there, and also the Angle and Bearing at every Station in that Field, by Prop 12, and measure the Distances and Offsets. Remove your Theodolite to ⊙ 4 in *A*, and take a Back-observation to ○ 3, (that being the Station next preceding that you are at, in your Field Book,) and then direct the moveable Sights to ⊙ 5 in the next Field *B*, so will the Index cut on the Limb the Angle, and the South Point of the Needle in the Box, will give the Bearing. In like Manner proceed, when you take the Angles, Bearings, Distances, and Offsets at the other Stations.

But there is a better and more expeditious Method of working with the Theodolite, which is

Thus;

Set up your Theodolite (suppose one of the best Sort, with Tooth and Pinion to both Motions) at ⊙ 1; fix the Index to o Degr. on the Vertex of the Arch, and bring the Bubbles on the Spirit-Levels to the Middle of their Tubes, so will the horizontal Hair in the Telescope, and the Limb of the Instrument be both perfectly level. Set the Index to 360 on the Limb, and turn the whole Theodolite about 'till the South

Point of the Needle stand directly at the Flower-de-luce (or 360 in the Box,) and fasten the Limb, then direct the Telescope to ☉ 2, and the End of the Index next you, will give on the Limb the Bearing, which also will be noted by the South End of the Needle in the Box. The Index remaining in this Position, erect your Theodolite at ☉ 2, and level the Telescope and Limb as before, then (by moving the Instrument about) turn back the Telescope to ☉ 1, and fasten the Limb, then the Telescope being directed to ☉ 3, the End of the Index which is next you will give on the Limb the Bearing, which also will be noted by the North End of the Needle in the Box, if no Mistake is committed, so will the Needle and the Index the one prove the other, and the Bearings will be all expeditiously and truly taken by the Index on the Limb, without depending in the least on the Needle. Thus proceed at every Station, and you will find one End or other of the Needle in the Box, always correspond with the Index on the Limb, at least so nearly as to prevent or discover any Error which might arise during the Course of the Survey. When the Instrument is brought to some Station already entered in your Field Book, in order to go round another Field, fix the Index to the Degree, &c. upon the Limb, of the Station preceding that you are at, and take a Back observation thereto, so will the Instrument retain its same parallel Position, and the Work may be carried on as before. A Field Book comformable to each Method begins in the next Page.

The

Sect III. Surveying *by the* Theodolite.

The First FIELD BOOK.

REMARKS	⊙	⊙ L	⊙	REMARKS.
	B	⊙ 1 264° 10' 0 290	25 28	In *A* *J* Jones's Ground. Hedge to *Jones*.
∠ 122° 10' B 264 10 ───── 386 20 180 00 ───── 206 20 = B	∠ B	⊙ 2 122° 10' 206 20 0 298	30 30	In Ditto G. Coles's Ground Hedge to *A*
∠ 76° 45' B 206 20 ───── 283 05 180 00 ───── 103 05 = B	∠ B	⊙ 3 76° 45' 103 05 0 155 290	33 30 31	In *A*. B Sand's Ground
∠ 98° 45' B. 103 05 ───── 201 50 180 00 ───── 21 50 = B	∠ B	⊙ 4 98° 45' 21 50 0 390 to ⊙ 1	30 35	In Ditto. Field B Hedge to Ditto Here *A* closes.
Return to ⊅ 181° 45' B 103 05 ───── 284 50 180 00 ───── 104 50 = B.	∠ B	⊙ + 181° 45' 104 50 0 30 290	34 30	In *A*. Corner Cross the Hedge into B B. Sand's Ground. Hedge to Sand's. Corner.

The First FIELD BOOK.

REMARKS	.	⊙L	O.	REMARKS
∠ 124° 40'		⌒ 5		In *B*.
B 104 50		124° 40'		
229 30	∠ *B*	49 30		
180 00		0		The Common.
49 30 = *B*				Hedge to *B*.
		400	24	
∠ 62° 45'		⊙ 6		In *B*.
B 49 30		62° 45'		
112 15	∠ *B*	292 15		
360 00		0	30	
472 15		210	32	
180 00		425	50	Close *B* at Corner of *A*.
292 15 = *B*.				Into Field *A*
		464		To ⊙ 1 in *A*.

The SECOND FIELD BOOK.

REMARKS	O.	⊙L	O	REMARKS.
		⊙ 1		In *A*.
	B	264° 40'		
		0	25	*J. Jones*'s Ground
				Hedge to *Jones*.
		290	28	
		⊙ 2		In Ditto.
	B	26° 20'		
		0	30	*G. Cole*'s Ground.
				Hedge to *A*.
		298	30	
		⊙ 3		In Ditto.
	B	103° 05'		
		0	33	*B Sand*'s Ground.
		155	30	
		290	31	

The

Sect. III. Surveying *by the* Theodolite.   331

The Second FIELD BOOK.

REMARKS	O.	⊙ L	O	REMARKS.
	B	⊙ 4 201° 50' o		In Ditto.
			30	Field *B*. Hedge to Ditto.
		390 To ⊙ 1	35	Close here *A*.
Return to	*B*	⊙ 4 284° 50' o		In *A*
		30	34	Corner. (into *B*. Cross the Hedge *B Sand*'sGround Hedge to *Sand*.
		290	30	Cornei
	B.	⊙ 5 49° 30' o		In *B*.
		400	24	The Common.- Hedge to *B.*
	B.	⊙ 6 112° 15' o		In *B*.
		210	30	
		425	32	(of *A*.
		464	50	Close *B* at Corner into Field *A*. to ⊙ 1 in *A*.

To draw the Plan.

This may be done two Ways; thus.

I. Draw *NS* for a Meridian, in which chuse any Point ⊙ 1 for your first Station; to which apply the Center of a Protractor, and lay down the Bearing at ⊙ 1 in your Field Book and draw the Line 1 2 = 290 Links.

Through ⊙ 2 draw another Meridian parallel to the former *NS*, and draw the Line 2 3, = 298, to make an Angle with the Meridian = the Bearing at ⊙ 2, and if the Line 2 3 cut the Limb of the Protractor at 122° 10′, (= Angle at ⊙ 2 in the Field Book) you may be assured your Work is so far right, but if it doth not intersect the Edge of the Protractor at the Degrees, &c. of the Angle, you may then conclude your Work to be wrong, which must be examined before you proceed further. Thus proceed at every Station 'till the Whole be protracted, after which lay down the Offsets and draw the Hedges, which will compleat the Plan.

The other Method (by much the best) is performed thus

II. Lay your Protractor (those are best having an open Center and a *Nonius*) on any Point ⊙, chosen at Pleasure; and moving its Index to the Degree, &c. of each Bearing in the second Field Book, point them severally off upon the Paper. Then take away your Protractor, and chuse some Point (⊙ 1) upon Paper, for your first Station, then lay the Edge of a Parallel Ruler on ○ and the Point numbered 1, extend its other Edge 'till it just touch ⊙ 1, and draw close thereby the Line 1 2 = 290 Links. Then apply the Edge of the Parallel Ruler to ⊙ and the Point 2, and its other Edge being extended to ⊙ 2, draw a Line as before, = Distance 298; thus proceed with every Bearing and Distance

The Angle included between any two Traverse Lines, according to this Method, may be had by subtracting the Bearing at the last preceding Station, from the

Sect III.   Surveying *by the* Theodolite.   333

the Bearing at the prefent Station, (if Subtraction can be made) and the Remainder is the prefent Angle, which if greater than a Semicircle (or 180°) is an outfide Angle, if lefs an infide One; and therefore the Line flowing from any Station, muft be drawn inwardly or outwardly, according as the Angle is lefs or greater than 180°. *Note,* If Subtraction cannot be made, add (or borrow) 360°, and then fubtract as above.

In my common Practice of Surveying (which is frequently after this Method,) I moftly mark the Bearings in the Field Book with the Letters *T* and *F*, fignifying true and falfe Bearing, as at every fecond Station from that I begin at, the Bearing is greater than it fhould be by a Semi-circle (or 180°); and this is occafioned by turning back the Telefcope, and looking in at the fame End at every Station. This might be eafily remedied by two Telefcopes, the one lying upon the other, and fo placed that the Axis of the one is exactly parallel to the Axis of the other, with their Eye-ends contrarily placed, fo that Obfervations might be made backward or forward, without fhifting the Inftrument or Index.

This Want is partly fupplied, by the plain Sights, which are at prefent fix'd upon the Telefcopes of our beft Theodolites, but greatly fhort in Point of Accuracy and Eafe, and is therefore worthy of our Inftrument-maker's Notice.

This Method of Protracting (or laying down Angles) from one Center, is but known to few Surveyors, and confequently has not been much ufed. It is of that Availment in the Practice of Surveying, that without it we are almoft rendered incapable of drawing a Plan of

any

any Size, with that Degree of Accuracy which is required, or might be wish'd for.

I have, I hope, sufficiently demonstrated every Branch of Practical Surveying, so far as relates to the measuring of Lines and Angles; and have also pointed out some of the best Forms of keeping a Field Book, which is one great Secret of Land-surveying; with all the Varieties of Protracting.

It is very easy to account for the Difficulty of closing a Plan, when we know that the Angles or Bearings have been protracted, according to the common Form before shewn, which is all the Method that has as yet been practised, by even the most noted and eminent of our practising Surveyors, for considering the great Nicety of pricking off Angles, and again the great Care and Exactness which is required in laying on the Protractor at every Station, makes it almost impossible but to commit an Error and if an Error (though never so trifling) should happen to be committed, either in the Angle or Distance, (but more especially in the Angle) that presently increases, and grows greater and greater, according to the Number of Bearings or Distances that immediately follow, after the Protraction of that Angle or Bearing, or the laying down of that Distance, where the Mistake was first entered

GENERAL PROBLEM.

To take the Plan of a Gentleman's Estate, Manor or Lordship.

In order to survey a Gentleman's Estate, it is necessary that the Surveyor be not only well skill'd in both

the

Sect III.   SURVEYING *by the* THEODOLITE.   335

the Theory and Practice of Surveying, but that he be well equipped with Inftruments fitting for his Purpofe, viz fuch as will meafure Lines, take and protract Angles or Bearings, and reduce Schemes or Plans.

The beft Inftrument for meafuring Diftances, is a ftrong four-pole Chain at $5\frac{1}{2}$ Yards to the Pole, as before defcribed The Perambulator is alfo an Inftrument for meafuring Diftances, being more expeditious than accurate, its greateft Ufe is in meafuring Roads, or in County Surveys

For meafuring of Angles, or taking the Pofition of Lines, no Inftrument whatever equals the Theodolite, of which there are various Sorts, as before defcribed

For protracting or laying down Angles, the only advantageous Inftrument, is a round Protractor with an open Center and a *Nonius*, by which Angles may be protracted to three Minutes of a Degree There are other Protractors of more fimple Conftruction, both circular and femi-circular; all of which have been already defcribed.

For laying down Diftances and pricking off Offsets, the Feather-edged Scales (already defcribed) deferve the Preference, as alfo doth the crofs-barr'd Parallel Ruler, for reducing irregular fided Figures to Triangles or Trapeziums.

EXAMPLE I

To take a Survey or Plan, of the Eftate of the Right Hon. H——, *Earl of* B——, *fituate at* A——, *in the Parifh of* L——, *and County of* N——.

Set up your Theodolite at *A*, in the Foot of the Lane, and (by Prop. 12) take the Pofition of the Line

AB, and measure its Length, with every particular Offset to the Right or Left, as they occur. Then remove your Instrument to *B* in in the Lane, and take as before the Position or Bearing of *BC*, with its Distance and Offsets. This done, remove your Theodolite to *C*, *D*, *E*, *F*, *G* and *H*, and repeat the Work as before, so will the Work of the first Field, viz. Alder Wood be finished. There are several other Particulars, which should have been noticed, such as the Names of the Fields, &c. on the Right and Left, and to which of them such and such particular Hedges, Walls, Fences, Ditches, &c. do belong, with other Particulars, which cannot be recited here, together with the Form or Method of disposing or ranging them in a Book kept for that Use, commonly called a Field Book, I say to make a Recital of all these, would in this Place be superfluous, as the Field Book directly follows, in which are contained all the Occurrences, which can possibly happen during the Survey; so that by examining the Field Book, and by comparing it and the Plan together, more Knowledge will be acquired, than can possibly be expected from a Number of tedious Repetitions.

Alder Wood being finished, you next remove your Theodolite to *F* in the Lane, from whence proceed as before, 'till Spring Close and the Rest of the Fields are finished.

Note, The Instrument used in this Survey, is a Theodolite with plain Sights, having its **Box** fixed to the Index.

Sect. III. SURVEYING *by the* THEODOLITE. 337

The FIELD BOOK.

A Survey of the Estate of the Right Hon. H———, *Earl of* B———, *situate at* A———, *in the Parish of* L———, *and County of* N———; *by* T——— B———, *Surveyor.*

REMARKS.	0	⊙ L	0	REMARKS.
				Monday, Nov 7, 1768.
		⊙ 1 *(A)*		In the Lane
	B	16° 00'		
J *Wilson's* Ground	10	0	10	Lord L——'s Ground
Hedge to *Wilson*.				Hedge to Lord
Against Hedge	10	15	10	Against Hedge
*B*e*la Holme*				*Alder* Wood
Hedge to *Holme*.				Hedge to *Alder* Wood
Corner	8	125	10	Corner
		⊙ 2 *(B)*		In the Lane
345° 30'		∠ 149° 30		
180 00	B	345 30'		
525 30		0		
16 00				
509 30	Cor. 12	138	10	Cor
360 00		145		
149 30 = ∠		○ 3 *(C)*		In Ditto
15° 30'		∠ 210° 00'		
180 00	B	15 30		
195 30		0		
360 00		150	8	Cor.
555 30	12	160		
345 30		⊙ 4 *(D)*		In Ditto.
210 00 = ∠		∠ 276° 50'		112° 20'
	B	112 20		180 00
Flatts	12	0		272 20
Hedge to Ditto				15 30
		8	9	Corner.
Cor.	10	128	10	Cor

X x 2 *The*

338 SURVEYING *by the* THEODOLITE. Book VIII.

The FIELD BOOK.

REMARKS	↩	⊙ L.	↪	REMARKS
86° 00' 180 00 266 00 112 20 153 40 = ∠ 1. Hedge Long Moor Hedge to Ditto	 ∠ B 8 10	☽ 5 (E) 153° 40' 86 00 0 55 70 126	 6	 Bye ⊙ for closing Long Moor
  185° 45' 180 00 365 45 86 00 Spring Close 279 45 = ⋝ H to Dit. Cor 28	 ⋝ B 12 8 30	⊙ 6 (F) 279° 45' 185 45 0 6 154 193	 	In Ditto. Cross the Hedge into *Alder* Wood
178° 00' 180 00 358 00 185 45 172 15 = ∠	 ∠ B 16	⊙ 7 (G) 172° 15' 178 00 0 198 212	 	In *Alder* Wood Into Lord *L—*'s Ground
266° 30' 180 00 446 30 178 00 268 30 = ⋝	 ⋝ B	⊙ 8 (H) 268° 30' 266 30 0 275 280 288	 14 13	In Lord *L—*'s Ground *Alder* Wood Hedge to Lord *L—*'s Cor close here. Into the Lane To ⊙ 1 in the Lane.

The

Sect. III. Surveying *by the* Theodolite. 339

The FIELD BOOK.

REMARKS	?	☉ L.	☉	REMARKS.
Return to		☉ 6 (F		In the Lane.
90° 30'	∠	184° 30'		
180 00	B	90 30		
270 30 Long Mooɪ	10	0		
86 30 Hedge to D				
18 30 = ∠		10	8	Againſt Hedge.
				Spring Cloſe.
				Hedge to Ditto.
Cor	14	126		
				Into Eaſtfield
		138		Bye ☉ for the Return to go round Long Moor.
		226	10	
184° 40'		☉ 9 (I)		In Eaſtfield.
180 00	⌐	274° 10'		
364 40	B	184 40		
90 30 *Bela* River	20	0		
274 10 = ∠	18	10		Croſs the Hedge into Spring Cloſe.
	5	106		
	17	182		
	4	285		
	14	394		Into Lord *L*—'s Ground.
	20	408		
271° 20'		☉ 10 (K)		In Lord *L*—'s Ground.
180 00	⌐	266° 40'		
451 20	B.	271 20		
184 40		0	14	Spring Cloſe.
266 40 = ⌐				Hedge to Ditto.
		194	15	Cloſe at Cor of *Alder* Wood.
		205		
				To ☉ 8 in L *L*—'s Ground.

The

Surveying by the Theodolite. Book VIII.

The FIELD BOOK.

REMARKS	O	⊙L	O	REMARKS
17° 50' Return to bye		⊙ at		138 in Line 6 9
180 00	∠	107° 20'		
197 50	B	17 50		
90 30		0		
107 20 = ∠ L.Moor	12	10		
Hedge to Ditto.				
		158	91	*Bela* River.
	11	220		
		230		
356° 00'		⊙ 11 (L)		In Eastfield
180 00	∠	158° 10'		
536 00	B	356 00		
17 50		0		
518 10	14	190		
360 00				
158 10 = ∠		⊙ 12 (M)		In Ditto
	∠	97° 00'		
273° 00'	B	273 00		
180 00		0		
453 00		15		
356 00				Into Long Moor
97 00 = ∠				*Powlands*
				Hedge to Ditto
		27	20	Cor
		144	8	
		255	15	
186° 50'		⊙ 13 (N)		In Long Moor
180 00	∠	93° 50'		
366 50		186 50		
273 00		0	15	Flatts
93 50 = ∠				Hedge to Long Moor.
		150	25	

The

Sect. III. Surveying *by the* Theodolite.] 341

The FIELD BOOK.

REMARKS	O.	L ☉	O	REMARKS
174° 45′ 180 00 354 45 186 50 167 55 = ∠	∠ B	☽ 14 (O) 167° 55′ 174 45 0 8 270 275	15 16	In Ditto Clofe here To bye ☉ at 70 in Line 5 6.
Return to 274° 10′ 180 00 454 10 273 00 181 10 = ∠	∠ B	☽ 13 (N) 181° 10′ 274 10 0 16 175 204 220 330	18 25 20 8	In Long Moor. Corner Into Flatts Long Acres Hedge to Ditto Bye ☉ for clofing L Acre Ag Hedge Broad Field Hedge to Ditto
172° 30′ 180 00 352 30 274 10 78 20 = ∠	∠ B	☉ 15 (P) 78° 20′ 172 30 0 147	15 17	In Flatts Scroggy Wood Hedge to Flatts

The

The FIELD BOOK.

REMARKS	⊙	⊙ L	⊙	REMARKS
188° 40' 180 00 ────── 368 40 172 30 ────── 196 10 = ∠ Flatts Hedge to Ditto	 ∠ B	⊙ 16 (♀) 196° 10' 188 40 0 196 210	 16	In Ditto Corner Into *Bela Holme*.
112° 20' 180 00 ────── 292 20 188 40 ────── 103 40 = ⌐ Close here	 ∠ B 14 15	⊙ 17 (R) 103° 40' 112 20 0 164 176		In *Bela Holme*. Into Lane To ⊙ 4 in the Lane.
Return to 271° 35' 16 00 ────── 255 35 = ⌐	 ⌐ B.	⊙ 1 (A) 255° 35' 271 35 0 13 272	 15 16	In the Lane *Bela Holme* Into *J. Wilson*'s Ground. Hedge to *J. Wilson*'s.

The

Sect. III. Surveying *by the* Theodolite.

The FIELD BOOK.

REMARKS	⊙	⊙L	⊙	REMARKS
180° 00″		⊙ 18 (S)		In *J Wilson*'s Ground
5 00	∠	273° 25′		
185 00	B	5 00		
360 00		o		
543 00 Cor	15	14		
271 35 (*le*		int		
273 25 = ⟶ H W				
Hedge to *B Holme*				
				In *B la Holme*
	15	265		
		273		
29° 30″		⊙ 19 (*T*)		In *Bal i Holme*
180 00	⟶	204° 30′		
209 30	B	29 30		
5 00		o		(Wood.
204 30 = ∠		56		Bye ⊙ for closing Hazzle
Ag Hedge	15	66		To ⊙ 17 (of Flatts
	20	280		*B la Holme* closes at Cor
259° 00′ Return to		⊙ 18 (S)		In *J Wilson*'s Ground.
180 00	∠	167° 25′		
439 00	B.	259 00′		
271 35		o		
167 25 = ∠		15	16	Corner
				Hazzle Wood
				Hedge to Ditto
		194	24	10
		375	15	Corner
		390		

Y y

344 SURVEYING *by the* THEODOLITE. Book VIII.

The FIELD BOOK

REMARKS	O	OL	O	REMARKS
356° 00'		⊙ 20 (V)		In *J Wilſon*'s Ground.
180 00	∠	277° 00'		
536 00	B	356 00		
259 00		0		
277 00 = ∠		17	10	Corner.
				On Weſt Field
		230	15	Cor
17° 40'		⊙ 21 (W)		In Weſt Field
180 00	∠	201° 40'		
197 40	B	17 40		
360 00		0		
557 40		19½	14	
356 00		⊙ 22 (X)		In Ditto
201 40 = ∠	⌐	248° 30'		
	B	86 10		
86° 10'		0		
180 00		12		
266 10		int		
17 40				In Hazzle Wood
248 30 = ∠				
Miles.				
Hedge to Ditto				
Cor	10	20		
Cor	15	167		
		180		
98° 45'		⊙ 23 (Y)		In Hazzle Wood
180 00	⌐	192° 35'		
278 45	B	98 45		
86 10		0		
192 35 = ∠	10	196		
				Into *Bela Holme*
		214		(17
				To Bye ⊙ at 56 in Line 19,

The

Sect III. Surveying *by the* Theodolite.   345

The FIELD BOOK.

REMARKS	O	⊙ L	O	REMARKS
	Return to	⊙ 22 (*)		In West Field
180° 05'		∠ 162° 25'		
17 40		B 0 05		
162 25 = ∠		0		
		10	15	A Hedge
				Scraggy Wood
				Hedge to Ditto
		314	18	
111° 30'		⊙ 24 (∠)		In Ditto
180 00		∠ 291° 25'		
291 30		B 111 30		
0 05		0		
291 25 = > S. Wood	12	15		Into Mires.
Hedge to Ditto				
Cor	14	310		
		318		
92° 50'		O 25 (7°)		In Mires
180 00		∠ 161 20'		
272 50		B 92 50		
111 30		0		
161 20 = ∠	16	184		
				Into Bela Holme
		205 to O	17	Mires close at Cor of
				B Holme and Flatts
351° 20'	Return to	⊙ 24 (∠)		In West Field
180 00		∠ 171° 15'		
531 20		B 351 20		
0 05	Ldn River	30	0	
531 15		10	15	A Hedge.
360 00				Scraggy Wood
171 15 = ∠				Hedge to Ditto.
		315	18	

Y y 2   *The*

346 SURVEYING *by the* THEODOLITE. Book VIII.

The FIELD BOOK

REMARKS	⊙	⊙ L	⊙	REMARKS
		⊙ 26 (B²)		In Ditto
	∠	293° 40'		
	B.	105 00		
		0		
		20		
		int		
105° 00'				In *Scroggy* Wood
180 00 Hud Ing	15	22		
285 00 H to Ditto				
360 00		35		Bye ⊙ for closing II In
645 00	15	195		
351 20	18	322		
293 40 = ∠				
		⊙ 27 (C-)		In *Scroggy* Wood
89° 00'	∠	164° 00'		
180 00	B	89 00		
269 00		0		
105 00 Ag Hedge		14		
164 00 = ∠ B Field				
Hedge to Ditto				
Close here S Wood	10	194		Cross the Hedge into
At Cor. of Flatts				the Line
		208		To ⊙ 15 in Flatts
3° 55' Return to		⊙ 12 (M)		In East Field.
180 00	∠	187° 55'		
183 55	B	3 55		
360 00		0		
543 55 Ag Hedge	18	20		
356 00 Powland's				
187 55 = ∠ H to D				
	6	223		
	10	255		

The

Sect. III.   SURVEYING *by the* THEODOLITE.   347

The FIELD BOOK

REMARKS	O	L	O	REMARKS
358° 30′ 180 00 538 30 3 55 534 35 360 00 174 35 = ∠	∠ B 10	◯ 28 (D²) 174° 35′ 358 30 0 175		In Ditto
270° 00′ 180 00 450 00 358 30 91 30 = ∠	∠ B	⊙ 29 (F²) 91° 30′ 270 00 0 10 258	 18 18	In Ditto Corner Into Powland's. Denton Holme Hedge to Powlands.
180° 45′ 180 00 360 45 270 00 90 45 = ∠	∠ B	⊙ 30 (F²) 90° 45′ 180 45′ 0 190 395 410	 15 15	In Powlands. Long Acres Hedge to Ditto. Cor. close here. Into Long Moor To ◯ 13 in L. Moor. P closes it the Cor. of L M and Flitts
180° 00′ Return to 1 30 181 30 360 00 541 30 Ag Hedge 358 30 D Holme 183 00 = ∠ H to D	∠ B 16 8	⊙ 29 (F) 183° 00′ 1 30 0 16 210		In East Field.
Corner North Common.	15	375 391		

The

348   SURVEYING *by the* THEODOLITE. Book VIII.

The FIELD BOOK.

REMARKS.	⊙	⊙L	⊙	REMARKS
260° 00′ 180 00 ———— 440 00 1 30 ———— 438 30 Cor. 360 00 ———— 78 30 = ∠	 ∠ B 15 16	⊙ 31 (G²) 78° 30′ 260 00 0 16 195		In Ditto Upon North Common
273° 30″ 180 00 ———— 453 30 260 00 ———— 193 30 = ∠	 ∠ B 15 10	⊙ 32 (H²) 193° 30′ 273 30 0 6 158		On North Common
167° 15′ 180 00 ———— 347 15 273 30 ———— 73 45 = ∠	 ∠ B 	⊙ 33 (I²) 73° 45′ 167 15 0 10 int 172 356 375	 10 18 10 	On North Common Cor of L A & *Swillands* In *Denton Holme*. Long Acres Hedge to Ditto Close at C of *Powlands* Into *Powlands* To ⊙ 30 in *Powlands*.
222° 50′ Return to 180 00 ———— 402 50 273 30 ———— 129 20 = ∠	 ∠ B 	⊙ 33 (I²) 129° 20′ 222 50 0 12 18 int 233	 + 10	On North Common. Into *Denton Holme* *Swillands* Hedge to Ditto In Long Acres

The

Sect. III. Surveying *by the* Theodolite   349

The FIELD BOOK.

REMARKS	O	⊙L	O.	REMARKS
171° 45′ 180 00 351 45 222 50 128 55 = ∠		⊙34(K²) ∠ 128° 55′ B 171 45 0 128 148 380	 15 14 10	In Long Acres Corner Bye⊙ for closing *Swirl*. Ag Hedge Broad Field. Hedge to Long Acres.
185° 45′ 180 00 365 45 171 45 194 00 = ∠		⊙35(L²) ∠ 194° 00′ B 185 45 0 194 218	 16	In Ditto Cor close here. Into Flatts (13 15. To bye ⊙ at 204 in L.
278° 15′ Return to 180 00 458 15 273 30 184 45 = ∠ Ag H *Scullards* Hedge to Ditto	 10 10 12	⊙33(I²) ∠ 184° 45′ B 278 15 0 14 164 326		On North Common.
262° 20″ 180 00 442 20 278 15 164 05 = ∠ Ag H Rough Pasture Hedge to Ditto	 17	⊙36(M²) ∠ 164° 05′ B. 262 20 0 175 190		On Ditto.

The

The FIELD BOOK.

REMARKS	O	☉ L	O	REMARKS
173° 25′ 180 00 353 25 20 20 0 0 =∠ Cor Swillands Hedge to Ditto	 <∠ B 14	☉37(N-) 91 05′ 173 25 0 14 90 160 226 334		On Ditto Into Rough Pasture
	10 18 11 15			
87° 00′ 180 00 267 00 173 25 93 35 =∠	 <∠ B.	☉38 (O-) 93° 35′ 87 00 0 16 int 165 316 333	 26 21 20	In Rough Pasture Corner Broad Field, H to D In Swillands C close here (34 35 To Bye Out 128 in L.
268° 30′ Return to 180 00 448 30 262 20 Rough Past 186 10 = ⇁ H. to D	 B 15 14	☉37(N-) 186° 10′ 268 30 0 350		On North Common.

Sect. III. SURVEYING *by the* THEODOLITE   351

The FIELD BOOK.

REMARKS	O	⊙L	O	REMARKS
171 20 180 00 ——— 351 20 268 30 ——— 82 50 = ∠		⊙39 (P-) 82° 50' B 171 20 0 14 98	 56 10 10	On Ditto Ed. River. Corner Into Rough Pasture Here the Hedge ends and *Eden* River be- comes the Fence
  264° 35' 180 00 ——— 444 35 171 20 ——— 273 15 = ⌐		208 364 ⊙40 (Q²) 273° 15' B 264 35 0 164 330 to 38	16 9 17 10 24	 In Rough Pasture Hard Ing. Hedge to Ditto. Rough Pasture Closes at the Corner of *Swillands* & Broad Field
178° 10' Return to 180 00 ——— 358 10 173 25 ——— 184 45 = ⌐ Cor Broad Field Hedge Ditto Cor	 20 28 14	⊙38 (O²) 184° 45' B 178 10 0 22 267 425 443 to	 ⊙27	In Rough Pasture Into Hard Ing Into *Scroggs* Wood Broad Field Closes at Cor of Hard Ing

The

352 SURVEYING *by the* THEODOLITE. Book VIII.

The FIELD BOOK.

REMARKS	☉	☉ I	☉	REMARKS.
176 50′ Return to		☉ 40 (2ª)		In Rough Pasture
180 0		185° 30′		
	B	176 50		
350 50		0		Eden River continues
171 20				the Fence
		18	6	Into Hard Ing
185 30 =		222	16	Here Eden River ceases
				to be the Fence
		295	19	Cor of Scroggy Wood
		304		Into Scroggy Wood
		320		To bye ☉ at 35 in
				Line 26, 27
				Hard Ing Closes at
				Cor of Screg Wood
	Return to	☉ 10		In Ld L——s Ground

Note, The Field Book might have been continued further, but the above containing all the Varieties that can possibly happen in that Survey, may be sufficient.

To draw the Plan

This is wholly performed by Prop. 16, to which I refer the Tyro for further Instructions.   FIG. 25

EXAMPLE II.

To take a Survey or Plan of the Manor or Lordship of W——, *in the Parish of* K—— S——, *and County of* W——, *the Property of the Honourable Sir* I—— L——, *Baronet*.

The

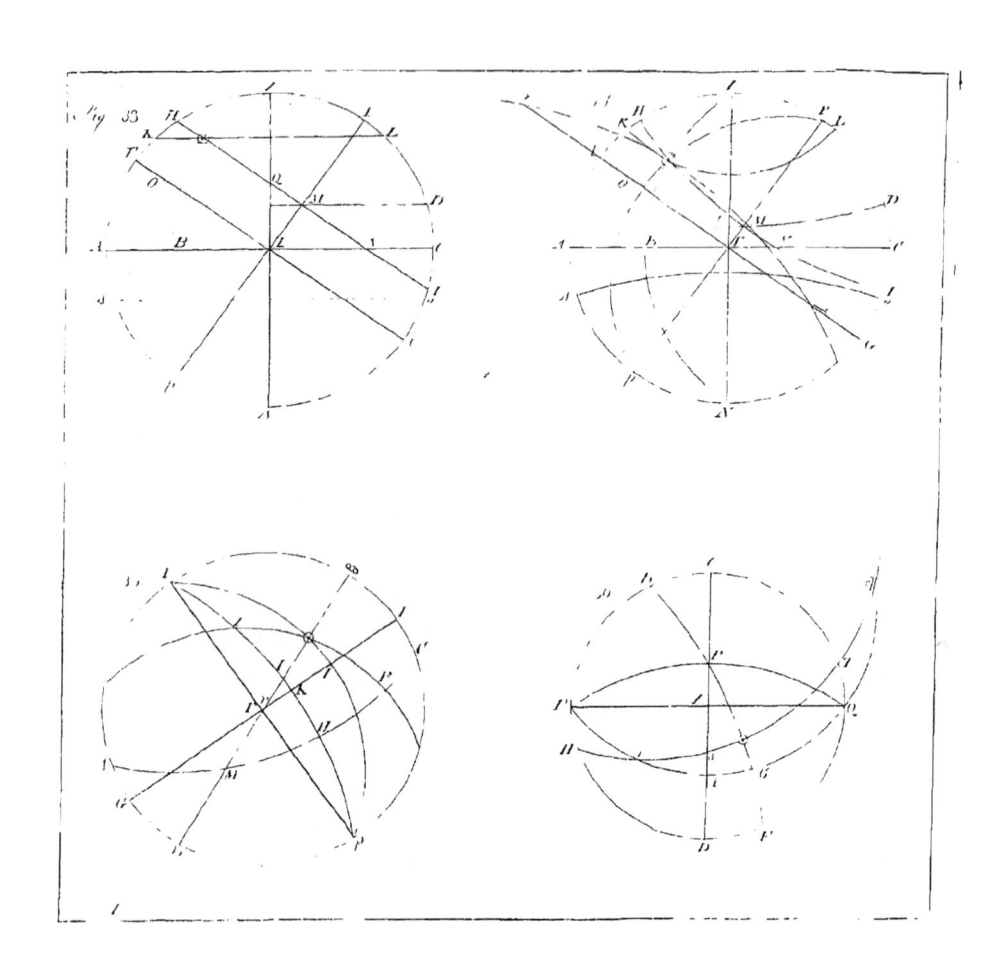

Sect. III.   SURVEYING *by the* THEODOLITE

The Work of this Example is performed by the latter Part of the Rule in Prop. 16.

Note, The Instrument used in this Survey, is a Theodolite of *Cole*'s Form, with Tooth and Pinion to the vertical and horizontal Motions.

The FIELD BOOK.

A Survey of the Manor or Lordship of W———, *the Property of the Honourable Sir* I——— L———, *Baronet; by* T——— B———, *Surveyor.*

FIG 26

REMARKS	⊙	⊙ L	⊙	REMARKS
Mr *I Wilson*'s Farm,		situate at ⊙ 1 (*A*)		W— *July* 25, 1769 In Sir P——— H———'s Ground
	T	355° 25'		
Hedge-buts to Turn-mire	24	25		
Turn-mire Hedge to Ditto				
	20	398		
	F	⊙ 2 (*B*) 183° 00'		In Ditto
		160		bye ⊙ for laying down *Eden* River
		180		to the River's Brink
		212		farther Side of Ditto.
Hedge-buts to *Bullas-how* Bullas-how Hedge to Ditto.	15	286		
		315		

Z z 2   The

354 Surveying by the Theodolite. Book VIII.

The FIELD BOOK

REMARKS	O	⊙ L O.	REMARKS
	T	⊙ 3 (C) 00° 00' 0	In Ditto.
	30	220	
		515	
	F	⊙ 4 (D) 173° 15' 0	In Ditto.
Hedge-buts to Riggs	18	22	
Riggs H to Ditto			
Hedge-buts to Riggs Lane	19	355	
	T	⊙ 5 (E) 6° 00' 0	In Sir P—— H—— Ground.
Hedge-buts to Long-fide	20	16	
Long-fide H to Dit	28	350	
	F	⊙ 6 (F) 169° 40' 0	In Ditto.
Hedge-buts to Long-fide North Moor	22	222	
		235	
	T.	⊙ 7 (G) 274° 30' 0	On North Common
Long-fide H to Dit	18	18	
Corner to Corner	15	205	
	15	600	

The

Sect. III SURVEYING *by the* THEODOLITE. 355

The FIELD BOOK.

REMARKS	O.	⊙ L	O	REMARKS.
	F.	⊙ 8 (*H*) 92° 30' o		On Ditto
Hedge-buts to Square Clofe	10	20		
Square Clofe Hedge to Ditto				
	20	295		
	15	555		
	T	⊙ 9 (*I*) 270° 30' o		On Ditto.
Hedge-buts to *Pow-lands*	10	25		
Hedge to Ditto				
Hedge-buts to *Pow-lands*	20	512		
Sand-field.				
		540		
	F.	⊙ 10 (*K*) 356° 35' o		On North Moor.
Corner	20	20		enter into Sand-field.
Powlands Hedge to Ditto				
	20	350		
	T.	⊙ 11 (*L*) 182° 22' o		In Sand-field.
	10	280		

The

356 SURVEING *by the* THEODOLITE. Book VIII.

The FIELD BOOK.

REMARKS	O	⊙L	O	REMARKS
	F	⊙ 12 (M) 1° 10' 0		In Sand-field
Hedge-buts to Long-tailbars Long tailbars Hedge to Ditto	10	14		
	20	274		
		310		to the Brink of *Eden* River
		340		to the farther Side of Ditto
		368		bye ⊙ for closing *Eden* River.
Hedge-buts to Ing. Ingmire H to Ditto	9	565		
		595		
	T	⊙ 13 (N) 168° 45' 0		In R *Adams*'s Ground
		488		
	T	⊙ 14 (O) 0° 50' 0		In R *Adams*'s Ground
Hedge-buts to Ing. *Toddl s* Hedge to *Adams*	22	25		
	30	240		
Hedge-buts to *Toddles* South Field	10	530		
		556		
	T	⊙ 15 (P) 84° 30' 0		In South Field.
Cornei *Toddles*, H to Ditto	20	15		
		410		

The

Sect III. Surveying *by the* Theodolite.

The FIELD BOOK

REMARKS	O	⊙L	O	REMARKS
	F	⊙16 (*Q*) 283° 30' o		In Ditto
Hedge-buts to B Field. Broad Field Hedge to Ditto	20	20		
Hedge-buts to Thoath Thoath. Hedge to Dit.	22 18	230 495 520		
	T	⊙17 (*R*) 91° 00' o		In Ditto.
Hedge-buts to Thoath. Turn-mire Hedge to Ditto.	9 20	190 400 425		
	F	⊙18 (*S*) 271° 30' o		in Ditto.
Corner	25 20	160 284 310		To ⊙1.
	F	⊙18- (*S*) 181° 40' o		in Ditto.
Thoath Hedge to Dit.	25 25	20 305	×	the H. into Turn-mire.
	T	⊙19 (*T*) 334° 00' o		In Turn-mire
Corner.	28	256 275	×	the H into *Bullas-how*.

The

The FIELD BOOK.

REMARKS.	O	⊙ L	O	REMARKS
		⊙ 20 (*V*)		In *Bullas-how*
	F	249° 10'		
		o	19	Turn-mire
				Hedge to *Bullas-how*.
		165	10	
		280		The River's Brink
		318		Further Side of the R
		405	20	20 Cor Close here.
		×		Hedge into Sir *P——*
				H——'s Ground.
		430		To ⊙ 3
		⊙ 17² (*R*)		In South Field
	T	17° 00'		
		o		
Corner	20	15	×	the H. into *Thoath*.
Broad Field				
Hedge to *Thoath*				
	20	200		
		⊙ 21 (*W*)		In *Thoath*
	T.	177° 30'		
		o		
Corner.	20	280	×	H. into *Bullas-how*.
		291		
		⊙ 22 (*X*)		In *Bullas-how*
	T.	78° 30'		
		o		19 *Thoath*.
				Hedge to *Bullas-how*
		250	20	Close here *Thoath* at
				Cor of Turn-mire
		275		to ⊙ 20.

Sect. III. Surveying *by the* Theodolite.

The FIELD BOOK.

REMARKS.	O	⊙ L	O.	REMARKS
	F	⊙ 14² (*O*) 271 30 o		In *R. Adams*'s Ground.
		20	×	Hedge into Ingmire. *Toddles*
				Hedge to Ingmire.
		320		Bye ⊙ for closing *Toddles* and Broad-field.
		332	18	Hedge-buts to Broad-field.
				Broad-field.
		470		Hedge into Stona
			×	Hedge to Stona
		495	20	
	T.	⊙ 23 (*T*) 91° 15' o		In Stona.
		185	29	
		450	20	Corner of Thorth.
			×	H into *Bullas-how*.
		470		to ⊙ 22
Return to	T.	315 169° 45' o		in Line 1 + 23
Broad-field		19	×	Hedge into *Toddles*.
Hedge to Ditto,				
Close at Corner	22	490	×	H into South-field
		508		to ☽ 16
				Close *Toddles* and Broad-field.
	F	⊙ 1² (*D*) 87° 30' o		in Sir *P— H—*'s G.
		18	20 ×	H into *Bullas-low* Riggs. Hedge to Dit
		432		

3 A

The FIELD BOOK.

REMARKS.	O.	⊙L	O	REMARKS
	T	⊙24 (Z) 257° 00′ 0 10 170 195 380	20 20 25	In *Bullas-how* bye ⊙ for clofing Riggs and Long-moor Hedge-buts to Long-moor Long-moor H to Dit.
	F	⊙25 (A¹) 352° 10′ 0 110 136 230 296 686 to ⊙ 22	24 20 × 7 20	In Ditto Hedge-buts to Stona. Stona. Hedge to *Bullas how* bye ⊙ for clofing Ingmire and Stona the River *Eden* *Bullas-how* clofes at the Cor of Thoath.
Long-t ulbu s Hedge to Ingmue Hedge buts to Long-moor Long-moor Hedge to Stona	T 20 28	⊙ 13² (N) 92° 00′ 0 20 325 480 510	×	In R. *Adams*'s Ground. Hedge into Ingmue

Sect. III. Surveying *by the* Theodolite.

The FIELD BOOK.

REMARKS.	O.	⊙ L	O	REMARKS
	F	⊙ 26 (B²) 268° 20' o 220		In Stona. × Eden River
Close *Bullas-how* and Stona.	22	466 484	×	H into *Bullas-low* to bye ⊙ at 136 in Line 25 22.
	F	⊙ 26² (B³) 350° 45' o 255 480 to ⊙ 23	25 30 26	In Stona Ingmire Hedge to Ditto. Close Ing at Cor next Broad-field, where Stona likewise closes
Corner Riggs. H. to Ditto.	T 10	⊙ 5² (E) 282° 30' o 20 25	12	In Sir *P— H—'s* G. Corner Long-side H. to Dit.
	12	292 ⊙ 27 (C²) 110° 50' o 320	10	in the Lane.
	F.			

3 A 2 *The*

The FIELD BOOK.

REMARKS	O	⊙L	O	REMARKS
		⊙28 (D²)		in Ditto.
	T	274° 30'		
		0		
Hedge-buts to Long-moor	10	20	22	Hedge-buts to Square-close
Long-moor H to Dit				Square-close
				Hedge to Ditto
	12	320	15	
		⊙29 (E²)		In the Lane.
	F	86° 00'		
		0		
	10	285	10	
		⊙30 (F²)		in Ditto
	T	178° 40'		
		0		
		8	24	
			×	H. into Long-moor.
				Powlands
				Hedge to Long-moor
		158		bye ⊙ for closing *Pow-lands* and Long-tail-bars.
		170	30	Hedge-buts to Long-tailbars.
				Long-tailbars
		375	20	
		608		into *Eden* River
		730	30	Close here
			×	Hedge into Stona
		760		to ⊙ 26
				Close Long-moor at it Cor of Ingmire

Sect. III. SURVEYING *by the* THEODOLITE. 363

The FIELD BOOK.

REMARKS	O.	⊙ L.	O	REMARKS.
	F	⊙ 8ᶻ (H) 358° 30′ 0		On North-moor
		15	×	Hedge into Long-fide. Square Clofe Hedge to Ditto
		202 425 455	30 26	Cor. Clofe here to ⊙ 28 in the Lane.
	T	⊙ 9ᶻ (I) 184° 30′ 0		On Ditto.
		15	26 ×	the Hedge into Square Clofe. *Powlands* Hedge to Ditto.
		470	22 ×	Corner Clofe Square Clofe the H in the Lane. to ⊙ 30 in the Lane.
		485		
	F.	⊙ 12ᶻ (M) 279° 00′ 10	12 ×	In Sand-field Hedge into *Powlands*. Long-tailbars Hedge to Ditto
		270 460	20 15 ×	Clofe here *Powlands* and Long-tailbars the Hedge into Long- moor
		490		to laſt ⊙ at 158 in Line 30 26

The

The FIELD BOOK.

REMARKS.	O	⊙ L	O.	REMARKS.
Return to		160		in Line 2 3 for laying down *Eden* River.
The River *Eden*.	T 20 15	127° 15' 0 150		
Return to		160		in Line 2 3
	T	307° 15' 0		
		140	8	*Eden* River.
		335	20	
		385	18	
	F	⊙31 (G²) 95° 15' 0		In *Bullas-low*.
		74	18	
		190	10	
		264	15	
	T.	⊙32 (H²) 287° 00' 0		in *Bullas-how*
		195	12	
		295	10	
		350	20	
	F.	⊙33 (I²) 125° 45' 0		In *Stona*.
		145	14	
		250		
		279	15	
	T	⊙34 (K²) 278° 00' 0		In *Long-moor*.
		100	20	*Eden* River.
		305	18	

The

Sect. III. Surveying *by the* Theodolite.   365

The FIELD BOOK.

REMARKS.	O	⊙ L.	O	REMARKS.
F.		⊙ 35 (L^2) 111° 40' 0 110 242 310 410	15 40	In Long-tailbars bye ⊙ at 368 in Line 12 13 to the River's Edge. Close here.

To draw the Plan.

Proceed in every Respect according to the Directions given in Prop. 16, and you will have a true Plan according to the Field Book. Fig. 27.

To find the Acres, &c contained in this Plan.

Reduce the several Fields in the Plan, into Triangles, or Trapeziums, or both, whose Area find by Prob. 27, 28 Book II. which are as follow.

AREAS.

	A	R	P.
Tarn-mire, reduced to the △ *ABC*.	1	3	16
Thoath, reduced to the △ *DEF*	1	2	39
Broad Field, reduced to the △ *GHI*	2	1	34
Toddles, reduced to the △ *KLM*	1	3	0
Ingmire, reduced to the △ *NOP*	2	1	10
Stona, reduced to the △ *QRS*	2	2	16
Bullas-how, reduced to the △ *TVW*	4	2	13
Long-tillers, reduced to the △ *XYZ*	2	1	37
Long-mroe, reduced to the △ *ADE*	4	1	04
Riggs, reduced to the △ *HGI*	2	1	33
Long-side, reduced to the △ *RDG*	3	0	02
Square Close, reduced to the △ *PBS*	2	1	31
Powlands, reduced to the △ *OLL*	2	3	20
	34	3	15

BOOK IX.

Altimetry; Longimetry; the Method of finding the horizontal Lines of Hills and Valleys, reducing of Plans from a greater Scale to a less, or from a less to a greater, County Surveying; the Method of taking the Perspective of any Gentleman's Seat or Building.

SECT. I.

Altimetry, or the Method of measuring accessible and inaccessible Altitudes.

PROP I.

To find the Altitude of the Tower AB. FIG. 28.

SET up your Theodolite at *C*, and take the Angle of Elevation $ACB = 45°$, measure the Distance from the Instrument at *C*, to *A* the Foot or Bottom of the Tower $= 59$ Feet. Then to find the Height of *AB*, make $AC = 59$, also draw *CB* to make an Angle with $AC = 45°$ (the Altitude) and draw the Perpendicular *AB* to cut *CB* in *B*. Then *AB* measured, is $= 59 =$ the Height of the Tower. Or the same may be performed by Case 3, of right angled plain Triangles.

But Altitudes are most commodiously taken by the best Theodolites thus

Set up your Theodolite *A* at the Distance of 100 Feet from the Bottom *B* of the Tower *BC*, and level

it

it there; then elevate the Telescope, till the horizontal Hair therein cut the Top *C* of the Tower, and the Index will cut off, among the Divisions on the vertical Arch, a Number of equal Parts, which added to *AD* (= *BG*) the Height of the Telescope from the Ground, will give *BC* the Height of the Tower.

Or thus.

The Instrument standing at *A* (= the Distance of 100 Feet from the Bottom of the Tower) direct the Telescope to *B* and *C* (the Bottom and Top of the Tower) and the Index will cut on the vertical Arch two Numbers, whose Sum or Difference (according as the Observations are both above or both below, or the one above and the other below the true Level of the Instrument) is the perpendicular Height of the Tower.

But provided the Distance of the Instrument from the Tower be not limited, then as 100 the Distance : the Altitude given by the Instrument the true Altitude. FIG 32

PROP. II

To find the Height of the Tower AB, *as also of the Spire* BC, *being inaccessible.* FIG. 28.

Chuse two Stations *D*, *E*; set up your Theodolite at *D*, and take the Angles *BDA*, *CDF*, also at *E* take the Angles *BEA*, *CEF*, and measure the Distance between the Stations *D*, *E*.

Then to lay this down upon Paper, draw *DE* = the Distance between the Stations; from *D* draw *DB* and *DC*, to make each an Angle with *AD* equal to to those taken by the Instrument, also from *E* draw

EB and EC, according to the Direction of the Angles BEA, CEF, to cut DB and DC (first drawn) in B and C; then is AB the Height of the Tower, and $FC - AB$ ($= Cd$) the Height of the Spire.

Or you may find the Altitudes by trigonometrical Calculation, for there are two oblique-angled Triangles DCE, DBE, in each of which are known all the Angles and the Side DE common to both, whence in the Triangle DCE, the Side DC may be found by Case 1 of oblique plain Triangles. Also in the right-angled Triangle DFC, we have the Hypothenuse DC and all the Angles, whence DF, and FC (= Height of both Tower and Spire are found by Case 3 right $\angle$ s; then again, in the oblique Triangle DBE, the Side DE and all the $\angle$ s are known, whence DB may be found. Then in the right-angled Triangle DBA the Hyp. DB and all the Angles are known, from whence (by Case 3, of right $\angle$ s) the Perp. AB is found = Altit. of the Tower. Then $FC - AB = Cd =$ Altitude of the Spire.

SECT. II

Longimetry, or the Method of measuring accessible and inaccessible Distances.

PROP. III

To find the Distance of the House C, from either of the Stations A, B, being inaccessible, by Reason of the Water D. FIG. 30.

AT each of the Stations A, B, take with your Theodolite the Angles BAC, ABC, and mea-
and

Sect. II.   LONGIMETRY.   349

sure the Distance AB. Then draw upon Paper a Line AB, which make = the Distance between the Stations; also from A and B draw AC, and BC, according to the Direction of the Angles BAC, ABC, their Point of Intersection C is the Place of the House, and AC and BC separately measured, is its Distance from each Station A, B. Also in the oblique Triangle ACB, all the Angles and the Side AB are known, from whence the other two Sides AC, BC are found by Case 1. oblique plain Triangles.

PROP. IV.

To find the Distance of two Houses C, D, being inaccessible to each other, and also to the Place where you are.

FIG. 31.

Chuse two Stations from whence you can see both the Houses C, D, with your Theodolite at A and B take the Angles CAB, DAB, and CBA, DBA, and measure the Distance between the Stations A and B. By the Help of these Angles and Distance construct the Triangles ABC, ABD, in each of which you have all the Angles and one Side AB (common to both) known, from whence, by Case 1. of Obliques, the Lengths of the Sides BC and BD, or AC and AD may be found. Then join the Points C, D, by which will be formed other two Triangles ACD BDC, in each of which are given two Sides and an included Angle, by which the third Side CD may be found by Case 3. of Obliques. On the Side CD measured on the same Scale the Diagram is drawn by, will give the Distance of the Houses C, D; in the Manner AC and AD, as also BC and BD measured as before, will shew the Distance of C and D from each of the Stations A, B.

PROP. V.

To take the Plot of a Field CDEFGH, *at a Distance from you.* FIG 33.

Take two Stations *A* and *B*, from each of which the several Corners of the Field may be seen, then with your Theodolite at *A* and *B*, take the Quantity of the Angles *CAB*, *DAB*, *EAB*, *FAB*, *GAB*, *HAB*, as also of the Angles *CBA*, *DBA*, *EBA*, *FBA*, *GBA*, *HBA*, and measure the Distance *AB*. Then Lines being drawing according to the Direction of their several Angles, and their Points of Intersection being joined by right Lines, will construct a true Plan or Draught *CDEFGH*.

SECT. III.

The Method of finding the Horizontal Lines of Hills and Vallies.

PROP. VI.

To find the Horizontal Line of an Hill. FIG 34.

PLACE a Mark *C* on the Top of the Hill, of equal Height with the Instrument at *D* and *E* (at the Bottom thereof on each Side) that is, the Mark *C* must be placed as high from the Ground, as the Telescope at *D*, *E*. Then take the Angles of Elevation *CDF*, *CEF*, and measure the Distance from *A* and *B* (the Foot of the Instrument) to the Bottom of the Staff *C*. Then in the two right angled Triangles

gles DFC, EFC, are all the Angles and the Hypothenuses separately given, whence the two Bases AG, GB, are found by Case 1. of right angled Triangles; then $AG + GB = AB =$ the horizontal Line of the Hill.

Prop. VII.

To find the horizontal Line of a Valley. Fig. 35

This is the Reverse of finding the horizontal Line of an Hill; for the Angles of Depression DAC, DBC being found, and the Distances from A and B to the Mark C being measured; we have as before, two right-angled Triangles, in which all the Angles and the Hypothenuses are known, from whence the horizontal Line AB may be found as before by Case 1. of right angled Triangles.

But the Work of this and the last foregoing Prop. may be much more commodiously performed by the best Theodolites, for the Telescope being elevated or depressed, till the horizontal Hair therein intersects the Objects C, C, Fig. 34, 35. the Index will cut off on the vertical Arch two Numbers, which being separately deducted out of each Chain's Length, in measuring up or down the Ascent or Descent, will give the horizontal Distance.

SECT. IV

Reducing of Plans from a greater Scale to a less, or from a less to a greater

PROP VIII

Let it be required to reduce the Plan AEGK to a Scale of Half the Size. FIG. 36, 37.

DRAW a Line NO through any Part of the original Draught (36) and make $KN = KO$, draw another Line NO, (37) and take KN or KO (36) in your Compasses, which make a parallel Radius to 10 10 on the Line of Lines on the Sector, then take the parallel Distance of 5 5, and set from K, to N and O (37). Take NA (36) in your Compasses, make that a parallel Radius to 10 10 on the same Line of Lines as before, and take the parallel Distance 5 5, with which (and one Foot on N) describe an Arch A (37), then make OA (36) a parallel Radius to 10 10, as before, and with the parallel Distance 5 5 (and one Foot on D) describe an Arch to cut the former in A (37). Again, make NB (36) a parallel Radius to 10 10, and with the parallel Distance 5 5 (and one Foot on N) describe an Arch B (37), also take OB (36) in your Compasses, and make it a parallel Radius of 10 10 as before, then with the parallel Distance 5 5 (and one Foot in O) cut the former Arch B in B (37), in like Manner project the other Points C, D, which being joined by Lines, constitutes a Draught of

Sect. IV. Reducing *of* Plans.

one Field. After the same Method must the other Fields be laid down.

There is another Method of reducing a Plan by geometrical Squares, but that being short, in Point of Accuracy, of the first Method, shall therefore be omitted.

There is another very good Method of reducing a Plan which does but consist of one Field, as suppose $ABCDE$ (Fig. 58), and is performed thus:

The Plan being to be reduced $\frac{1}{4}$ Part less, divide any one of its Sides EA into four equal Parts, and set one of these Parts from A to F, from E draw EB, EC, and from F draw FG parallel to AB, which will cut EB in G, also from G draw GH parallel to BC, to intersect EC in H, and lastly, draw HI parallel to CD, to cut ED in I, then is $EFGHI = \frac{1}{4}$ Part less than $ABCDE$, or $= \frac{3}{4}$ Parts thereof.

Or by the Sector thus.

Make EA a parallel Radius of 4 4 on the Line of Lines, then take the parallel Radius 3 3 and set from E to F, and draw the parallel Lines FC, GH, HI as before. Or thus. Make EA, EB, EC, ED respectively equal the parallel Radius 4 4, then take the parallel Radius 3 3, and set from E to F, G, H, I, which Points being joined, produce the Plan $EFGHI$, proportional and similar to the original $ABCDE$.

SECT.

SECT. V.

County Surveying.

COUNTY Surveying is performed in all Respects like unto the Method made use of in Surveying and Plotting a Gentleman's Estate, and the Instructions given in Sect. 3. Book 8. are here sufficient for our Purpose.

For *AGKP* may be said to represent some County, and the several traverse Lines therein may be supposed to denote so many Highways, or public Roads leading to and from some City, Town, Village, Church, Castle, or other memorable Monument within the County (the Hedges in the Plan being in this Case considered as nothing.)

Then, with your Perambulator for measuring Distances, and Theodolite for taking the Position of Lines and the Bearings of remarkable Objects, proceed to take the Out-bounds first, leaving a Mark at the Crossing of any Road, &c. which is to be returned to · As suppose beginning at *A*, you measure forwards (the Position of *AB* being first taken) to ☉ 2 which is at *B*; from thence you proceed along the Line *BC*, and at ☉ you meet with a Road coming in on the left Hand Side, which may be denoted by *RO*, where observe to leave a Mark.

Then measuring forward to ☉ 3, another Road comes in, where place a Mark as before. From thence proceed to *D*, where another Road occurs, as also doth another at *L* From *E* proceed to *H*, where

ano-

Sect. V. COUNTY SURVEYING. 375

another Road comes in, and from H to I, and so on from Station to Station until the Circuit closes at A where you first began.

The Out-side Bounds being thus taken, you next return to some one of the Marks left at the Crossing of some Road, as suppose to S, from whence you measure along the Road till you come to V, where you enter another Road, and leaving a Mark as before, pursue your Course along the Road VC to C, and one Part of the County is set off. Then returning to the Mark R, proceed from thence to W and X, where a Mark being left, pursue your Course to the Mark V, and so is another Part of the County finished.

Returning to O, measure forwards til you fall in with a Road at Q, where leaving a Mark, proceed as before to Y, where you meet with another Road, and a Mark being left as usual, pursue your Course to X which closes another Part of the County.

Again return to the Mark D, and measure from thence to Z, Q, A^2, $\odot$, and X, which finishes another Part of the County. Then return to $\odot$ in the Road AX, and going from thence to B^2, you close another Part of the County at Y, and returning to B^2 proceed along the Road $B^2 N$, to N, which finishes another Part of the County.

Return to the Mark E, and measure forwards to C^2, D^2, and $\odot$ in the Line ZA^2, which closes in another Part of the County. Then return to D^2, and pursue your Course to E^2, F^2, and so on to B^2, where another Part of the County closes.

Then returning to D^2, measure from thence to H, which will close another Part of the County. Also re-
3 C turn

576 COUNTY SURVEYING. Book IX.

turn to Γ^2, and from thence proceed to the Mark I, so will another Part of the County be set off. Lastly, return to M, and proceed from thence to the Mark $\odot$ in the Line $\Gamma^2 B^2$, which closes the Whole.

As you are measuring along from Station to Station, you may take the Bearings of any remarkable Objects, such as Churches, Castles, Towers, &c. which may offer themselves to your View. Then to lay down the several Rivers, measure along the Sides thereof, beginning at their Entrance into the County, or at the Place of their Exit, and so pursuing the Course thereof, as far as the Limits of the County extend. The Method of the Field Book is the same as already shewn, Sect. 3 Book 8. As to the Method of Protracting, that is the same as already shewn in protracting the Survey of a Gentleman's Estate. FIG. 26.

As for Cities or Towns of Note, these must be distinguished in the Plan, by some particular Mark or Character, and the Name of the City, &c. written close beside it. But any Country-town or Village may be denoted in the Plan with a Point only, as thus ( ) and its Name placed close to it.

Roads that have Hedges on the Sides thereof, must be distinguished by black parallel Lines, but such as are open, and have no Hedges, Walls, &c on the Sides thereof, may be denoted by pricked Lines. If the Road go through a Wood, it must be distinguished in the Plan, by a Number of Trees drawn on all Sides thereof, or if it be a Road going over a Mountain, shadow the Mountain pretty strong at the Bottom, letting it grow lighter till you come to the Top.

Rills may be distinguished by small Lines, Brooks
by

by double Lines, and Rivers by several Lines, also the Name of the River must be inserted in the Plan

Having surveyed all the public Highroads, and Rivers of Note, you must in like Manner survey all private Roads, Bridle-roads, and Foot-paths; as also the several small Rills, Rivulets, &c. which being done, and neatly introduced into the Plan, will greatly tend to the Beauty and Ornament thereof. FIG. 26.

SECT. VI.

The Method of taking the Perspective of any Gentleman's Seat or Building.

BY Perspective we are to understand the Method of projecting upon any Plane, any Front, or Part of a Building, in such Sort that the Representation thereof upon the said Plane, shall be every Way similar to the Appearance of the Building itself. For the Magnitude of any Object is determined by Lines or Rays of Light proceeding therefrom, and meeting one another in the Eye of the Observer, where an Angle is formed either great or small, according to the Distance of the Object from us; hence it is, that every Object which appears under a great Angle, is always greater than one which appears under a less Angle, and the farther any Object is removed from the Eye, the less is the visual Angle, and vice versâ. It is also further to be observed, that the Shape of Objects will vary according to the different Planes they are projected upon, though the Distance from the Eye be be neverthelefs the fame, for the Reprefentation of the Front of any Houfe, &c upon a plane Parallel to itfelf, is quite different from that upon a plane Oblique thereto, as is evident from Fig 70, 71 where the Front *PK* is widely different from the Front *PQ*, being projected upon different Planes

Room will not permit me to handle this Subject in as copious a Manner as perhaps fome few of the Curious may expect, what I fhall here do, is to lay down a practical Method of Perfpective by the Theodolite only, without the Affiftance of any other Inftrument, except a Scale and Compaffes, a Sector, Protractor, and parallel Ruler, thefe being the Inftruments that every Surveyor either is, or ought to be equipped with.

Example I

Let *K a* reprefent a Building, the Perfpective of which is required to be taken from *T*, the Place of Obfervation, upon a Plane parallel to the Front *PK*. Fig. 70.

The Method of performing this by *Cole*'s beft new-improved Theodolite, is as follows

Find the Bearing of the Front *PK*, to which add or fubtract 90 Degrees, and you will have the directing Number, which keep, then remove your Theodolite to *T*, the Place of Obfervation, level it there, and bring the Index to the Beginning of the Divifions on the Limb, and the Inftrument being levelled as aforefaid, the Telefcope will ftand at the Beginning of the Divifions on the vertical Arch, then bring the Needle to the directing Number, and fecure the Inftrument in this Pofition, which is now adjufted and fit for Obfervation   Di-

Sect VI *of* Perspective 37)

Direct the Telescope to the Point *P* in the Building, and the Index will cut, among the Divisions on the Limb, 20 Feet, and on the vertical Arch 15 Feet. Depress the Telescope to *W*, and the Indices will cut the same as before on the Limb, and $6\frac{1}{4}$ Feet on the vertical Arch

Direct the Telescope to *K* in the Building, and the Index will cut on the vertical Arch $44\frac{1}{2}$ Feet. In like Manner direct the Telescope to *A, B, C, D, E, F, G, H, M, O, Q, N*, and the Indices will give on the Limb and the vertical Arch, as in the following Table.

For the returned Front *a W*, find as before the several Points *a, b, c, e, g, i, l, n, d, f, h, k, m, o*, whose Distances are as in the following Table. In like Manner you may find as many Points as you have Occasion for

To draw the Plan.

Draw *XT* and *CV* perpendicular to each other, let *C* denote the Center of the Plan or Picture, and *CV* the horizontal Line, from these two Lines must every Part of the Building be laid down, according to their apparent Distances therefrom

N.B. By the Center of the Plan or Picture is meant that Point in the Plane thereof, to which a Line drawn from the Eye is perpendicular to the said Plane.

Then make $CZ = 20$ Feet, and $CX = 15$, from *X* draw *XP* parallel to *CV*, and from *Z* draw *ZP* parallel to *XT*, to cut each other in *P*, whence the perspective Appearance of the Point *P* is found. In like Manner may the perspective Appearance of any other Point be found

Again, make $ZW (= CS) = 6\frac{1}{4}$ Feet, because the
Ob-

Obfervation was downwards, which gives the Point W, therefore the Line PW in the Plan, is the Reprefentation of the Line PW in the Building. Make ZA, ZB, ZC, ZD, equal their refpective Heights in the Table.

For the Point K, make $CL = 44\frac{1}{2}$, and through L draw ELK perpendicular to CV, alfo draw AE, BF, CG, &c. limiting the Tops and Bottoms of the Doors, Windows, &c. After this Method may every other Part of the Front PK be laid down.

For the returned Front aW, becaufe C is the Center of the Picture; draw PC, AC, BC, CC, DC, determining the Heights of the Windows, &c. The Points a, b, c, e, &c. may be all laid down according to their refpective Dimenfions in the Table, and fo the Breadths of the feveral Windows, &c. may be determined.

Thus may any other Window, Door, Chimney, &c. be laid down according to their apparent Magnitudes, without fo much as meafuring a fingle Line.

That this Compendium of Perfpective may be more ufeful and better underftood, I fhall infert a few neceffary Theorems of Dr *Brook Taylor*, felected from Page 155, 156, 157, of *Warner*'s Surveying.

THEOR. I. All the Lines of any Object (as in a Module or Building) which are parallel to one another, and to the Picture, will be reprefented by Parallels on the Picture.

THEOR. II. All Lines parallel to the Module or Building, which are perpendicular to the Picture, will, if continued run to the Center of the Picture, tho' thefe Parallels be or be not all in the fame Plane.

THEOR.

Sect. VI. *of* PERSPECTIVE. 381

THEOR. III All Lines in the Module or Building, perpendicular to the Plane of the Horizon, will be in the Picture perpendicular to the horizontal Line, and these three Theorems are sufficiently visible in the preceding Example.

THEOR. IV. All Lines in the Module or Building, parallel to one another, and to the Plane of the Horizon, but oblique to the Picture, will meet in some one Point of the horizontal Line CV. Thus the parallel Lines in the Front Wa, meet in the Point V, and those of the Front PQ, meet in the Point Y. These Points V and Y are (by Dr *Taylor*) called the vanishing Points of these Parallels.

THEOR. V. All the Lines of an Object which are parallel to one another, but oblique to the Picture, and not parallel to the Plane of the Horizon, will be represented by Lines meeting in a vanishing Point, found by the Intersection of the Picture and a Line drawn from the Eye parallel to those parallel Lines. But this vanishing Point will not be in the horizontal Line, but either above or below it.

THEOR. VI The Shadows of all parallel Lines made by the Intersection of the Sun's Rays, will, on the Ground, be parallel, and consequently in the Picture, either be parallel, as in Theor. I. or else meet at a Point in the horizontal Line, as in Theorem II.

The last Example may be performed another Way, by one of the best new-improved Theodolites, thus

The Bearing of the Front, and the directing Number being found as before, and the Instrument duly adjusted at T, by fixing the Index to 360 on the Limb, and the Telescope to 0° on the vertical Arch, and bringing the Needle to the directing Number; direct the Telescope to P in the Building, and the Index will cut on the Limb 21° 50', and the Telescope on the vertical Arch 16° 30', which enter as you see in Table II with the Mark ᴠ, denoting Elevation; then depress the Telescope to W, and the Indexes will give 21° 50' on the Limb, and 7° 00' on the vertical Arch, which because it is an Angle of Depression must be noted with the Mark ᴧ, after this Method take the Angles of $A, B, C, \&c$ I have, to avoid Confusion, only taken a few Angles, by which the Reader may readily discover how all the rest may be found.

To draw the Plan.

Through C the Center of the Picture draw CV the horizontal Line, and ICT perpendicular thereto; make $CT = CV =$ any Distance, according to the Size the Plan is to be With the Center of your Protractor at T, prick off the Angle $CTZ = 21°$ 50', and draw the Line TZ to cut the horizontal Line CV in Z; apply the Center of the Protractor to V, and lay down the Angle $XVC = 16°$ 30', draw VX to cut the perpendicular Line XT in X, through X draw XP parallel to CV, also from I draw ZP parallel to CX, to cut XP in P. After the same Manner may be found the Point W, with all the rest of the Points $A, B, C, \&c$ Fig. 70.

But this may be done more expeditiously by a Sector thus. Make $TC (= VC)$ a parallel Radius of 45 : 45 on the Line of Tangents, take the parallel Tangent of 21° 50' and set from C to Z, as also the parallel Tangent of 16° 30' and set from C to X; then the paral-

rallel Tangent of 16° 30′ and set from C to X, then the parallel Lines Z P, X P being drawn, will intersect each other in the Point P, after the same Manner may the other Points A, B, C, &c be found with Ease and Expedition.

TABLE I.

Horizon Distance	Vertical Distance	
20	15	P \
—	9¼	A \
—	6	B \
—	1	C \
—	3¼	D \
—	6	W /\
44½	9¼	E \
—	6	F \
—	1	G \
—	3¼	H /\
—	6	K /\

TABLE II.

Horizon Angles.	Vertical Angles.	
21° 50′	16° 30′	P \
— —	10 15	A \
— —	7 00	B \
— —	1 10	C \
— —	4 00	D /\
— —	7 00	W /\
42 00	10 15	E \
— —	7 00	F \
— —	1 10	G \
— —	4 00	H /\
— —	7 00	K /\

EXAMPLE II

Let aQ be a Gentleman's House, the Perspective of which is to be taken on a Plane oblique to the Fronts PQ, aW, from T the Place of Observation. FIG 71.

Plant the Theodolite and a Staff in the Line SW, which is the Ground Line of the Picture, or at equal Distances from it.

Note, If the Obliquity of the Plane of the Picture with either Front be given, the Ground Line of the Picture, in which (or parallel to which) the Instrument

ment and Staff are fixed, muft be fet off to make an Angle with the ground Line of the Front, equal to the Quantity of the given Obliquity. This done, find as before the directing Number, and plant your Theodolite at the defigned Station *T*, which adjuft as before in the laft Example. Direct the Telefcope to the feveral Points *P*, *A*, *B*, *W*, &c. in the Building, and the Indices will note among the Divifions on the Limb and vertical Arch, the Diftances of thefe Points.

To draw the Plan.

Affume any Point *C* for the Center of the Picture and draw *C V*, *C X* perpendicular to each other. Then lay down as before in the laft Example, the Line or Coin *PW*, with the feveral Points *A*, *B*, &c. and alfo the Line *a b*. Draw *P a*, *W b*, which produce till they meet in *V*, which is called the vanifhing Point. Alfo *PR*, *WQ* being produced, interfect each other in the vanifhing Point *T*, in the horizontal Line *VC* continued, then proceed with the Fronts *P Q*, *a W* as before in the laft Example, ufing the vanifhing Points as you did the Center of the Picture.

This may alfo be performed according to the fecond Method in the laft Example, only you muft find the Bearing and directing Number of the Ground Line of the Picture, inftead of the Front.

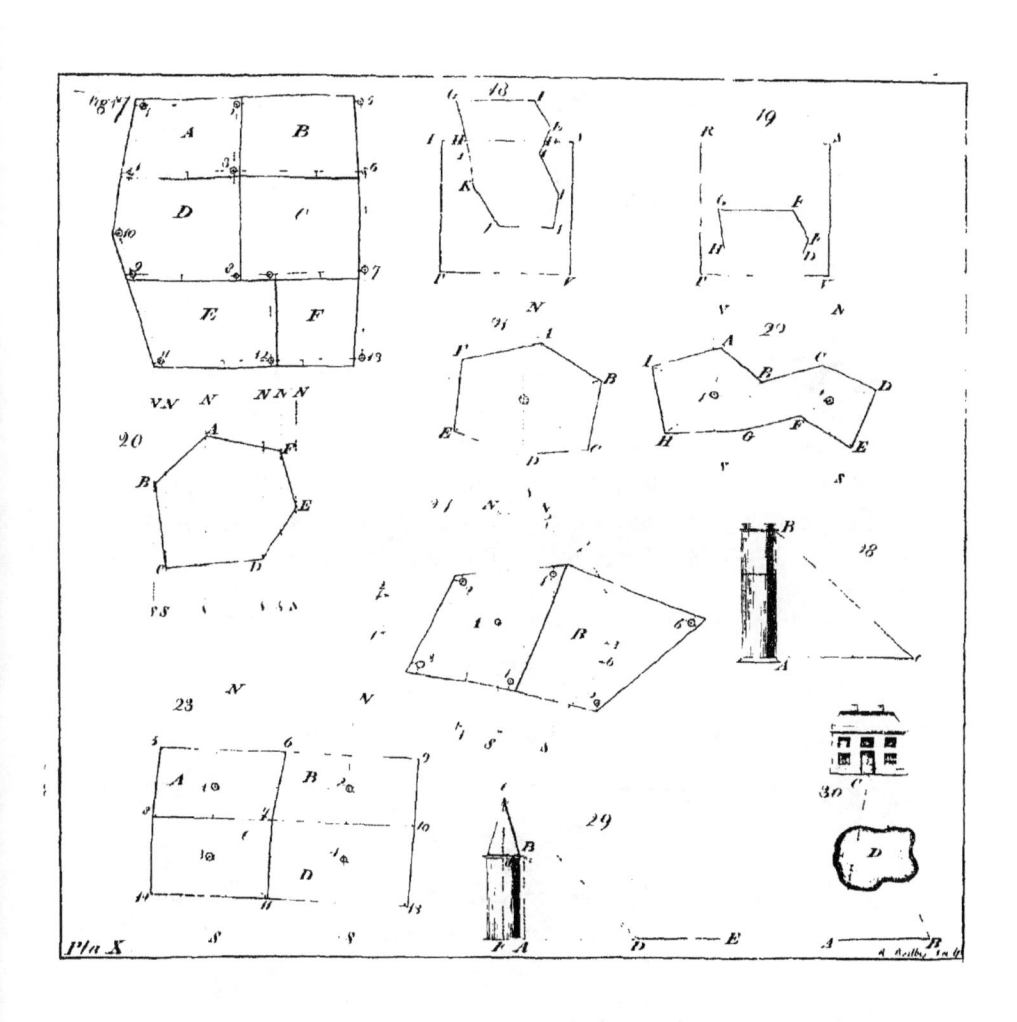

BOOK X.

Division of Ground in every Part, the Theory and Practice of Levelling; the Method of finding the Variation of the Compass, the Manner of Washing or Colouring of Maps or Plans

DEFINITION.

DIVISION of Ground is a very useful and necessary Branch of practical Surveying, teaching us to divide any Plot or Draught into any Number of Parts equal or unequal, according to any assigned Proportion, and according to the Quantity and Quality of the Ground about to be divided

SECT. I
Division of Ground in every Part.

PROP. I.

To reduce any Number of Acres, Roods, and Perches, into square Links.

RULE.

IF the Number of Roods given, be 1, 2, or 3, add 40, 80, or 120 to the given Number of Perches, that Sum multiply by 625 (= the square Links in one square

square Perch) that Product if it consists of 5 Places of Figures, write after the Acres, but if it doth not consist of so many Figures, the Deficiency must be supplied by annexing Cyphers on the left Hand; and then the same being placed after the Acres, will give the Number of square Links required

Example I.

Reduce 6 A 2 r 18 p into square Links
80 + 13 × 625 = 61250 square Links.
Then 661250 = square Links in 6 Acres 2 r. 18 p

Example II.

Reduce 4 A o r o8 p. into square Links.
8 × 625 = 5000, then o5000 placed after the 4, will give 405000 square Links.

Example III.

Reduce 10 A. o r. 1 p. into square Links
Ans. 1000625 square Links.

Example IV.

Reduce 18 A. 3 r 12 p into square Links.
Ans. 1882500 square Links

Prop. II.

To lay out any Number of Acres, &c (*suppose* 28 *Acres* 3 r. 24 p) *in Form of a Square* ABCD   Fig 39

Reduce the Acres, &c into square Links by Prop. I, extract the square Root of their Sum (= 2890000), whose

Sect. I.   DIVISION *of* GROUND.   387

whofe Root (= 1710) is the Side of the required Square, on which (by Prob IX Book I) draw a Square *ABCD*, and it is done.

PROP. III.

To lay out any Number of Acres (fuppofe 34 Acres 2 r. 1856 p) in Form of a Parallelogram ABCD whofe Length AD (= BC) = 2340 Links FIG 40

Divide the Area 34 Acr 3 r. 18·56 p. by the propofed Length 2340 Links, and the Quote 1490 will be the Breadth, with the Length 2340 and the Breadth 1490, draw (by Prob. X Book I) the Parallelogram *ABCD*. Or fuppofe the Breadth be given inftead of the Length, then the Area divided by the Breadth quotes the Length, by which you may draw the Parallelogram as above

PROP. IV.

To lay out any Number of Acres (fuppofe 13) in a Triangle ABC, having its Bafe AC given and equal to 25 Chains FIG 41.

Divide 260 fquare Chains (the double Area) by 25 Chains (the Length of the Bafe *AC*) and the Quotient 10·40 is the Length of the Perpendicular *BD*. Or fuppofe *BD* = 10 40 Chains given, then $\frac{260}{1040}$ = 25 Chains the Length of the Bafe *AC*, by which you may draw the Triangle *ABC*.

PROP. V.

388   DIVISION of GROUND.   Book X.

PROP. V.

To find a Triangular Field ABC *containing* 650 *square Chains, between two Persons* A, B, A *to have* 213, *and* B *the Remainder* 437, *let* A's *Part lie towards the Corner* A, *and* B's *next the Corner* C, *and both to enter at one Gate* B *in the Corner of the Field* FIG 42.

By the Sector.

Take AC in your Compasses, and make it a ‖ Radius to 650 650 on the Line of Lines, then take the ‖ Distance 213 213 and set from A to D, and draw the Line BD for the divisional Line of the Field, so shall the $\triangle ABD$ be $= 213$ Chains the Share of A, and the $\triangle DBC = 437$ the Share of B.

ARITHMETICALLY.

The Area being $= 650$, of which A is to have 213, and B the Remainder 437, therefore it will be, as the Area of the $\triangle ABC$ 650 Length of AC 52 Area of the $\triangle ABD$ 213 · Length of AD $17\frac{26}{650}$, then make $AD = 17\frac{26}{650}$, and draw the divisional Line or Hedge BD, as before

PROP VI.

Let ABC *be a Triangular Field, which is to be divided between two Persons* A, B, *and both to enter at one Gate,* D, *at or near the Middle of the Hedge* BC; *now suppose the Content of the Field* $=$ 2800000 *square Links, of which let* A *have* 800000, *and* B *the Remainder* 2000000. FIG. 43.

By

Sect. I.   DIVISION of GROUND.   389

By the Sector.

Draw DA from the Gate D to the opposite Corner A, also draw $EF \parallel$ to AD to cut AB in F, then draw DF for the divisional Line or Fence; so is the $\triangle DBF = 800000$ the Share of A, and the Trapezium $DFAC = 2000000$ the Share of B.

ARITHMETICALLY.

The Area of the Triangle ABC being found $= 2800000$, and the Area of the Triangle $DBF = 800000$ square Links, and the Length of $AB = 2400$ Links, $BD = 1000$, and $BC = 2360$, then will BE be $= \frac{800000}{2800000}$ of BC, but $\frac{800000}{2800000}$ is $= \frac{2}{7}$ in its least Terms, and therefore BE is $= \frac{2}{7}$ of BC, $= \frac{2}{7}$ of $2360 = 674\frac{2}{7}$, then to find the Point F to which the Line of Division is to be drawn, the Proportion is (by Prop. XII. Book II *Emerson*'s Geom) as $BC = 2360$ $BA = 2400$ $BE = 674\frac{2}{7}$ $BF = 1618\frac{2}{7}$; then make $BF = 1618\frac{2}{7}$, and draw the divisional Line DF, as before.

PROP. VII.

To divide a Field in Form of a $\triangle$ ABC, between two Persons A, B, *by a Line parallel to one of its Sides* AB, A *to have* 620000, *and* B *the Remainder* 1517500 *square Links.* FIG 47.

By the Sector.

As the divisional Line is to be parallel to AB it is plain it must cut the other two Sides AC, BC. Then (by Prop. V.) divide AC in Proportion as 2137500 620000,

620000, which will give the Point D. With $\frac{1}{2} AC$ for a Radius defcribe the Semicircle AEC, and from D erect the Perpendicular DE, to cut the Semicircle in E. Take CE in your Compaffes, and fet from C to F, alfo from F draw $FG \parallel AB$, which will cut BC in G, fo will the $\triangle CFG$ be $= 620000 =$ the Share of A, and the Trapezium $ABGF = 1517500$ fquare Links the Share of B.

ARITHMETICALLY.

Divide AC ($= 2850$) in Proportion as $2137500 : 620000$, which will give $CD = 826\frac{3}{4}$, then find a mean Proportion between 2850 ($= AC$) and $826\frac{3}{4}$ ($= CD$) which will be 1534.92 ($= CE$); then make $CF = 1534.92$, and draw FG as before.

Now to fet this off in the Field, meafure with your Chain from C towards A and B, and at the End of 1534.92 Links place a Mark F, as alfo at 1340 fet another Mark G, then run a ftraight Line between the two Marks, cutting an Hole in the Ground at the End of each Chain, &c. which will be a Guide for making the Fence.

PROP. VIII

Suppofe a Field in Form of the $\triangle$ ABC, *whofe Area is* $= 1925000$ *Acres, from one Side* ($=$ BC) *of which,* 752000 *Acres are to be fet off in a Trapezium, the divifional Line being to be drawn parallel to the Side* BC. FIG. 44.

By the Sector.

It is plain from the Figure, that the Line of Divifion

Sect. I.   DIVISION *of* GROUND.   391

sion will cut the Sides AB, AC. Then from the Area of the △ ABC (= 1935000) subtract the Area of the Trapezium $BCFG$ (= 752000) the Remainder 1183000 is the Area of the △ AGF.

Then divide AC in proportion as 1935000 : 1183000, which will give the Point D; then with $\frac{1}{2} AC$ for a Radius, describe the Semicircle AEC, and draw $DE \perp$ to AC, to cut the Semicircle in E; make $AF = AE$, and from F draw FG parallel to CB, to cut AB in G, compleating the Trapezium $BCFG$, whose Area is = 752000 Acres as was required.

ARITHMETICALLY.

From the Area of the △ ABC take the Area of the Trapezium $BCFG$, the Remainder is the Area of the △ AFG = 1183000, as above. Then divide AC (= 1800) in proportion as 1935000 : 118300, and you will have $1100\frac{22}{43}$ = Length of AD; also find a mean Proportion between 1800 (= AC) and $1100\frac{22}{43}$ (= AD) and you will have 1407, which set from A to F, and draw the Parallel FG.

PROP. IX.

Let ABC *be a triangular Field to be divided among five Persons in such Manner, that every one shall have the Benefit of a Fountain* D, *in the Hedge* AC; *required the Position of each Person's Share* FIG. 45.

Draw BD from the Corner B to the Fountain D, and divide the Base AC into five equal Parts in G, H, E, F, from each of those Points, and parallel to *BD*, draw *G I*, *H K*, *E L*, and *F M*, dividing the Sides of the △ in *I, K, L, M*, then from *D*, to each of these Points draw the Lines *D I*, *D K*, *D L*, and *D M*, which will divide the given △ *A B C* into five equal △s *A D I*, *I D K*, *K D L*, *L D M*, and *M D C*, each of which is the distinct Share of each Person.

Prop. X

Suppose a Field in Form of the Trapezium ABCE, *containing* 42 *Acres, which is to be divided between two Persons* A B, *A being to have* 12 *Acres, and* B 30, *and both to enter at one Gate* A, *A's Part or Share being to lie next the Hedge* AE. Fig 46.

Reduce the given Trapezium *ABCE*, by Prob. 21. Book 1 to the Triangle *EAF*. Divide the Base *EF* in proportion as 42 : 12 by Prop 5. which will give the Point *D*, to which draw the Line *AD*, so is the △ *ADE* = 12 Acres the Share of *A*, and the Trapezium *ABCD* = 30, the Share of *B*.

Prop. XI

Suppose a Field in Form of a Trapezium ABCD, *whose Content is* = 56·92500 *Acres, which is to be divided between two Persons* A, B, *by a Fence drawn from the Gate* F *where both Parties are to enter*, A *being to have* 33·35000 *Acres laid off towards the Side* AD. Fig 50.

Reduce *ABCD* to the △ *EFG* (by Prob. 21. Book 1) and divide the Base *EG* in proportion as 56·92500 : 33·35000 (by Prop 5) and draw the divi-

sional

Fig 25

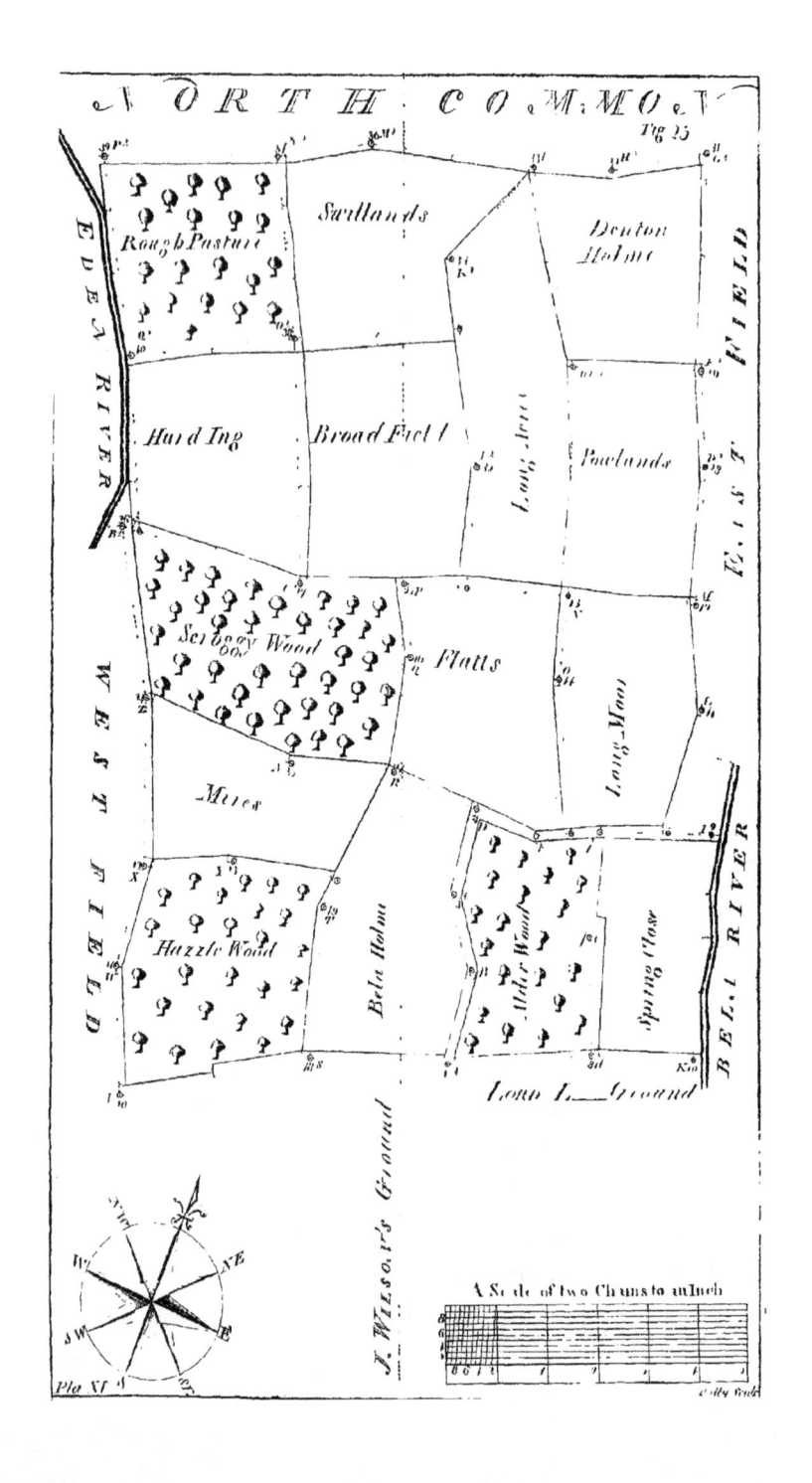

NORTH COMMON

Rough Pasture · Swillands · Denton Holme

Hard Ing · Broad Field · Long Acre · Powlands

EDEN RIVER

Scroggy Wood · Flatts · Long Moor

Mires

Hazzle Wood · Bela Holme · Alder Wood · Spring Close

WEST FIELD

EAST FIELD

BELA RIVER

J. Wilson's Ground

Long L— Ground

A Scale of two Chains to an Inch

fional Line FH, fo fhall the Trapezium $ADHF$ be $= 33.35000$ Acres the Share of A, and the Trapezium $FBCH = 23.57500$ Acres $=$ the Share of B.

Prop. XII.

Let A B C D E F G *be an irregular Parcel of Ground, whofe Area is* $= 110.42025$ *Acres, which is to be divided between two Perfons* A, B; *of which* A *is to have* 53.47025 *Acres, and* B *the Remainder* 56.95000; *the Line of Divifion to be drawn from the Corner* A, *and the* 53.47025 *Acres to be laid off next the Corner* B Fig. 48.

Firft divide the Plot into Triangles or Trapeziums; then beginning with the Trapezium $ABCD$, find the Area of it $= 41.80025$, which being lefs than $53.47025 (= A$'s Share) add thereto the Area of the next $\triangle ADE = 19.32000$, and the Sum 61.12025 being greater than 53.47025 by 7.65000, cut off from it (by Prop. 5) the $\triangle AEH$ whofe Area is $=$ that Excefs, fo is AH the true Line of Divifion, making $ABCDH = 53.47025$ Acres the Share of A, and $AHEFG = 56.95000$ Acres the Share of B.

Prop. XIII.

Let ABCDE *be a Field given, from which* 16.18500 *Acres are to be fet off in fuch Sort, that the Fountain* ☉ *at or near the Middle thereof, may be in common to both Parcels.* Fig 49.

The 16.18500 Acres being to be fet off towards the fide AB, draw a Line A ☉ for one of the divifional

fional Lines, then draw $B \odot$, and calculate the Area of the $\triangle A \odot B$ (by Prob. 28. Book 2) = 10 02000 Acres, which being less than 16 18500, add thereto the Area of the next $\triangle B \odot C$ = 9 42500, and the Sum 19 44500 being greater than 16 18500 (= the Acres required to be set off) cut off the Excess 3 26000 (by Prop. 5) from the $\triangle B \odot C$, and draw the divifional Line $\odot F$, so shall $ABF \odot$ be = 16 18500 Acres, as was required.

P R O P. XIV.

Let DEFG *be a Pasture belonging to three Persons* A, B, *and* C, *which is to be divided among them according to the Number of Grasses each Person hath Now suppose the whole Number of Grasses to be* 18, *of which* A *hath four,* B *six, and* C *eight, and the Ground upon View appears to be all of equal Goodness or Quality, required the Position and Number of Acres of each Person's Share.* FIG 51.

In a Work of this Kind the Surveyor must, along with the Proprietors (or Persons concerned in the Affair) walk over every Part of the Ground about to be surveyed, in order to examine the Qualities thereof. And if the Ground in every Part thereof, be found to be of equal Goodness (as we will suppose it to be in the present Case) then there is no more to be done, but to take a general Survey of the Whole, according to some of the Methods before given, a true Plan of which must be obtained, and the same carefully and accurately divided, as shall be shewn more fully hereafter. But if the Ground be found of different Qua-

lities

Sect. I DIVISION *of* GROUND.   395

lities (as it almost frequently is) then every Part must be staked out, and the whole surveyed as so many different Parcels or Inclosures, a true Plan of which must be drawn. Then let the Surveyor require the Proprietors or Commissioners, to value each of the different Parcels of Ground so staked out as above, and that they do it very judiciously. As to the Rates or Values, it is no ways material what Sums are made Use of, provided there be but a just Proportion, according to the Difference in the Qualities of the Ground, for it is all the same, whether the Rate be 5*l.* or 5*s.* or 5*d* per Acre, so as there be but a just Equality in the Ratios.

The Values or Rates being obtained, calculate by the Rule of Proportion, the Amounts of the Values of the several Parcels of Ground, according to their respective Rates, whose Sum shall be the Value of the Ground which is to be divided.

Then calculate each Person's Share of the said Value, which is readily done by the Rule of Proportion, saying as the Total of the Grasses &c. . Total of the Values . each Part its Grasses, &c. his Share of the Value or whole amount. Or thus, as the Total of the Grasses, &c. Total of the Values . 1 Grass, &c. its Share or Part of the whole amount. The Value or Share of Money belonging to 1 Grass being thus determined, if by it be multiplied each Person's Grasses, the Product will be his Share of the Value or Amount, according to his Grasses.

Each Persons proportional Share in Money being thus determined, the next Thing to be done is to give him Land equal in Value thereto, but before that can be be done, it muſt be conſidered in what Sort of Ground ſuch Share will fall, which being known, the Number of Acres thereto belonging may be readily found, by ſaying as the Total Value of the Ground ſuch Share ſhall fall in : the Acres contain'd therein . each Perſon's Share in Money . his Share in Land. Theſe ſeveral Shares thus diſcovered, muſt be ſet off in the Plan, as ſhall be ſhewn more fully hereafter.

But in the preſent Caſe, the Ground within the Plan is all of one Quality or Sort; therefore the Quantity is only to divide, without conſidering the Quality at all, and therefore ſuppoſing upon a Survey, the Content of the whole Paſture = 37·05650 Acres, then by the Rule of Three ſay, as 18 (= the Graſſes) 37·05650 (= Acres in the whole) . 4 (= *A*'s Graſſes) : 8·23478 (= *A*'s Share of Acres), in like manner *B*'s Share is found = 12·35216 Acres, and *C*'s = 16·46956 Acres, then 8·23478 + 12·35216 + 16·46956 = 37·05650, a Proof of the Calculation.

Then ſet off each Perſon's Share in the Plan thus. Draw a Line at Pleaſure through the Plan, as the Line *H I*, which muſt be ſo drawn, as that the Area of the Space cut off by it, may be as nearly equal as poſſible to the propoſed Quantity, that is, as near it as you can imagine, then compute the Area of the Part *D E H I* = 6·80258 Acres, which being leſs then 8·23478 (= *A*'s Share) by 1·43220, divide the ſaid Deficiency by 1540 (= Length of *H I*), and the Quotient is 93; then drawn *K I* ‖ to *H I*, at 93 Links Diſtance from it, which will be the diviſional Line in the Plan, ſufficiently near the Truth But to be more exact, find the Area of the Space *H I L K* = 1·42755; which being

ſome-

Sect. I.   DIVISION *of* GROUND.   397

somewhat lefs than 1·43220, divide the Difference 465 by the Length of $LK = 1530$, and the Quote 0·3 Links added to 93 (= the firft Breadth), the Sum 93·3 Links is the corrected Breadth; therefore if a Line KL be drawn parrallel to HI, at 93·3 Links diftance from it, it will be the true divifional Line in the Plan

Then for *B*'s Share, draw $PM \parallel KL$ at any fuppofed Diftance, and compute the Area of the Part $KLPM = 10·33616$ Acres, which being lefs than 12·35216 by 2·01600, draw another Line $RO \parallel PM$, and find the Area of the Part $PMOR = 3·39200$, which being greater than 2·01600 by 1·37600, divide the Excefs 1·37600 by 1600, ($= RO$) and the Quotient is 86; therefore draw $QN \parallel RO$ at the Diftance of 86, which is the Line of Divifion in the Plan. Then compute the Area of the remaining Part $NFGQ$, left for *C*, and if it amount to 1·646956 Acres, the Work of Divifion is truly performed, but if it amount to either more or lefs than 1·646956, there is a Miftake committed in the Work, which muft be corrected before you can have a true Plan.

The Plan being divided, the next Work is, to fet off the feveral Shares on the Ground, in doing of which there is not the leaft Difficulty, for taking your Plan into the Field or Pafture, meafure the Diftance in the Plan betwen ⊙1 and the Point $a = 525$ Links, then meafure in the Field from ⊙1 towards ⊙2, and at the Diftance 525 place a Mark, through which the divifional Line is to be drawn from another Mark hereafter to be placed on the oppofite Side of the Ground. Then meafure the Diftance in the Plan from ⊙3 to *b* = 200 Links, (*b* being the Point of Interfection between

the

the divisional Line $Q N$ and the traverse Line 2, 3, and in like manner as before, measure from ⊙3 in the Ground towards ⊙2, and at the End of 200 Links place a Mark in the Ground, by which the next divisional Line is to be drawn. After the same Manner measure the other Distances 8 c, 10 d, in the Plan, and fix Marks as before. Lastly run straight Lines across the Field between the Marks a, d, and b, c, making Holes and driving in Plugs at the End of every 2, 3, &c. Chains, so is the Work of Division fairly compleated.

If the Distances be such, as that the Mark d cannot be seen from the Mark a, or the Mark c from the Mark b, being prevented by the Interposition of some Hill, &c, then take your Theodolite and fix it up (suppose at a) in the Ground, and set the Index on the Limb to the Degree, &c. of the ∠ 1 a d, then directing the fixed Sights to ⊙1, look through the moveable Sights and order an Assistant to place a Poll in such Direction, that the vertical Hair shall cleave the same, then if you can from that Poll fairly discern the Mark d, continue the same straight Line thereto; but if the same cannot as yet be seen, then have Recourse to your Theodolite again, and proceed as before.

If it be a Theodolite of the best Sort, fix the Index to 360 on the Limb, and take a Back-sight to ⊙1, then fix the Index to the Degree, &c. of the ∠ 1 a d; and looking through the Telescope, direct your Assistant to place a Poll as before.

Note, When you make the general Survey observe to mark and Number every Station.

Having been very full and copious in this Prop. in demonstrating the best Method of Dividing of Ground

ac-

Sect. I.   DIVISION of GROUND.   399

according to Quantity and Quality, I shall therefore for the future be as concise as may be, inserting only the calculative Part of the Work.

PROP. XV

Let DEFG be a common Field, and the Property of three Persons A, B, C; which is to be divided among them according to the yearly Value of their Estates, now supposing A's Estate worth 25l. a Year, B's 35l. a Year, and C's 40l. a Year; required the Number of Acres each Person hath, and the Position of their Shares   FIG. 52.

The Content of the whole Field being = 33.42490 Acres, as found by a general Survey; and the Amount of the yearly Values of the Estates of A, B, and C, being = 100l.

Then $\frac{33.42490 \times 25}{100}$ = 8.35622 Acres = A's Part.

$\frac{33.42490 \times 35}{100}$ = 11.69872 Acres = B's Part.

$\frac{33.42490 \times 40}{100}$ = 13.36996 Acres = C's Part.

Then by the last Prop set off $DEHI$ (in the Plan) = 8.35622 Acres = A's Share, and $IHOP$ = 11.69872 Acres = B's Share; so will $POFG$ be = 13.36996 = C's Share.

The Plan being divided, set off each Person's Share in the Field, by Prop. 14.

PROP. XVI.

Let DEFG be a common Pasture, which is to be divided according to Quantity and Quality, among three

3 F   Persons

Perſons A, B, and C, *according to the Number of Graſſes each Perſon hath*, let A's Graſſes be 45, B's 34, *and* C's 21, *and the Ground of two Sorts; required the Poſition of each Perſon's Share* FIG 53.

Let $GLKF$ be 113 Acres, 2 r 30 7926 p = the Area of the better Sort of Ground, and $DEKL$ = 51 Acres, 1 r. 17 3624 p. = Area of the worſe Sort then 113 Acres, 2 r 30 7926 p + 51 Acres, 1 r 17 3624 p = 165 Acres, or 8 1550 p. = Area of the whole Paſture. Then 113 Acres, 2 r 30·7926 p. at 20 *l* an Acre, is = 2273 84907 2 *l*. = Value of the better Sort of Ground, and 51 Acres, 1 r 17 3624 p at 15 *l* an Acre, is = 770·377728 *l* = Value of the worſe Sort, then 2273 849072 + 770 377728 = 3044 22680 *l* = Value of the whole Paſture

Then 45 + 34 + 21 = 100 = Number of Graſſes; alſo $\frac{3044\ 22680 \times 45}{100}$ = 1369 90206 *l*. = A's Share of the whole Value, and $\frac{3044\ 22680 \times 34}{100}$ = 1035 037112 *l*. = B's Share, and laſtly $\frac{3044\ 22680 \times 21}{100}$ = 639 287628 *l* = C's Share. Now A's Part falling entirely among the good Land, $\frac{113\ 692453750 \times 1369\ 90206}{2273\ 849072}$ = 68 Acres, 1 r 29 2165 p = A's Part or Share = $GNMF$.

Then 2273 849072 — 1369 90206 = 903 947912 *l*. = remaining Part of the better Sort of Ground, which is leſs than 1035 037112 *l* (= B's Share of the Value) by 131 090100 *l* therefore $\frac{131\ 090100}{15}$ = 8 Acres, 2 r 38 2944 p which laid to the Part $NLKM$, will

give

Fig 26

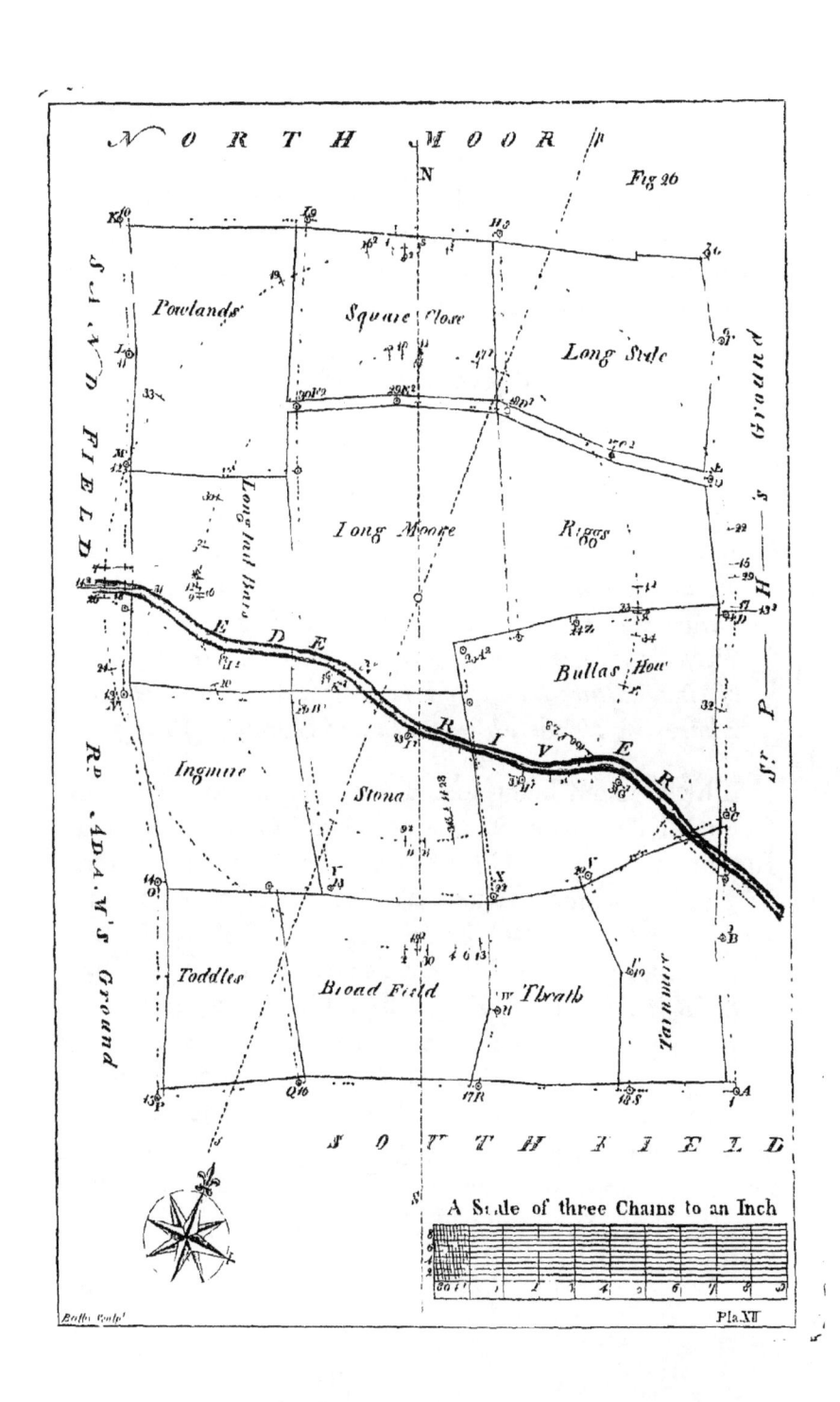

give 53 Acres, 3 r 29 8705 p. = *NIHM* = Share or Part of *B*   Then the remaining Part *IDEH* = 42 Acres, 2 r 19·0680 p. = the Share of *C*. The Plan being divided, set off each Person's share in the Ground, by Prop 14.

Prop. XVII

Suppose ABCD *a common Pasture, which is to be divided among five Persons according to the Quantity and Quality of the Ground. Let* A *have an Estate worth* 80l *a Year,* B *an Estate worth* 98l. *a Year,* C *an Estate worth* 37l. *a Year,* D *an Estate worth* 88l *a Year, and* E *an Estate worth* 97l *a Year, each Person's Share to be in Proportion to the yearly Value of his Estate, required the Position of the several Shares, with the Acres contained therein.* Fig. 54.

The Ground being staked out by the Proprietors or Commissioners, is of three Sorts, viz Good, Bad, and Indifferent, let *AEFGHD* be = 93 Acr   2 r. 17 6128 p. of good Land, also *EIKWH* = 79 Acr. 1 r. 2·9760 p. of bad Land; and *IBCZK* = 56 Acr. 3 r. 33·4848 p. of indifferent Land; then *AEFGHD* + *EIKWH* + *IBCZK* = *ABCD* = 229 Acr 3 r. 14 0736 p. Then 93 Acr. 2 r. 17·6128 p. at 20l an Acre, is 1872 2016 0l. = Value of the good Land, 79 Acr. 1 r 2·9760 p. at 10l. an Acre, is 792·68600l. = Value of the bad Land, and 56 Acr 3 r. 33 4848 p. at 15l an Acre, is 854 38920l = Value of the indifferent Land, whose Sum 3519 27680l = Value of the whole Pasture.

Then

Then $80 + 98 + 37 + 88 + 97 = 400$; and therefore $\frac{3519\cdot27680 \times 80}{400} = 703\cdot85536\,l. = A$'s Share of the Value, $\frac{3519\cdot27680 \times 98}{400} = 862\cdot22816\,l. = B$'s Share of the Value, $\frac{3519\cdot27680 \times 37}{400} = 325\cdot533104\,l. = C$'s Share of the Value, $\frac{3519\cdot27680 \times 88}{400} = 774\cdot240896\,l. = D$'s Share of the Value, $\frac{3519\cdot27680 \times 97}{400} = 853\cdot424624\,l. = E$'s Share of the Value; the Sum of these is $3519\cdot27680\,l.$ the same as before.

Then A's Part happening to be entirely among the good Land; $\frac{703\cdot85536}{20} = 35$ Acr. o r. 30·84288 p set off by Prop 14, will give $AMND =$ the Share of A.

After A's Share cometh in B's, therefore draw OP parallel to MN, as near as you can imagine where the divisional Line will fall: and as the said Line OP takes in two Sorts of Ground, viz. good Land and bad, find the Area of each Sort separately, and you will find $MEPN = 42$ Acres, 3 r. 32·822528 p and $EOV =$ o Acres, 1 r. 9·92000 p the Amount of these at their respective Rates of $20\,l.$ and $10\,l.$ per. Acre is $862\cdot22816\,l. =$ the proportioned Share of B. But if the said Amount had been greater or less then $862\cdot22816\,l$ then a Part must be taken from, or added to the Part first taken, and then find the Area and Amount as before; and if the Amount still differ from the proportioned Share required, add or deduct as before, 'till you make it correspond therewith.

Then, to lay off C's Share, draw QR, and find the Area of $VXRP = 13$ Acres, 3 r. 25·027392 p.
and

Sect. I.   DIVISION *of* GROUND.   403

and of $OQXV = 4$ Acres, 2 r 38·47488 p theAmount of these, according to the Rates of 20 *l*. and 10 *l*. an Acre, is 325·533104 *l*. = the proportioned Share of C, so shall $OQRP$ be = C's Share of Ground

For *D*'s Share, draw ST, so shall $QSTR$ consist of three Sorts of Ground, viz. $XGHR = 1$ Ac. 2 r. 8·92 p. $QSLZH = 68$ Acres, o r 14·558336 p and $LTZ = 4$ Acres, o r. 23·637344 p the Amount of these according to the Rates of 20 *l* 10 *l* and 15 *l*. per Acre, is = 774·240896 *l* = proportioned Share of *D*, so is $QSTR =$ *D*'s Share or Part set off

The remaining Part $SBCT$ is left for C, which consisteth of 6 Acres, or. 20·022784 p of bad Land (= $SIKL$), and 52 Acres, 3 r. 9·847456 p of indifferent Land (= $IBCTLK$), the Amount of these according to the Rates of 10 *l* and 15 *l*. per Acre, is 853·424624 *l*. = *E*'s proportioned Share of Money.

The several Shares of good Land, bad Land, and indifferent Land being summ'd up, are 93 Acres, 2 r. 17·6128 p. of good Land, 79 Acres, 1 r 2·9760 p. of bad Land, and 56 Acres, 3 r 33·4848 p of indifferent Land, which being equal to the Quantities first found, is an undoubted Proof of the Truth of the whole Performance.

The Plan being divided as above, lay off each Person's Share thereby in the Ground, according to Prop. 14

Before the Conclusion of this Sect. I shall give the Reader two Forms of Awards, used in the Division of Commons, &c.

The

The Award of the Division of the Common or Tract of Waste Ground, belonging to the Township of C——, commonly called C———— Moor.

To all to whom these presents shall come; We T—— I—— of P—— in the County of C—— Yeoman, L— F—— of T—— in the county of W—— Yeoman, and I—— G—— of A—— in the said County of W—— Gentleman, send greeting; Whereas there is a large Tract of Common or Waste Ground lying and being within the Manner of C—— in the Parish of B—— and County of W——, commonly called and known by the Name of C—— Moor, whereof R— M— of A— in the said County of Westmorland Clerk, is Lord, and L—— H——, I—— H——, the younger, R—— H——, I—— S——, H— A—— and Margaret his Wife, I—— A——, I—— W—— and Agnefs his Wife, I—— H—— the elder, L—— I——, H—— H——, R—— S——, I—— D——, and I—— P——, are severally poffeffed of Freehold or Customary Estates within the said Manner of C——, in Respect thereof, they are respectively entitled to Right of Common upon the said Tract of Common or Waste Ground as appendant or appurtenant to their said several Estates, and apprehending it would be a general Benefit to each and every of them, if the said Tract of Common, or Waste Ground was divided among them according to their several Rights, Privileges, and Emoluments thereon, so as each and every of them might have, hold, and enjoy their respective Rights and Interests in it severally, and might also hedge up and inclose the same, Did by

their

their Article of Agreement bearing Date the 22d Day of February 1768, feverally agree with each other, that the faid Tract of Common or Wafte Ground fhould be furveyed and divided among them, according to their refpective Rights, Privileges, and Emoluments thereon, fo as each Perfon interefted might enjoy his, her, or their refpective Rights in it feverally, and might alfo inclofe and improve the fame. And whereas they the faid R— M—, L— H—, I— H— the younger, R— H—, I— S—, H— A— and Mary his Wife, I— A— I— W—, and Agnes his Wife, I— H—, the elder, L— I—, H—— H——, R—— S——, I—— D——, and I—— P——, in order to carry the faid Divifion into Execution, did by their faid Article of Agreement among other Things covenant and agree with each other, to give and grant, and did thereby give and grant full Power and Authority to furvey, divide, fet out, and apportion to each and every of them their refpective Shares, Rights, Privileges, and Emoluments in and upon the faid Common or Wafte Ground, unto the faid T—— I——, L—— F——, and I—— G——, or any two of us, Referees indifferently chofen to furvey and divide the fame, and to fettle other Matters and Things touching the faid Divifion and Inclofure, as by the faid Article (Reference being thereunto had) may more fully and at large appear. Now know ye, that we the faid T— I——, L—— F——, and I—— G——, taking upon us the Burden of the faid Survey and Divifion, and the other Powers vefted in us by Virtue of the faid Article, and having fully confidered the Quantity, Conveniency, and Contiguity of each and every Part of

the

the said Common or Waste Ground, and also heard the Alligations of all and every of the said Proprietors, and caused a true and perfect Plan of the said Common or Waste Ground to be made, which is hereunto annexed, and declared by us to be Part of this our Award, do make and publish this our Award in Manner and Form following, that is to say, We do set out and apportion to each and every of them their respective Shares as followeth. Unto the said R—— M—— as Lord of the Manner of C——, and as such Owner of the Soil of the said Tract of Common or Waste Ground, in Lieu and full Satisfaction of his Right of Common which he hath upon the said Common or Tract of Waste Ground in Respect of his Demesne and other Lands lying and being within the said Manor of C—— (except such particular Rights and Privileges as are herein-after reserved unto him as Lord of the said Manor All those two Parts and Parcels of the said Common or Waste Ground, as the same are out on the said Common, and distinguished in the said Plan with the Letters *A, B*, containing together   Acres, Roods, and   Perches, the one of which said Parcels is bounded on the East by a Common or Tract of Waste Ground belonging to the Township of B——, on the South West by the antient Inclosures belonging to the Township of C——, and on the North West by the Share or Part herein-after set out unto the said I—— D——. The other of which said Parcels is bounded on the North East, by the said Common belonging to the Township of B——, and the antient inclosed Lands of the said L——H——, on the South East by the Shares herein-after set out unto the said L—— H——,

Sect. I.   DIVISION *of* GROUND.   407

H——, and I—— S——, on the South West by the River E——, and the antient inclosed Lands belonging to the Township of C——. Unto the said I—— D—— in Lieu and full Satisfaction of all his Common Right in and upon the said Common or Waste Ground, All that Part and Parcel thereof as the same is marked out on the said Common, and distinguished in the said Plan with the letter C, containing   Acres   Roods and   Perches, and bounded on the South East by the Share or Part herein-after set unto the said R —— M ——, on the North East by the said Common belonging to the Township of B——, on the North West, by the Share herein-after set out unto the said H——A——, and on the South West, by the ancient inclosed Lands belonging to the Township of C—— unto, &c.

   H —— A —— and Margaret his Wife, idem.
   I —— P ——, idem.
   R —— S ——, idem.
   L —— I ——, idem.
   H —— H ——, idem
   R —— H ——, idem.
   I —— H ——, idem.
   L —— H ——, idem.
   I —— H —— the younger, idem.
   I —— S ——, idem
   I —— W —— and Agnes his Wife, idem.
   I —— A ——, idem.

And we the said T—— I——, L—— F——, and I— G—, do order, direct, and appoint that there be a Road eleven Yards broad (exclusive of Ditches) from the Gate called G—— Gate leading on to the said Common, along the high End or South East End of the

3 G   antient

antient Inclosures belonging to the said Township of C———, untill it arrive at the Share herein before set out unto the said L——— I———, as the same is described in the said Plan with the Letter *A* to the Letter *B*, for the Use and Benefit of the several Persons, their Heirs and Assigns, who have Shares or antient inclosed Lands abutting or joining upon the same, and also for the Use of the said L——— I——— his Heirs and Assigns to occupy the Share herein-before set out unto him. And also that there be a Road from the said Gate called G——— Gate, through the Share of the said R——— M——— untill it arrive at a Parcel of antient inclosed Land belonging to the said L——— H——— his Heirs, and Assigns to occupy the said Parcel of Ground, as the same is described in the said Plan from the Letter ( ) to the Letter ( ), and also that there be a common foot Road from the Road herein before first set out, through the Share of the said I——— D——— along the North West Side thereof, until it arrive at the said Common called B——— Moor, as the same is described in the said Plan from the Letter ( ) to the Letter ( ) and also that there be a common High Road from the Turnpike Road twenty Yards broad (exclusive of Ditches) to the said Common called B———Moor, between the Shares of the said R——— M———, and L———H———, as the same is set out on the said Common, and described in the said Plan from the Letter ( ) to the Letter ( ), and also that there be a common High Road eleven Yards broad (exclusive of Ditches) from the said Turnpike Road to the South East Corner of the Share herein-before set out unto the said L——— A———, and from thence along the East or South East Side of the said I——— A———'s

Fig. 27

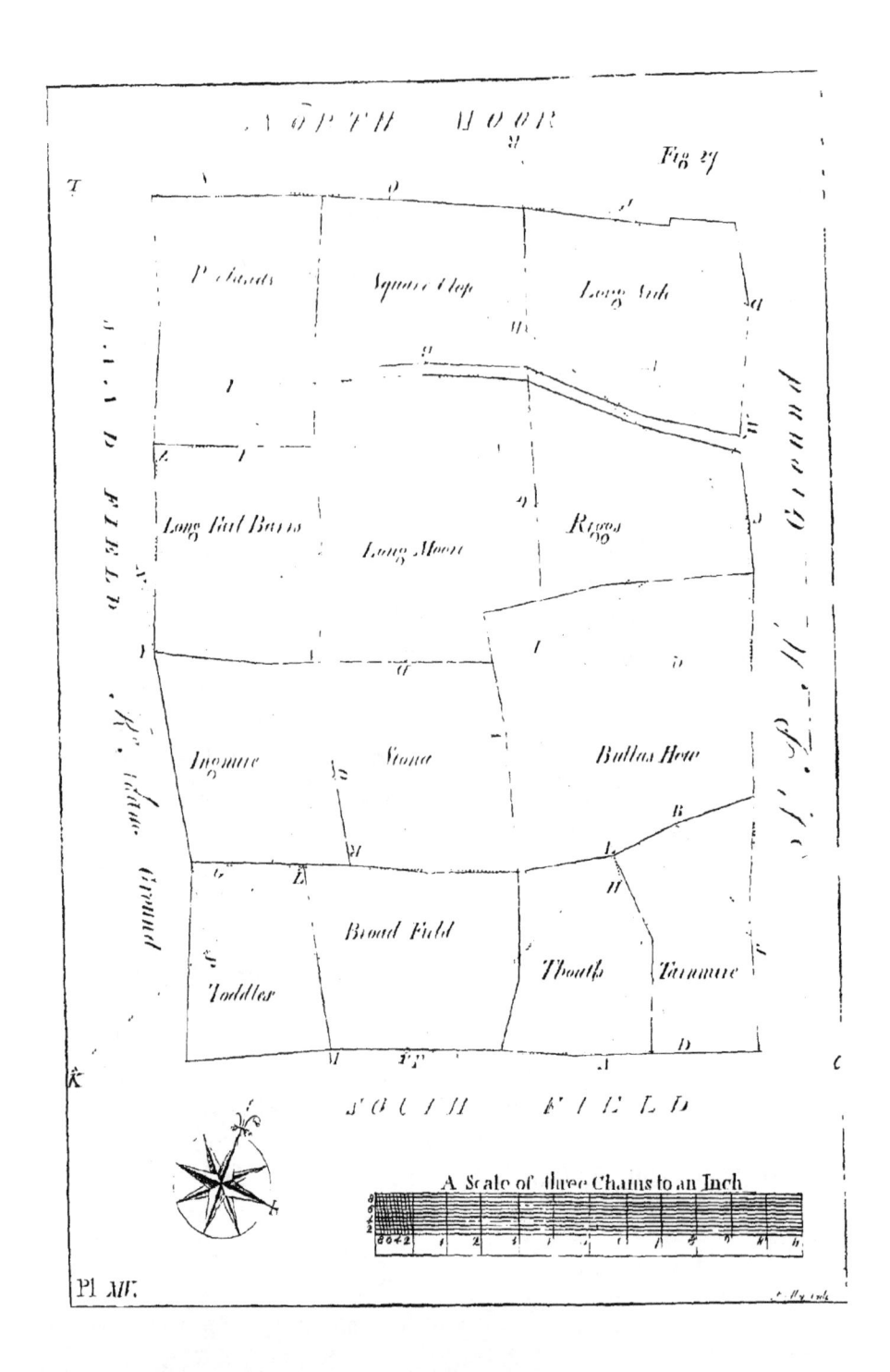

NORTH MOOR

Pighteads | Square Flat | Long Sick

Long Flat Butts | Long Moor | Riggs

Inemire | Stone | Bullas How

Toddles | Broad Field | Thoath | Tarnmire

SOUTH FIELD

A Scale of three Chains to an Inch

Pl. IV.

Sect. I. DIVISION *of* GROUND. 409

A ——'s Share, until it arrive at the North East Corner thereof, and from thence along the North West End of the said Share, until it arrive near the North West Corner of the said Share, and from thence along the old Road to the River E ——, as the same is set out on the said Common, and described in the said Plan from the Letter ( ) to the Letter ( ), and so to the Letter ( ), and so to the Letter ( ), and so to the Letter ( ), and also that there be a sufficient Road seven Yards broad, from the Road last set out, through that Part of the Share herein-before set out for the said R —— M ——, adjoining O ——'s Farm, until it arrive at the Inclosures called E ——, and from thence along the Side of the said Inclosures until each Person who has antient Fields lying there, can go into their several Inclosures, as the same is described in the said Plan, from the Letter ( ) to the Letter ( ), and so to the Letter ( ), and so to the Letter ( ), and so to the Letter ( ), for the occupying the said Fields, but for no other Use, Intent or Purpose whatsoever. And also that there be an Occupation Road from the above Road, leading down the East or North East Side of the Share herein before set out unto the said I —— A ——, for the occupying such antient inclosed Lands belonging to the Township of C ——, as lie adjoining upon the North West Side of the said I —— A ——'s Share, as the same is described in the said Plan, from the Letter ( ) to the Letter ( ), and also that there be an Occupation Road five Yards and a half broad, through a small Parcel of the said Common herein-before set out unto the said I —— H —— from S —— House belonging to the said L —— H ——, along the North East End of an antient Inclosure belonging to the said I —— H ——, to an

3 G 2 Inclo-

Inclosure belonging to the said L—— H——, for the Benefit of the said L—— H—— his Heirs and Assigns to be used on all Occasions as an Occupation Road, but for no other Use or Purpose whatsoever, as the same is described in the said Plan, from the Letter ( ) to the Letter ( ); and that all the Public Roads herein-before set out, be for ever hereafter maintained and repaired in such Manner, and by such Ways and Means as the Law in that Case hath provided, and that all the Occupation Ways be for ever hereafter maintained and repaired by the several Persons, their Heirs and Assigns, who have Lands herein-before set out unto them, in Proportion to their Properties in the said Premises And we the said T—— I——, L—— F——, and I—— G——, do hereby order, direct and appoint that the said R—— M—— his Heirs and Assigns do make, erect, and set up good and sufficient new Ditches, Hedges, or Fences upon the said Common between his Share and B—— Moor, and between his Share and the Share of the said I—— D——, and also between his Share and the Share of the said I—— S——, and also between his Share and all Places where he adjoins upon any High Road herein before set out, as the same is marked in the said Plan with the Letter ( ), and plant the same with good Quick Thorn Plants, after the Proportion of five to each Yard (if he make the said Fences of Earth); and that he, his Heirs or Assigns, for ever hereafter maintain and repair the same that Mr D—— make between his Share and B——Moor, and between his Share and H——A——'s Share; that H——A—— and Margaret his Wife make between their Share and B——Moor, and P——'s Share that

I——

Sect I. DIVISION *of* GROUND. 411

I——P——make between his Share and the Share of W——S——, and B——Moor That L—I— make between his Share on the North West Side and Mr H———'s Share, and Brampton Moor: That Mr H—— of Bondgate, make between his Share and the Turnpike Road, and between his Share and R———H———'s Share, and B——— Moor, and down the Syke between his Share and that of L———I———: That R———H——— make between his Share and the Turnpike Road, and also between his Share and B———Moor, and between his and I———H———'s Share: That I———H——— make between his Share and the Turnpike Road, and B——— Moor, and Mr L———H———'s Share, and also between his Share and Mr L———H———'s Share, and the Turnpike Road where the small Piece is set out to, on the West Side of the Turnpike Road That L———H———make wherever he adjoins upon any Roads, and between his Share and B———Moor, and between his Share and the Share of the said I———A———: That I———S——— make between his Share and Mr L———H———'s Share, and wherever he adjoins upon any Road. An we the said T— I—, L—F—, and I—G———, do also order, direct and appoint that such of the abovesaid Hedges, Ditches, or Fences as are to be made of Earth and planted with good Quick-Thorn Plants of five to each Yard, be erected and made on or before the 1st Day of April 1769, and be all set upon the Grounds of the several Persons who are herein before ordered to erect the same, without any Allowance from his Neighbours for, or in Respect of any Hedge or Ditch thereto belonging And that no Goods of any Kind be turned loose into any of the abovesaid Lanes, but that the Grass
grow-

growing therein be from Time to Time eaten in such Manner, and by such Ways and Means, as a Majority in Value of the said Proprietors, their Heirs or Assigns, shall order and direct And whereas in the abovesaid Article of Argument it is provided, that the abovesaid Division, or any Thing therein contained, shall not extend, or be construed to extend to defeat, lessen or prejudice the Right, Title, or Interest of the said R———— M————, his Heirs or Assigns, as Lord of the Seigniories and Royalties incident and belonging to the same Manor, but that the said R———— M————, his Heirs and Assignees, shall and may from Time to Time and at all Times for ever hereafter hold and enjoy all Rents, Services, Courts, Perquisites, and Profits of Courts, Goods and Chattles of Felons and Fugitives, Dividends, Waifs, Estrays, and all other Royalties, Privileges, and Appurtenances, as Lord of the said Manor, incident or appendant, belonging or appertaining, in as full and ample Manner as he the said R———— M————, his Heirs and Assigns could or might have held the same in Case such Agreement or the said intended Division had never been made We the said T———— I——, L—— F————, and I———— G————, do order, direct and appoint that nothing herein contained, or in the above Division, shall be construed, deemed, or taken to deprive the said Lord of C————for the Time being, his Heirs or Assigns, or any of them, of any of the Rights, Privileges, Franchises, Royalties, or other Emoluments to him or them belonging, but that the said Lord or Lords of the said Manor enjoy all the above Manerial Rights in as full, large, and ample Manner as if no Division of the above Premises had ever taken Place (any Thing herein contained to the contrary thereof

in

Sect. I.   DIVISION *of* GROUND.   413

in any wife notwithstanding). And we do also order, direct, and appoint, that immediately after the signing of this our Award, all Right of Common upon the abovesaid Premises shall cease, and all and every the abovesaid Persons, and their Heirs and Assigns, who have Shares herein-before set out unto them, shall enjoy the same in Lieu and full Satisfaction and Compensation of all Right of Common heretofore used and enjoyed by them or any of them, or by their or any of their Ancestors And that all and every of the abovesaid Persons do severally and respectively release to each other all Rights and Privileges upon all and every Part of the said Premises (except the Share or Part herein before severally set out unto them, and that the said R—— M—— do convey all and every the above Shares herein-before respectively set out unto the abovesaid Persons to hold severally to them, their Heirs and Assigns for ever, in Fee Simple, reserving to himself as Lord of the said Manor, all the above Manerial Rights, in as full and ample Manner as if no Division of the Premises had ever taken Place And whereas in the above said Article it is agreed by and between the said R—— M——, Lessee of the Tythes of C——, under the Dean and Chapter of C——, and the said several Proprietors who have Shares herein-before set out unto them, that the abovesaid Premises shall be free and clear of and from the great Tithe of Corn, for and during the Term of six Years from the signing of this our Award, and that the said Proprietors should pay such a Sum as is stipulated in the said Article for the said Tithe of the Township of C—— for and during the said Term of six Years We do therefore in

Pur-

Purfuance of the faid Article, order, direct, and appoint that the faid Premifes, as alfo the Townfhip of C—— be freed, difcharged, and exonerated of and from the faid Tithe for and during the Term aforefaid, and that the faid Proprietors or Land-Owners do give Security to the faid R—— M—— (if required) for the Payment of fuch Sum as is ftipulated in the faid Article, in Lieu of the Tithe, as well of the antient inclofed Lands, as of the faid Common lately divided   And we do alfo order, direct, and appoint that no Sheep be put into any Part of the Premifes hereinbefore fet out and divided, for and during the Term of nine Years from the Date of thefe Prefents. And laftly, we do afcertain the Cofts of furveying, dividing, fetting out and apportioning the above Premifes to each and every of the Proprietors, and of every other Matter and Thing relating to the fame, at the Sum of   and do order
within the Space of   from the Date hereof, to collect the fame from the above Proprietors, in Proportion to their refpective Rights and Properties in the above Premifes, and they to pay the fame when due and owing; In Witnefs whereof &c. &c.

The

Sect I.   DIVISION of GROUND.   415

The Award of the Division of the Common Pasture called D—— W——, situate in the Parish of D—— and County of W——.

To all to whom these Presents shall come; We A—— H—— of C——, in the Parish of K——, and County of C——, Clerk, and T—— I—— of P—— in the Parish of P——, and County aforesaid, Gentleman, send greeting. Whereas W—— W——, Esq, I—— F——, E—— E——, R—— B——, I—— E—— Son of T——, T—— W——, I—— E—— Son of W——, W—— R——, M—— A——, I—— P——, W—— D——, F—— H——, T—— Y——, R—— D——, I—— E——, W—— R——, and W—— R—— the younger, being jointly seized and possessed of a large Tract or Parcel of Ground or stinted Pasture called D—— W——, lying and being in the Parish of D——, and County of W——, and having enjoyed the same by stinting, according to the respective Number of Cattle-gaits they severally possess therein, and apprehending it would be a general Benefit or Advantage to all the Persons interested, if the said Parcel of Ground or stinted Pasture called D—— W——, was divided among them according to their respective Rights, Privileges and Emoluments therein, so as each Person might have, hold, and enjoy their respective Rights, and Interests therein severally, and might also hedge up and inclose the same, did by their Articles of Agreement, bearing Date the thirtieth Day of November, in the Year of our Lord one Thousand seven Hundred and sixty-three, severally agree with each other, that the said Pasture called D—— W—— should with all

3 H   con-

convenient speed be surveyed, and divided among them according to their respective Rights, Privileges, and Emoluments therein, so as each Person interested might enjoy his, her, or their respective Rights and Privileges therein severally, and might also inclose and improve the same. And whereas they the said W——— W———, &c. in order to carry the said Division into Execution, did by their said Articles of Agreement, among other Things covenant and agree with each other, to give and grant, and did thereby give and grant full Power and Authority to survey, divide, set out, and apportion to each and every of them, their respective Shares, Rights, Privileges and Emoluments in and upon the said Pasture, unto us the said A——— H———, and T——— I———, Referees indifferently chosen to survey and divide the same, (due regard by us being had to the Quantity and Quality of the same) and other Matters and Things touching the Division of the said Pasture, as by the said Articles (Reference being thereunto had) may more fully and at large appear. Now know ye that we the said A——— H——— and T——— I——— taking upon us the Burden of the said Survey and Division, and the other Powers vested in us by Virtue of the said Articles, and having fully considered the Quantity, Quality, Convenience and Contiguity of each and every Part of the said Parcel of Ground or stinted Pasture, and also heard the Allegations of all and every of the said Proprietors, and caused a true and perfect Plan of the said Pasture to be made, which is hereunto annexed, and declared by us to be Part of this our Award, Do make and publish this our Award in Manner and Form following, that is to say, We do set

our

Fig. 70

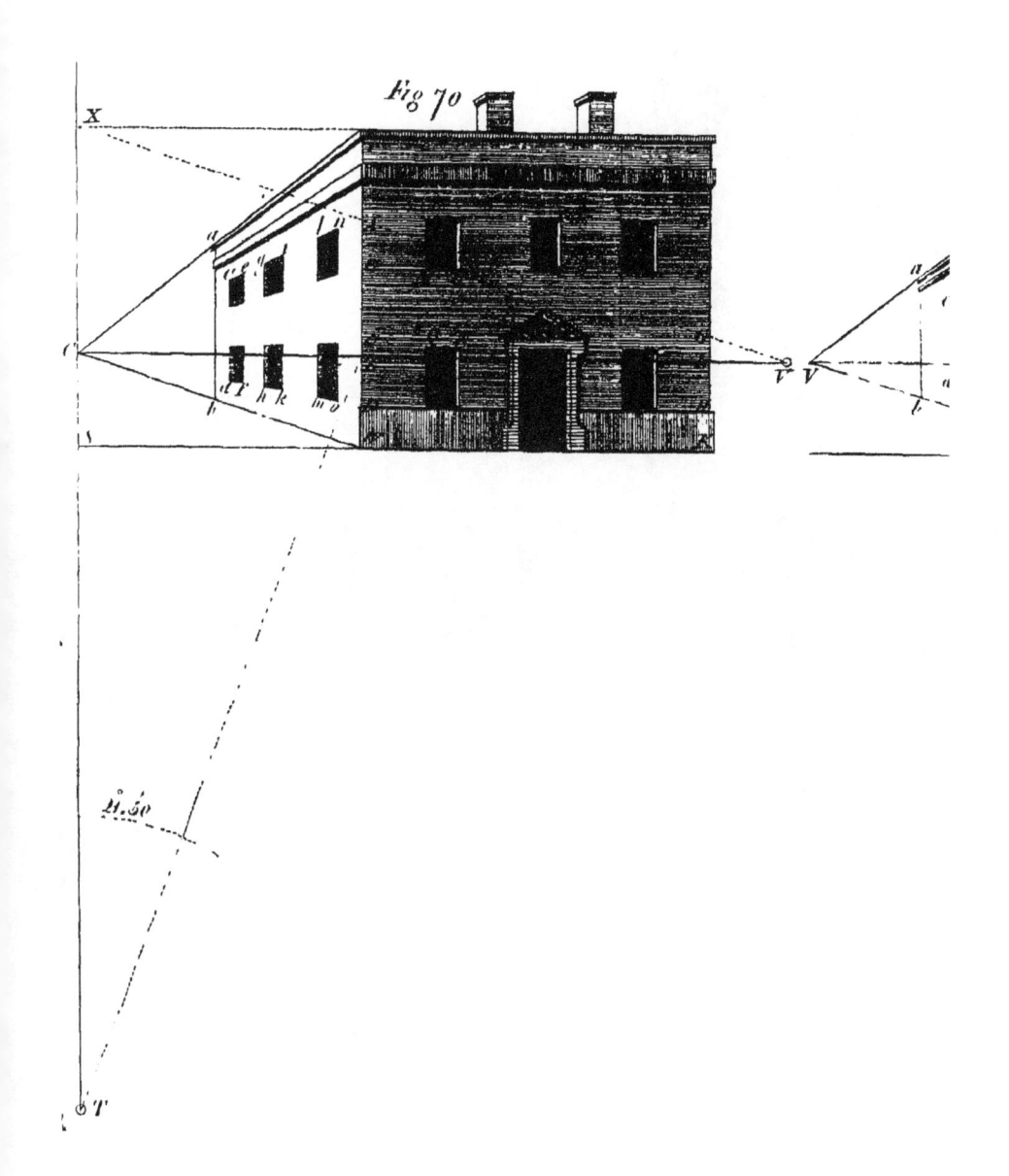

Pla. XVII.

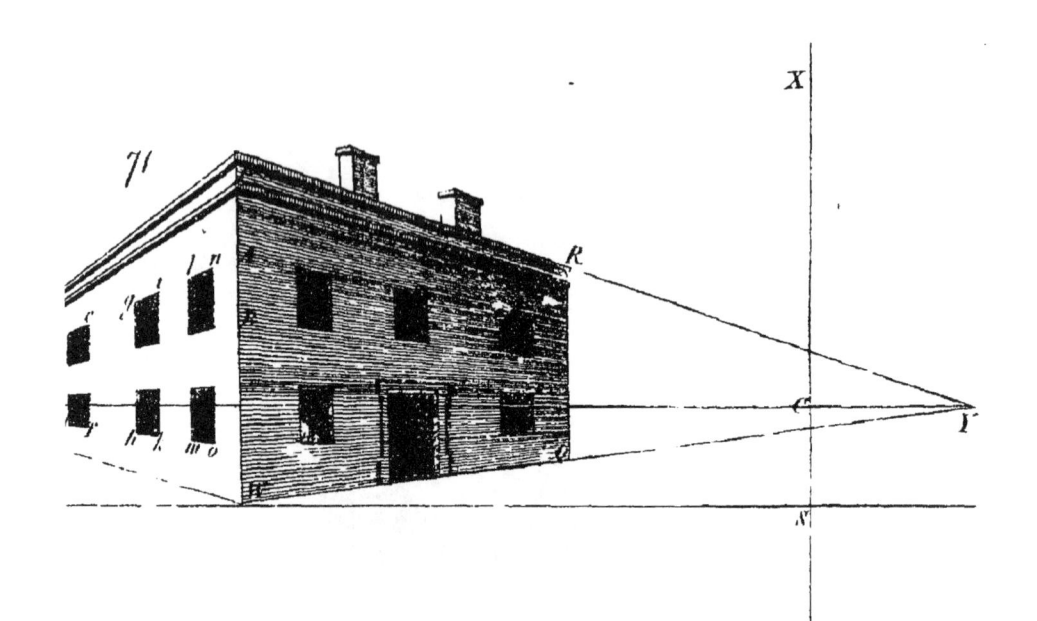

Sect I   DIVISION *of* GROUND.   417

out and apportion to each and every of them their respective Shares as followeth. Unto the said W—— W——, Esq, as Owner of 50½ Cattlegaits in and upon the said stinted Pasture in Lieu and full Satisfaction thereof, and of all his Right, Title, Interest and Privilege thereon (except a divided Share of a Moss in the said Pasture, and all Rents, Royalties, Franchises, Rights, Privileges, and Jurisdictions heretofore or now due, or payable to the said W—— W——, as Lord of the Manor of D—— aforesaid, out of, in, or from the said Pasture called D—— W——, as the same is set out on the said Pasture, and marked in the same Plan with the Letter *A*, containing   Acres, &c and bounded on the *N E.* and *S E.* by the ancient inclosed Grounds of the said W—— W——, Esq, on the *S W.* by the Common and inclosed Grounds belonging to the Township of B——, and on the *N W.* by the Road herein-after set out Unto the said I—— E——, the elder, as Owner of two Cattlegaits in and upon the said stinted Pasture, in Lieu and full Satisfaction thereof, and of all his Right, Title, Interest and Privilege thereof (except as is herein-after set forth) all that Part or Parcel thereof as the same is set out on the said Pasture, and marked in the said Plan with the Letter *B*, containing   Acres   Roods   Perches, and bounded on the *N. E* by the ancient inclosed Lands of the said W—— W——, Esq, on the *S E* by the aforesaid Road, on the *S. W.* by the Share or Part herein after set out to the said I—— E——, on the *N W* by a Part of the said Pasture herein-after set out for a Free-stone Quarry: Unto the said I—— E——, the Son of W——, as Owner of two Cattlegaits in and

3 H 2   upon

upon the said stinted Pasture, in Lieu and full Satisfaction thereof, and of all his Right, Title, Interest and Privilege therein (except as is hereafter set forth) all that Part or Parcel thereof, as the same is set out on the said Pasture, and marked in the said Plan with the Letter *C,* containing   Acres, and bounded on the *N E* by the Share or Part herein-before set out unto the said I—— E——, on the *S. E.* by the said Road, on the *S W.* by the Share or Part herein-after set out unto the said F—— H——, on the *N. W.* by a Part of the said Pasture herein-after set out for a Free-stone Quarry · Unto the said F—— H——, as Owner of two Cattlegaits in and upon the said stinted Pasture, in Lieu and full Satisfaction thereof, and of all his Right, Title, Interest, and Privilege thereon (except as is herein-after set forth) all that Part or Parcel thereof, as the same is set out on the said Pasture, and marked in the said Plan with the Letter *D,* containing   Acres, and bounded on the *S E* by the abovesaid Road, on the *N. E.* by the Share or Part herein-before set out unto the said I—— E—— the elder, and E —— Son of W——, on the *N. W.* by the Rivulet called M—— Beck, or a stinted Pasture callest M—— Park, on the *S W* by the Share or Part herein-after set out to the said E—— E——. Unto the said E—— E——, as Owner of four Cattlegaits in and upon the said stinted Pasture in Lieu and full Satisfaction thereof, and of all his Right, Title, Interest, and Privilege thereon (except what is herein-after set forth) all that Part or Parcel thereof as the same is set out in the said Pasture, and marked on the said Plan with the Letter *E,* containing   Acres, &c and bounded on the *S. W.* by the

Share

Share or Part herein-after set out unto the said W―― D――, on the *N W* by the abovesaid M―― P――, or Rivulet called M―― Beck; on the *N E.* by the Share or Part herein-before set out unto the said F―― H――, on the *S E* by the above Road, Unto the said W―― D――, as Owner of three Cattlegaits in and upon the said stinted Pasture, in Lieu and full Satisfaction thereof, and of all his Right, Title, Interest, and Privilege therein (except what is herein-after set forth) all that Part or Parcel thereof, as the same is set out on the said Pasture, and marked on the said Plan with the Letter *F*, containing   Acres, and bounded on the *S E.* by the above said Road, on the *S W* by the Share or Part herein-after set out unto the said I―― F――; on the *N W* by the abovesaid M―― Beck or M―― Park, on the *N E* by the Share herein-before set out unto the said E―― E――. Unto the said I―― F――, as Owner of six Cattlegaits in and upon the said stinted Pasture, in Lieu and full Satisfaction thereof, and of all his Right, Title, Interest, and Privilege thereon (except as is herein-after set out) all that Part or Parcel thereof, as the same is set out on the said Pasture, and marked on the said Plan with the Letter *G*, containing   Acres, &c and bounded on the *N. E.* by the Share or Part herein-before set out unto the said W―― D――, on the *N W.* by the said M―― Beck and M―― Park and the ancient inclosed Lands of the said W―― W――, Esq, and W―― E――, on the *S W.* by the Share or Part herein-after set out unto the said R―― D――; on the *E* by the abovesaid Road, on the *S. E.* on one Part by the

above-

above-said Road, and on another Part by Part of the Share herein-after set out unto the said W—— R—— the younger and M—— A—— Unto the abovesaid R—— D—— as owner of two Cattle-gaits in and upon the said stinted Pasture, in Lieu and full Satisfaction thereof, and of all his Right, Title, Interest, and Privilege thereon (except what is herein-after set out) all that Part or Parcel thereof, as the same is set out on the said Pasture, and marked on the said Plan with the Letter *H,* containing   Acres, &c and bounded on the *N E* by the Share or Part herein-before set out unto the said I—— F——, on the *S. E.* by Part of the Share herein-after set out unto the said W—— R—— the younger, and M—— A——; on the *S. W.* by the Share or Part herein-after set out unto the said W—— R——, on the *N. W.* by an ancient Inclosure called M——: And whereas the said T—— Y—— and R—— B—— each Owner of two Cattle-gaits upon the said stinted Pasture, have since the signing of the abovesaid Articles, agreed to let their Shares or Proportions lie together undivided, We do therefore set out to them as Owners of four Cattle-gaits in and upon the said stinted Pasture, in Lieu and full Satisfaction thereof, and of their Rights, Titles, Interests, and Privileges thereon (except what is herein-after set out) all that Part or Parcel thereof, as the same is set out on the said Pasture, and marked on the said Plan with the Letter *I,* containing   Acres, &c. and bounded on the *S* and *S. W.* by the Common and ancient inclosed Lands of B—— aforesaid, on the *N.* by that Part of the said Pasture formerly divided among the Proprietors of Cattle-gaits in the said Pasture,

and

Sect I.   DIVISION *of* GROUND.   421

and set apart and used as a Peat-moss, on the *E.* by Part of the Share herein-after set out unto the said W—— R—— the younger, and M—— A——, and the abovesaid Road: And whereas since the signing of the abovesaid Article, the said W—— R—— as Owner of two Cattle-gaits, and the said M—— A—— as Owner of three Cattle-gaits, have agreed to let their Shares lie together undivided, we do therefore set out to them as owners of five Cattle-gaits in and upon the said stinted Pasture, in Lieu and full Satisfaction thereof, and of all their Rights, Titles, Interests, and Privileges thereon (except what is herein-after set out) all that Part or Parcel thereof as the same is set out on the said Pasture, and marked in the said Plan with the Letter *K*, containing   Acres, &c and one Part of it bounded on the *E.* and *S. E* by the abovesaid Road, on the *S W.* by the abovesaid Moss and Share herein before set out unto the said T—— Y—— and R—— B——, on the *N. W.* by the Share or Part hereinafter set out unto the said W—— R——, the other Part bounded on the *E.* and *S E* by the above-said Road; on the *N W.* by the Shares herein-before set out unto the said I—— F—— and R—— D——, and on the *S. W* by the Share or Part herein-after set out unto the said W—— R——, and adjoining upon the first Part herein-before set out to the said W—— R—— and M—— A——. Unto the said W—— R——, as Owner of five Cattle-gaits, in and upon the said stinted Pasture, in Lieu and full Satisfaction thereof, and of his Right, Title, Interest, and Privilege thereon (except what is herein-after set out) all that Part or Parcel thereof, as the same is set out on the

said

said Pasture, and marked in the said Plan with the Letter *L*, containing   Acres, &c and bounded on the *E* and *N E.* by the Share or Part herein-before set out to the said R——— D——— and Part of the Share herein-before set out to the said W——— R——— the younger, and M——— A———; on the *S. E.* by the other Part of the Share herein-before set out to the said W ——— R——— the younger, and M——— A———; on the *S W.* and *N. W* by the said Moss and said Inclosure called M———· And we the said A——— H——— and T——— I——— do order, direct, and appoint that the Parcel of Ground marked in the said Plan with the Letter *M*, and lying at the *N. W* Ends of the Shares herein-before set out unto the said I——— E——— the elder, and I——— E——— Son of W———, be set apart for the Sake of getting Stones upon, for the Use of the said W——— W——— and such of the several Persons herein-before mentioned to be Proprietors of the stinted Pasture, to be used within the Manor of D———, as shall obtain the Licence and Consent of the said W——— W——— his Heirs or Assigns to get Stones there; And also for the Use of such other Persons as shall obtain the Licence and Consent of the said W——— W——— his Heirs or Assigns to get Stones there (such other Persons making a reasonable Recompence and Satisfaction to the respective Owners of the Grounds through which they may pass, for any Damage which may be done by bringing the Stones from the Quarry thereon, and that there be a Road to the same, from the Road herein-after set out, down by the *N W.* side of the Share of W——— W———, through the Share of the said E——— E———,

till

Sect. I.   DIVISION *of* GROUND.   423

till it come to the Corner of the said F—— H——'s Share, where the Road to the said Ground set apart for such Quarries enters the said Share of F—— H——, and then along the said old Road heretofore used for the Sake of leading Stones from the said Quarry Ground, but to be used on no other Account whatsoever than for leading Stones from the said Quarry Ground. But that the said I—— E—— the elder, and I—— E—— Son of W——, their Heirs and Assigns, solely enjoy the Herbage of the said Ground so set apart for Quarry-ground. And we the said A—— H—— and T—— I—— do also order, direct, and appoint that every Person enjoy their respective Shares of the said Peat-moss next adjoining to the Liberties of B——, in the County of Westmorland aforesaid, as the same has heretofore been divided among them, and they had formerly enjoyed the same. And also that there be an High-way $6\frac{1}{2}$ Yards broad, from the Gate called B—— Gate, marked in the said Plan with the Letter *N*, along the *S. E* Side of the Share herein-before set out to the said W—— W——, Esq; to S—— or Place marked in the said Plan with the Letter *O*; and also that there be an Highway $6\frac{1}{2}$ Yards wide (exclusive of Ditches) from a Place called W—— Gate, or Place marked in the said Plan with the Letter *P*, along the *N W* Side of the said Share herein-before set out to the said W—— W——, Esq; on the Outside of the said Share, until it reach a Place called B—— Steps, or Place marked in the said Plan with the Letter *Q*, and there lead out upon the said Common of B——. And that there be an Occupation Way from the Place called W—— Gate, or Place marked in the said Plan

with

with the Letter *P*, along the Leafes Foot, through the Share or Part herein-before set out to the said W—— W——, Esq, to B—— Gate, or Place marked in the said Plan with the Letter *N*, for the Use of the above Proprietors that have any Shares of the abovesaid Pasture, and occupy the same from the Town of D——, but for no other Use, Intent, or Purpose whatsoever, and also that there be an Occupation Way through the Shares herein before set out unto the said W—— R—— and M—— A—— and W—— R——, from the abovesaid Highway leading from W—— Gate to B—— M——, from the Place marked in the said Plan with the Letter *R*, to the abovesaid Peat-mofs, and so along the abovesaid Peat-mofs Head, and through the Share of the said W—— R—— in a convenient Direction, until it arrive at the Gate into M—— abovesaid, for the Sake of leading Peats, and occupying the abovesaid Peat-mofs, and also for occupying the abovesaid Field or Inclosure called M——; and an Occupation Way for the abovesaid W—— R—— on all Occasions, to his Share of the said Pasture, but for no other Use or Purpose whatsoever. And also that there be an Occupation Way through the Share or Part herein-before set out unto the said I—— F——, to the Share or Part herein before set out to the said R—— D——, as the same is described in the said Plan, from the Places therein marked with the Letter *S* to the Letter *T*, from the said Highway leading from the said W—— Gate to B—— M—— at B——Steps, for the Use of the said R—— D——, but for no other Use, Intent, or Purpose whatsoever. And we the said A—— H—— and T—— I—— do also

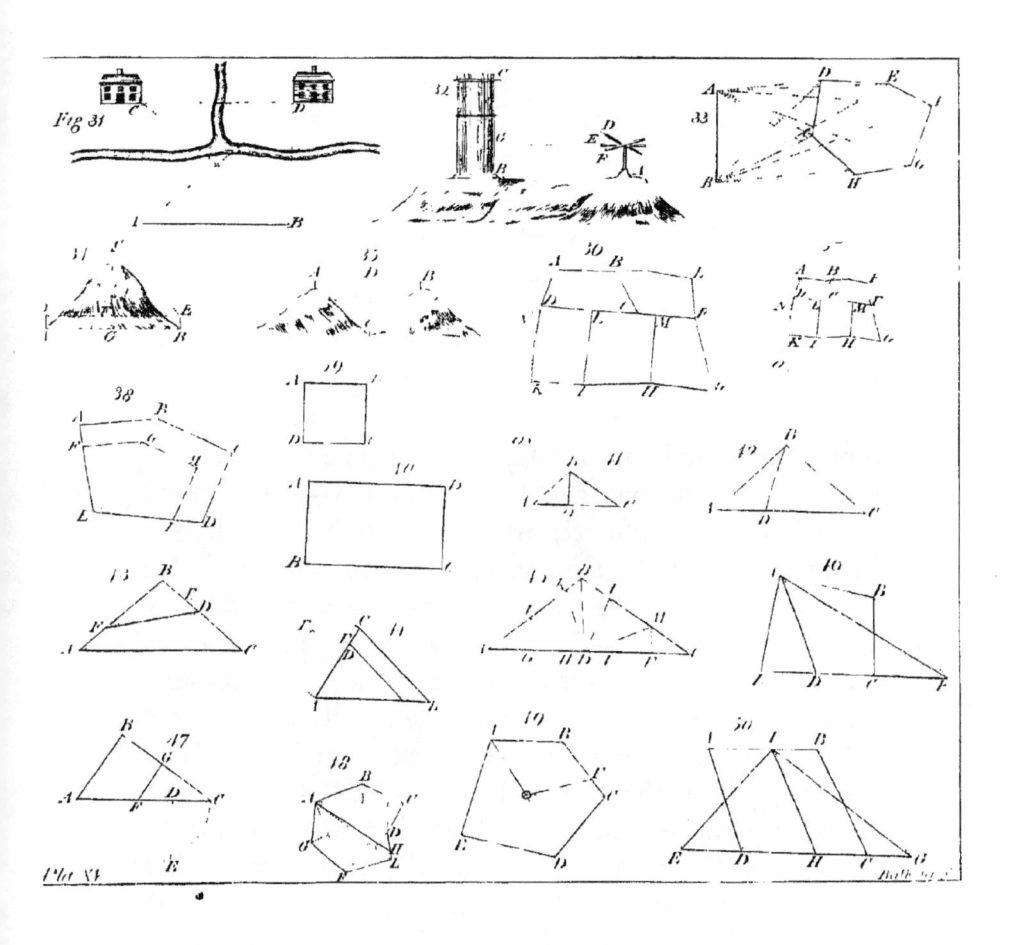

Sect. I.   DIVISION *of* GROUND.   425

alſo order, direct, and appoint, that the ſaid W—— W——, Eſq, his Heirs or Aſſigns, do make, erect, and ſet up good and ſufficient Hedges or Fences upon the ſaid Paſture, from the above ſaid W—— Gate to B—— Steps, along the *N. W* Side of the Share herein-before ſet out to him, between his ſaid Share and the aboveſaid Road leading from the ſaid W—— Gate to B—— Steps, as the ſame is marked in the ſaid Plan with the Letters *a a a*, and for ever hereafter maintain and repair the ſame And that the ſaid I—— E——, his Heirs and Aſſigns, make, erect, and ſet up good and ſufficient Hedges or Fences upon the ſaid Paſture, between his Share and the Share of the ſaid I—— E——, and alſo along the ſaid Road Side leading down to B—— Steps, as far as his Share goes, as the ſame is marked in the ſaid Plan with the Letters *B B B*, and for ever hereafter maintain and repair the ſame And that the ſaid I—— E—— his Heirs or Aſſigns, make, erect, and ſet up good and ſufficient Hedges or Fences upon the ſaid Paſture, on the *S W.* Side of his Share, between his Share and the Share of the ſaid F—— H——, and againſt the ſaid Road as far as his Share adjoins upon the ſame, as the ſame Hedges are marked in the ſaid Plan with the Letters *C C C*, and for ever hereafter maintain and repair the ſame And that the ſaid F—— H——, his Heirs or Aſſigns make, erect, and ſet up good and ſufficient Hedges or Fences upon the ſaid Paſture, between his Share and the Share of the ſaid E—— E——, and alſo againſt the ſaid Road as far as his Share goes, as the ſaid Hedges are marked in the ſaid Plan with the Letters *D D D*, and for ever maintain and repair

3 I 2   the

the fame: and that the faid E—— E——, his Heirs or Affigns, make, erect, and fet up good and fufficient Hedges or Fences upon the faid Pasture, between his Share and the Share of the faid W—— D——, and also against the faid Road as far as his Share adjoins thereon, as the fame are marked in the faid Plan with the Letters *E E E*, and for ever hereafter repair and maintain the fame: And that the faid W—— D——, his Heirs or Affigns, make, erect, and fet up good and fufficient Fences or Hedges upon the faid Pasture, between his Share and the Share of the faid I—— F——, and also against the faid Road as far as his Share adjoins thereon, as the fame are marked on the faid Plan with the Letters *F F F*, and for ever hereafter repair and maintain the fame. And that the faid I—— F——, his Heirs or Affigns, make, erect, and fet up good and fufficient Hedges or Fences upon the faid Pasture, between his Share and the Share of the faid R—— D——, and betweenn his Share and the Share of the faid W—— R—— the younger, and M—— A——, and also against the faid Road as far as his Share adjoins thereon, as the fame are marked in the faid Plan with the Letters *G G G*, and for ever hereafter repair and maintain the fame. And that the faid R—— D——, his Heirs or Affigns, make, erect, and fet up good and fufficient Hedges or Fences upon the faid Pasture, between his Share and the Share of the faid W—— R—— the younger, and M—— A——, and also between his Share and the Share of the faid W—— R——, as the fame are marked on the faid Plan with the Letters *H H H*, and for ever hereafter maintain and repair the fame. And that the

faid

Sect. I.   DIVISION *of* GROUND   427

said T—— Y—— and R—— B—— make, erect, and set up good and sufficient Hedges or Fences upon the said Pasture, between the said Shares and the abovesaid Moss, and between their said Shares and the Share of the abovesaid W—— R—— and M——A——; and also between their Share and the abovesaid Road as far as their Shares adjoin thereon, as the same are marked in the said Plan with the Letters *I I I*, and for ever hereafter maintain and repair the same. And that the said W—— R—— the younger, and M——A——, their Heirs and Assigns, make, erect, and set up good and sufficient Hedges or Fences upon the said Pasture, between their Shares and the abovesaid Peat-moss, as the same are marked on the said Plan with the Letters *K K K*, and for ever hereafter maintain and repair the same: And that the said W—— R——, his Heirs or Assigns, make, erect, and set up good and sufficient Hedges or Fences upon the said Pasture, in all Places between his Share and the Shares of the said W—— R—— the younger, and M——A——, and also between his Share and the abovesaid Peat-moss, as the same are marked in the said Plan with the Letters *L L L*, and for ever hereafter maintain and repair the same And we do also order, direct, and appoint that all the abovesaid Hedges or Fences be set upon the Grounds of the Persons who are herein-before ordered to erect the same, without any Allowance from his Neighbours for or in Respect of the said Hedges or Fences or Ditches thereto belonging, and that all the abovesaid Hedges or Fences be made and compleated. on or before the   next ensuing And also that all and every of the abovesaid Owners or Pro-

prietors

prietors of the said stinted Pastures do for ever hereafter make and repair such Parts of the ancient Outfences belonging to the said Pasture, as shall lie opposite to their respective Shares thereof (except the Out-fence at the Foot of the Leases which we do also order to be repaired for ever hereafter by the said I—— E—— the elder, and I—— E—— Son of W——, their Heirs and Assigns) as far as his Share adjoins thereon; and the said W—— W—— as far as his Share adjoins thereon, each of them the said I—— E—— the elder, and I—— E—— Son of W——, W—— W—— their respective Heirs or Assigns having allowed by the several Persons who formerly had Dots or Shares of Fence adjoining upon their respective Shares of Common, or their respective Heirs or Assigns, the Sum of One Shilling per Rood, to be paid unto them within one Month next after the signing of this our Award; and also that the Gate called B—— Gate, and the Gate called S—— Gate be hung, and for ever hereafter maintained by the said W——W——, Esq; and that the Gate called W—— Gate be hung, and for ever hereafter maintained by the Persons living in D——, and enjoying any Part of the abovesaid stinted Pasture, in Proportion to their respective Rights in the said Pasture, and that the Gate at the Foot of the Road herein-before set out at B—— Steps be hung and for ever hereafter maintained by the said T—— Y——, R—— B——, W—— R—— the younger, M—— A——, and W—— R——, their Heirs and Assigns, in Proportion to their respective Rights and Interests in the said Pasture. And we do also order that the abovesaid Highways be for ever
here-

Sect. I.   DIVISION of GROUND.

hereafter repaired by the Persons, their Heirs or Assigns, that have herein-before Lands set out to them in the said Pasture, in Proportion to their respective Rights and Interests therein, and that no Goods be turned loose into the abovesaid High-roads, but that the Grass growing in the said Roads be eaten by each Person at the Ends of their respective Fields by Tethering or Herding. And we do also order that all the Gates across any of the Occupation Ways herein-before set out be hung, and for ever hereafter maintained by the respective persons, their Heirs or Assigns, that are herein-before ordered to make and repair the respective Hedges or Fences through which the said Roads shall pass, (except the Gate leading out of the Share of the said I——F——, into the Share of the said R—— D——, as the same is marked in the said Plan with the Letter ( ), which we do order to be hung and for ever hereafter repaired by the said R—— D——, his Heirs or Assigns And whereas in the abovesaid Articles of Agreement it is provided and declared, that nothing therein contained shall extend, or be construed to deprive the Lord of the Manor of D—— aforesaid for the Time being, his Heirs or Assigns, or any of them, of all or any of the Rights, Privileges, Franchises, Royalties, or other Emoluments to which he or they might be hereby intitled in or from the said Tract of Ground called D—— W——, or from the Owners or Proprietors thereof, or from any of them, in Case these Presents had not been made in anywise however, any thing therein contained to the contrary thereof in anywise notwithstanding. And we the said A—— H—— and T—— I—— do therefore order, direct

direct, and appoint that nothing herein, or in the abovesaid Division shall be construed, deemed, or taken to deprive the said Lord of D—— for the Time being, his Heirs or Assigns or any of them, of any of the Rights, Privileges, Franchises, Royalties, or other Emoluments to him or them belonging, (any thing herein contained to the contrary thereof in anywise notwithstanding) And lastly, we do ascertain the Costs of surveying, dividing, setting out, and apportioning to each and every of the above Proprietors, and of every other Matter and Thing relating to the same, at the Sum of   and do order   within the Space of   from the Date hereof, to collect the same from the above Proprietors, in Proportion to their respective Number of Cattle-gaits upon the said Pasture, or in Case of Refusal by any Person, to take proper Methods for Recovery thereof, or for enforcing the said Article, and to pay the same when due and owing, with all convenient Speed, In Witness &c.

SECT. II.

The THEORY *and* PRACTICE *of* LEVELLING.

TO demonstrate the Theory upon which the Practice of Levelling is founded; let DAE be an Arch of the Earth, and F its Center from F draw the right Line FA, and through A draw $BC \perp FA$, which is a Tangent, also from the Center F draw FB, FC, to intersect the tangential Line in B and C. Then because a true or real Level is every where equally distant from the Earth's Center, therefore it must either be an Arch DAE thereof, or some other Arch parallel thereto. BC being $\perp$ to AF, is the apparent Level at A, and therefore if a Glass Tube be filled with Water, Spirits of Wine, or other Liquid, all but a small Space left for a Particle of Air, and placed at A in the Direction of the Line BC, the Liquid will equally possess every Part thereof, and the Bubble of Air will rest in the Middle of the Tube, but if the Tube be elevated or depressed above or below the said Direction, the Liquid (as being the heavier Fluid) will all descend into the lower Part of the Tube, and the Bubble of Air will be forced thereby into the higher. FIG 56.

The Point B being further removed from the Earth's Center than the Point A, it is plain, that if a Particle of Water, &c. be laid at B, it will (by the Power of Gravity) slide along the inclining Plane BA; and when arrived at A, will become quiescent.

Sup-

Suppose the Arch $AE =$ one Mile, then is $BE =$ 7.409 Inches $=$ the Difference between the Radius FA and the Secant FB, which is readily known by the Logarithmic Canon. But the Descent of $7\frac{1}{2}$ Inches in a Mile is too little for the conveying of Water, and therefore to give the Water a proper Velocity, it has been found by Experience, that 12 or 15 Inches per Mile, below the apparent Level AB, is only sufficient.

If B is a Spring or Fountain Head, then BG is the apparent Level or Position of the Horizon; and therefore directing the Telescope to A, you find the $\angle GBA$, which is ever equal to the $\angle BFA$; or if the Arch AE be $=$ one Mile, the $\angle EFA$ is found by Calculation $= 0°\ 00'\ 52''$; and therefore in the right-angled plain Triangle BAF, there are given all the Angles, and a Side or Leg FA ($=$ Earth's Semidiameter), by which the Hypothenuse FB may be found, then $FB - FE = BE = 7.409$ Inches as before. And therefore whenever the Distance is one Mile, you must deduct 7.409 Inches from the Height given by the Telescope, which will reduce it to a true Level, but instead of 7.409 Inches, you may in common Practice use eight Inches and therefore at the Distance of each Mile measured upon the Earth's Surface, you may deduct eight Inches from the horizontal Level, and the Remainder will be the true Level.

It has been proved to a Demonstration, that there is a Necessity for making an Allowance for the Earth's Curvature, and as Distances are most frequently measured by a four Pole Chain at $5\frac{1}{2}$ yards to the Pole, I have therefore calculated the following Table, which shews by Inspection the Allowance in Inches for every Chain from one to 100. As

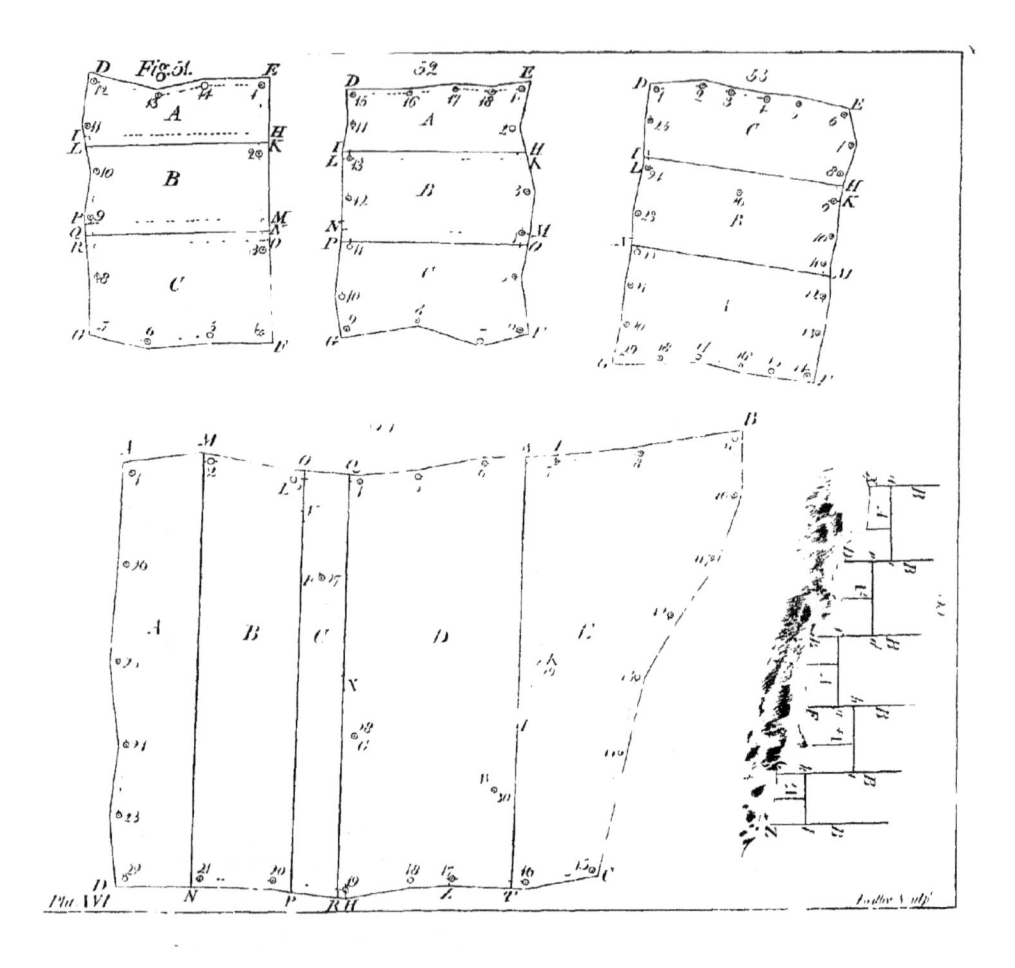

Sect. II.   *of* LEVELLING.   433

As to the practical Method of Levelling, the following Example will render it plain and easy, provided you be furnished with a good Spirit-level, or a Theodolite of the best Construction, and two Staves, the Staves ought to be each ten Feet long, and divided (first) into ten equal Parts, and numbered 1, 2, 3, &c to 10, being the Feet, each of these must be again divided into twelve equal Divisions, and numbered 1, 2, 3, &c to 12, by which the whole Staff is divided into 120 equal Divisions, which are Inches, each of these are again to be subdivided into ten equal Parts, being the Tenths of an Inch; so that by these Divisions each Staff will be divided into 1440 equal Parts. Each Staff must likewise have a Vane to slide up and down, the better to distinguish the Divisions in Time of Practice.

EXAMPLE.

Let *X* be a Fountain, from whence Water is to be conveyed to a Cistern *Z*, required the Descent, or how much *Z* is lower than *X*. FIG 55.

Set one Staff at *X*, and another at *D*, and order an Assistant to stand at each, then erect your Theodolite or Level at *A* (about the middle Way between the two Levelling-Staffs), and adjust it there; then direct the Telescope to the Staff *B X*, and order your Assistant by a Signal, to slide the Vane up or down, till the horizontal Hair in the Telescope cut the Middle thereof, and then let him mark the Place *a* upon the Staff, so is $Xa =$ the Height of the Level at *X*, which write in a Book or Paper   Then direct the Telescope forward to the Staff *B D*, and cause your Assistant to slide the Vane up

3 K 2   or

or down, till the horizontal Hair cut the Middle of the Vane as before, so is $Dc=$ the Height of the Level there, which write in your Book or Paper as before; then measure the Distance from the Instrument A to each Staff which write in proper Form in your Field Book or Paper, the Back Dimensions must be inserted in the Columns titled Back-Sights, and the Fore-Observations in the Columns titled Fore Sights. Then take up the Staff BA, and remove it to E, and set up your Instrument at A^2, then turn back the Telescope to the Staff BD, and find the Altitude De; also direct the Telescope to the Staff BE, and take the Altitude Ed; measure the Distances AD, AE Then the Instrument being removed to A^3, A^4, and A^5, find the Altitudes, and measure the Distances as before. The several Altitudes given by the Instrument, as also the corrected Altitudes, with the several Distances measured by the Chain are as specified in the following Field-Book.

Note The Field-Book is divided into two large Columns, each of which is subdivided into three more, the first Column on the left Hand containeth the Distances in Links, and is titled on the Top Dist Link. the second contains the apparent Altitudes in Inches, and is titled on the Top Altit Inch the third contains the corrected Altitudes, and is titled on the Top. Correct Inch. The two large Columns are the one titled on the Top Back-Observat. in which are inserted the Back-Observations, and the other Fore-Observat. and contains all the Fore-Observations.

The

Sect. II.   *of* LEVELLING.   435

The FIELD BOOK.

Back Observat.				Fore Observat.		
Dift	Altit	Correct	Dift	Altit	Correct
Link	Inch.	Inch	Link	Inch	Inch.
800	36 0	35 92	550	82 0	81 96
650	49 5	49 45	660	91 8	91 74
472	28 2	28 17	760	50 0	49 93
645	76 8	76 75	502	138 4	138 37
490	55 75	55 72	460	61 0	60 97
3057		246 01	2932		422 97
2932					246 01
5989				Defcent	176 96

Now add the Numbers in the Back-Sight Column (marked Correct Inch) into one Sum, and the Numbers in the Fore-Sight Column (marked Correct Inch) into another Sum, and fubtracting the lefs from the greater, the Remainder will be the Afcent or Defcent: So in this Example the Sum of the Back-Obfervations is 246 01 Inches, or 20 Feet 6 01 Inch. and the Sum of the Fore-Obfervations 422 97 Inch. or 35 Feet 2 97 Inch. then Difference 14 Feet 8 96 Inch is the Defcent, which is fo much as Z is lower than X. Alfo the Sum of the Back-Diftances added to the Sum of the Fore-Diftances, will give 5989 Links or 59 Ch. 89 Links = the Diftance between X and Z, fo that the Defcent in 59·89 Ch. is 14 Feet 89 Inch.

TABLE

TABLE of CURVITURE.

Chain	Inches	Chain	Inches	Chain	Inches	Chain	Inches
1	0 00125	14	0 24	27	0 91	40	2 00
2	0 005	15	0 28	28	0 98	45	2 28
3	0 01125	16	0 32	29	1 05	50	3 12
4	0 02	17	0·36	30	1 12	55	3 78
5	0 03	18	0 40	31	1·19	60	4 50
6	0·04	19	0 45	32	1 27	65	5 31
7	0 06	20	0 50	33	1 35	70	6 12
8	0 08	21	0 55	34	1·44	75	7 03
9	0 10	22	0 60	35	1·53	80	8 00
10	0 12	23	0 67	36	1 62	85	9 03
11	0 15	24	0 72	37	1 71	90	10 12
12	0·18	25	0 78	38	1·80	95	11 28
13	0 21	26	0 84	39	1 91	100	12 50

N. B The Numbers of this Table are calculated upon the well known Principle, That the Subtenses *E B* and *D C* of the tangential Angle, are as the Squares of their respective Arches *A E*, *A D*, that is $EB : DC :: AE^2 : AD^2$.

SECT. III.

The Method of finding the Variation of the Compass.

AS the Variation of the Mariner's Compass is of the utmost Importance in the Art of Navigation, it
is

is also highly requisite to be known in the **Practice of Surveying** For how is it possible that the true or real Situation of a Gentleman's Estate, &c should be known, so long as the Variation of the Magnetic Needle remains a Secret, and the true Meridian of the Place not known.

The several Bearings given by the Needle are not to be accounted as true Bearings, and therefore after a Plan is projected thereby, it is requisite that a true Meridian Line be drawn therein; which Meridian must intersect the Magnetic Meridian (or Meridian the Plan is laid down by), making an Angle therewith of so many Degrees, &c. as the Variation is found to be.

I shall now shew two Methods of finding the Variation of the Needle, viz. instrumentally and trigonometrically.

Example I

Let it be required to draw a true Meridian to the Plan $AGKP$. (Fig. 26.)

First, Instrumentally by the best Theodolite.

Set up your Theodolite in any Part of the Ground the Plan is drawn for, and find the Sun's apparent Altitude ($= 49°\ 00'$) about 9 or 10 o'Clock in the Forenoon, and also its Magnetic Azimuth ($= 142°\ 30'$) at the same Time, keep the Index fixed at this Altitude, or otherwise write the Degrees, &c thereof, upon a Piece of Paper, and keep by you till the Afternoon. Let the Instrument remain in the same Place, and in the same Position 'till the Afternoon, and if the Index belonging the Telescope hath not

not been shifted, (if it hath, fix it to the same Elevation as before), watch 'till through the Eye Glass of the Telescope you observe the Intersection of the cross Hairs to cut the Sun's Center, and the Index will give on the Limb the Sun's Magnetic Azimuth (= 253° 50'). The two Azimuths being thus found, the Variation of the Needle may be readily known by the following

R u l e.

Add the Half-Difference of the two Azimuths to the less Azimuth, that Sum (if less than 180°) subtract from 180°, and the Remainder is the Variation East, but if the said Sum exceed 180°, deduct 180° therefrom, the Remainder is the Variation West.

And therefore $\frac{253° 50' - 142° 30'}{2} + 142° 30' =$ 198° 10', then 198° 10' — 180° = 18° 10' the Variation West

Secondly, Trigonometrically by Means of the Sun's true and Magnetic Azimuth

This is a Branch of Surveying that requires a perfect Knowledge in the Doctrine of spherical Triangles, and also a little Acquaintance with a few of the first Problems in Astronomy But as few Surveyors can boast of these Qualifications, I shall therefore for the Benefit of such, insert the Analogies and Calculations at full of a few Examples, in a very plain and simple Manner, which I intend as a Specimen of the Form hereafter to be followed But for those conversant in the Doctrine of the Sphere and spherical Triangles, let them consult *Prob. XIX, XX, B. VI.*   As

Sect. III. *of the* COMPASS.

As the Sun's true Altitude is of the utmost Importance in this Particular, I shall therefore shew the Method of finding the same at any Hour of the Day, when the Sun's Body can be seen.

To find the Sun's true Altitude.

Take the Altitude of the Sun's lower or upper Limb by a Quadrant or good Theodolite; to or from this apparent Altitude (according as you observe the Sun's lower or upper Limb) add or subtract 16' (the Sun's apparent Semidiameter), the Sum or Difference is the apparent Altitude of the Sun's Center: Then out of the Table of Refraction take the Quantity of the Sun's Refraction according to his Altitude, which subtracted from the apparent central Altitude, will give the true Altitude.

EXAMPLE II.

Suppose the apparent Altitude of the Sun's lower Limb $= 46° \ 12' \ 16''$, required his true Altitude.

$46° \ 12' \ 16'' =$ the app. Altitude.
$ \ 16 \ 0 =$ Sun's Semidiam. add.

$46 \ \ 28 \ \ 16 =$ app. Altit. Sun's Center
$ \ \ 0 \ \ 46 =$ Refract. subtr.

$46 \ \ 27 \ \ 30 =$ Sun's true Altitude.

EXAMPLE III.

Suppose the apparent Altitude of the Sun's upper Limb $= 44° \ 14' \ 30''$; required its true Altitude.

```
54° 14' 30" = app. Altit. Sun's upper Limb
    16  00  = Sun's app. Semid  subtr.
───────────
53  58  30  = app. Altit. Sun's Center.
     0  36  = Refraction substract
───────────
53  57  54  = Sun's true Altitude.
```

The Method of finding the Sun's true Altitude being thus shewn, the Variation of the Needle is easily discovered by the following.

Rule.

First find the Sun's magnetic Azimuth, and for the same Time calculate his true Azimuth, by Prob 19, 20 *B VI* the Difference of these two Azimuths is the Variation.

Note. To find the Sun's true Azimuth, there must be given the Latitude of the Place, the Sun's Declination, and Altitude; or the Latitude of the Place, the Sun's Altitude, and Hour of the Day. An Example of each follows.

Example IV.

Suppose in the Latitude of 54° 25' North, the Sun's true Altitude by Observation is 49°, and his Declination North 23° 29', required his true Azimuth at the Time of this Observation.

Operation.

Complement of the Latitude	35° 35'
Complement of the Sun's Declination	66 31

Com-

Pl. XVII

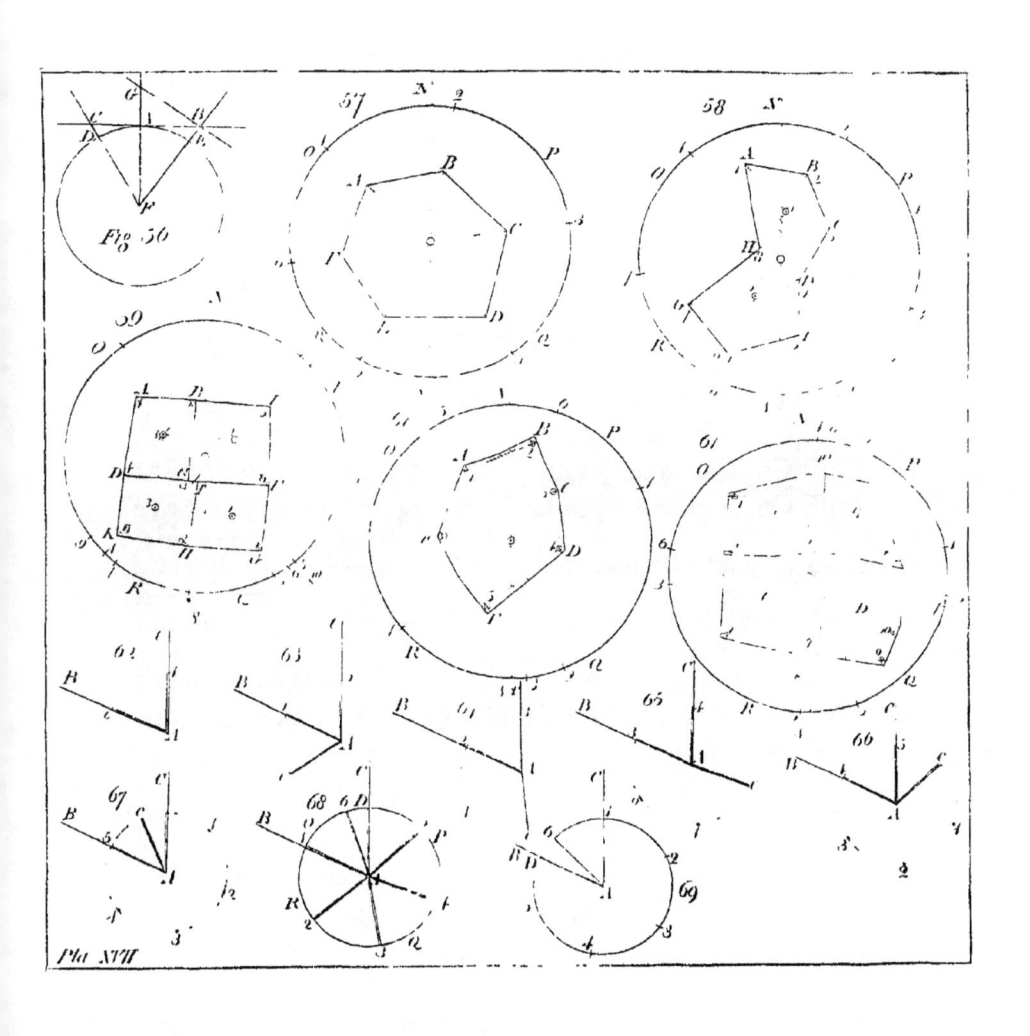

Sect III.   *of the* COMPASS.   441

Complement of the Sun's Altitude — — 41° 00′
Sum of the 3 Sides   —   —   —   143   06
Half Sum   —   —   —   —   71   33
Compl. Latit. subtract   —   —   35   35
Difference   —   —   —   —   35   58

Half Sum   —   —   —   —   71° 33′
Compl. Altit. subtract   —   —   41   00
Difference   —   —   —   30° 33

Then proceed thus;

Compl of Lat S   35° 30′   Co. Ar. 0·235162
Compl Sun's Altit. S.   41 00   Co. Ar. 0·183057
Diff Co. Lat and ½ Sum S. 35 58   —   9·768871
Diff. Co. Altit and ½ Sum S 30 33   —   9·706112

Sum of the Logarithms   —   —   19·893202

Half is the Sine of 62° 10′   — —   9·946601

which doubled is 124° 20′ = the Sun's true Azimuth from the North, whose supple 55° 40′ is the Azimuth from the South.

EXAMPLE V.

Suppose the Latitude and Altitude the same as before, and the Time of Observation 9 Hours, 35 min. 11 sec 52 thirds in the Forenoon; required the Sun's true Azimuth

Radius   —   —   90° 00′ 00″ = 10·000000
Tan. Hour from Noon   36 12 02 = 9·864532

3 L 2   Sin.

Sin. of the Latitude — 54 25 00 = 9·910235

Cotan. — — — 59 14 00 = 9 774767

Then,

Tan. Latitude — 54° 25′ — Cotan. 9 854603
Cof — — — 59 14 — — 9 708882
Tan. Sun's Altit. — 49 00 — 10 060837

Cof. — — 65 06 — — 9 624322

Then 59° 14′ + 65° 06′ = 124° 20′ = the Sun's true Azimuth, the same as before.

Or,

The Sun's Azimuth may be found, by having his Altitude, Declination, and Hour of the Day given. And therefore supposing Things as before, the Analogy is,

Cof. Sun's Altitude   49° 00′ 00″ Co. Ar 0 183057
S. Hour from Noon   36 12 02 — — 9·771355
Cof. Sun's Declinat.   23 29 00 — — 9·962453

S. Sun's Azim. from South 55° 40′ — 9 916865

Whose Supplement 124° 20′ is the Azimuth from the North, and the same as before.

Then reckoning both Azimuths from the North, observe the following

RULE.

In the Forenoon, the true or Magnetic Azimuth being greatest, the Variation is accordingly East or West, in the Afternoon West or East.

The

Sect III.   *of the* COMPASS.   443

The Sun's $\begin{cases} \text{True Azimuth} & 124°\ 20'\ N.\ \text{Easterly.} \\ \text{Magnetic Azim.} & 142\ \ 30\ \ \ N.\ \text{Easterly.} \end{cases}$

Subtracted gives the Variation   18 10   West.

Having thus shewn how to find the Variation of the Needle instrumentally and trigonometrically, by Means of an Azimuth, I shall next shew how the same may be found by Means of an Amplitude.

Example VI.

Suppose the Latitude and Declination the same as before, required the Variation of the magnetical Needle

First find the Sun's magnetic Amplitude at his Rising or Setting, and at the same Time calculate his true Amplitude, then if the true Amplitudes agree, there is no Variation, but if they differ (as most frequently they do), their Difference is the Variation Then reckoning both the Amplitudes from the North (like as the Azimuths), observe the following

Rule.

At Sun Rising, the true or magnetic Amplitude being greatest, the Variation is accordingly East or West; at Sun Setting West or East.

Then to find the Sun's magnetic Amplitude by the best Theodolite, proceed thus

Adjust the Instrument for taking an Observation, then looking at the Sun just as he rises, through the Eye-Glass of the Telescope, observe that the horizontal Hair therein do cut the Sun's Center, then will the Index give on the Limb 64° 57' = the Sun's magnetic

netic Ampletude from the North, whose Complement 43° 13' is the Amplitude from the East Northerly, but if the magnetic Amplitude from the North be above 90 and less than 180, subtract 90 from it, the Remainder is the Amplitude East Southerly, also if the magnetic Azimuth from the North exceed 180 and be less than 270, subtract it from 270, and the Remainder will be the Amplitude West Southerly, but if the Amplitude from the North be greater than 270, and less than 360, subtract 270 from it, and the Remainder is the Amplitude West Northerly. The magnetic Amplitude being thus found, the true Amplitude is readily discovered by Prob. 7, *B.* VI. The Anology follows.

ANALOGY.

As Cos Latitude — — 54° 25' — — 9 764838
To Radius — — 90 00 — — 10 000000
So S. Sun's Declen. — — 23 29 — — 9 600409
To S Sun's Amplit — — 43 13   9 835571

Whose Complement 46° 47' is the Sun's true Amplitude from the North.

The Sun's { Magnetic Amplitude.   64° 57'   *N* East.
          { True Amplitude.   46   47   *N.* East.

Their Diff is the Variation   18   10   West.

The Variation of the Needle being thus found by any of the fore-mentioned Methods, you may readily draw a true Meridian to the Plan, by drawing a Line *ps* to make an Angle of 18° 10' with the Meridian the Plan was laid down by, observing to have the North

End

End of the true Meridian, to the Right (or East) of the magnetic Meridian, because the Variation is West; but if the Variation had been East, the North End of the true Meridian must have been to the Left (or West) of the magnetic Meridian.

SECT. IV.
The Method of Washing or Colouring Maps or Plans.

AS to the Preparation of Colours, there is little Occasion to give any Directions thereupon, as any Colours (especially such as are used by Surveyors) may be had from any Colour-Shop. But as Allum and Gum-Water (especially the latter) are constantly used in Colouring, I shall therefore only give Directions for forming these, and so proceed to shew the Method of Washing, or laying on Colours.

I. *To make Allum-Water.*

To a Gallon of Water add one Pound of Allum beat to Powder, mix these well together, and boil the Mixture a considerable Time, till the Allum be quite dissolved, take it off the Fire, and when cold, bottle it up for Use.

Note, If with this you wet your Paper before you lay on the Colours, and then let it be perfectly dry, it will not only keep them from sinking into it, but will also add a Lustre and shining Beauty when laid on.

II. *To make Gum-Water.*

Beat the clearest and best Gum Arabic into small Pieces, which bind up in a fine linen Rag, hang this in clear Spring-Water 'till the Gum be all diffolved; then put your Finger into the Water, and if you feel it too ftiff or glutinous, add more Water, if otherwife add more Gum, 'till it be of a fufficient Stiffnefs.

Note, With this Water you mix and temper moft of your Colours that are not of a gummy Nature.

III. *The Method of Wafhing, or Laying on Colours.*

Having the Plan of a Gentleman's Eftate, &c. to wafh, firft begin with one of the Fields, and dipping your Pencil in the Colour you defign to ufe, draw it along on the Infide of the Lines, making the coloured Part of an equal Breadth; you may make it either broader or narrower, according to the Size of the Field; then dip a clean Pencil in fair Water, and draw it along on the Infide of the coloured Part, wafhing down the Edge that the Colour may fade or die away down to the Paper, and appear ftrong next the Lines. It is cuftomary with Surveyors to wafh each Field with one intire Colour This is left to the Difcretion of the Surveyor.

THE

THE
NEW ART
OF
SURVEYING,
By the Plain Table.

CONTAINING,

A New Method of Surveying and Planning by that Inftrument, by which the Angles (or rather Bearings) are taken and protracted at one and the fame Inftant in the Field, and thereby the Trouble and Inconvenience of fhifting the Papers entirely removed; fo that the Bearings (though never fo many) may be all protracted upon one Sheet of Paper in a manner different from any as yet practifed by that Inftrument.

By THOHAS BREAKS.

THE NEW ART OF SURVEYING,

By the Plain Table.

ALL the Methods of Surveying by the Plain Table hitherto practised or treated of by Authors on that Subject, are not only flow and tedious, but likewise liable to many and great Errors, so that this Instrument (once so famous) is in a Manner totally rejected by the Ingenious. But the Method here to be advanced is such, that by a Plain Table only of very simple and ordinary Construction, actual Surveys may be made with that Accuracy, Correctness, and Expedition, as with a Theodolite of the best and most modern Invention.

SECT. I

Surveying and plotting of Fields by the Plain Table.

Prop. I.

To take the Plot of a Field A B C D E F *from one Station therein.* Fig. 57.

Chuse any Station from whence you can see every Corner of the Field, and place a Mark at each, which number with the Figures 1, 2, 3, &c. At this Station erect

450 *The* New Art *of* Surveying,

erect your Plain Table covered with Paper, and if it hath a Box and Needle, bring the South Point of the Needle to the Flower-de-luce (or 360) in the Box; then draw a Circle *O P Q R* upon the Paper, as large as it will well contain, through whose Center ☉ draw the Line *N S* parallel to that Side of the Table which is parallel to the Meridian Line in the Box; this will be the Meridian of the Plan. On the Center ☉ move the fiducial Edge of the Index 'till you observe through the Sights the several Marks *A, B, C,* &c. in the Corners of the Field, and the Edge thereof will cut the Circle in the Points 1, 2, 3, &c. Then having taken and likewise protracted the several Bearings, the Distances are next to be measured, but the Method of doing that, as also the Form of the Field-Book have been sufficiently shewn in the fore Part of this Work, where the Uses of the Theodolite and Plain Table have been particularly demonstrated.

To draw the Plan.

Through the Center ☉ and each of the Marks 1, 2, 3, &c. draw the Lines ☉*A*, ☉*B*, ☉*C*, ☉*D*, ☉*E*, ☉*F*, and make each equal to its respective Distance in the Field, join the Points *A, B, C,* &c. and the Plan is finished.

Prop II.

To take the Plot of a Field A B C D, *&c. from several Stations* Fig 58.

Having chosen the necessary Stations in the Field, and drawn the Circle *O P Q R* (which you must ever observe

Sect. I. *by the* PLAIN TABLE. 451

obferve to do in every Cafe), fet up your Inftrument at the firft Station, and bring the Needle to the Meridian (which is called adjufting the Inftrument), move the Index on the Center ☉, and take an Obfervation at *A, B, C,* ☉ 2, *H,* and the fiducial Edge thereof will interfect the Circle in 1, 2, 3, &c. Then remove your Inftrument to the fecond Station in the Field, and applying the Edge of the Index to the Center ☉ and the Mark ☉ 2 in the Circle, take a Back Sight to the firft Station, and faften the Table in this Pofition, then move the Index on the Center ☉, and direct the Sights to the remaining angular Marks, fo will the fiducial Edge thereof cut the Circle in the Points 4, 5, 6, &c. The feveral Diftances being meafured with a Chain, the Work in the Field is finifhed.

Note, In the laft Prop I omitted the Field-Book, referring to Specimens formerly given, but confidering that a Field-Book is of the utmoft Advantage to Tyros, I fhall therefore, in order to exercife the young Surveyor in this new, accurate, and expeditious Method of Surveying, infert the Field Book belonging to every particular Survey. The Field-Books belonging to Prop I, II, are as below.

The FIELD-BOOK *to* Prop. I.

N°.	Dis
	Links
1	700
2	595
3	650
4	800
5	764
6	700

The

The FIELD-BOOK to Prop. II.

N°.	Dist	N°	Dist
	⊙1		⊙2
1	520	3	
2	344	4	370
3	360	5	470
⊙2	730	6	550
8	386	7	550
		8	

To draw the Plan.

Having chosen ⊙1 upon Paper to represent the first Station in the Field, lay the Edge of a Parallel Ruler to ⊙ and the Mark 1, and extend the other Edge 'till it touch (or lay upon) ⊙1, and close by its Edge draw a Line 1 1 = 520. Then lay the Ruler as before to ⊙ and the Mark 2, and extending the other Edge to ⊙1, draw thereby the Line 1 2 = 344, which gives the Corner *B*, as the Line 1 1 does the Corner *A*. After the same Manner project ⊙2, together with the Corners *C H*. Again, apply the Edge of the Ruler to ⊙ and the Point 4, and extend the other Edge 'till it touch ⊙2, and draw the Line 2 4 = 370, which will give the Point or Corner *D*. Thus project the remaining Corners *E, F, G*, and the Plan is ready for closing.

Sect. I.   *by the* Plain Table.   453

Prop. III.

To take the Plot of several Fields A B C D, B E F I, D I H K, *and* I F G H, *from Stations chosen at or near the Middle of each.* Fig. 59.

Adjust your Plain Table at the first Station in *A B I D*, and draw the protracting Circle and Meridian *N S*; then by Prop. I. project the Angles or Corners of *A B I D, B E F I,* and also the 2d Station, into the Points 1, 2, ⊙2, 3, 4, 5, 6. Again, erect your Instrument at the 1st Station, and lay the Index on the Center ⊙ and the Mark ⊙2, and direct the Sights (by turning the Table) to the 2d Station, then move the Index till you observe the 3d Station, and the Edge thereof will cut the Circle in ⊙3. Then remove the Instrument to the 3d Station, lay the Index on the Center ⊙ and the Mark ⊙3, and take a Back Observation to the first Station; after which by the last Prop. find the Points 7, 8, ⊙4, 9 in the Circle *O P Q R*. As to the measuring of Distances both in this and the two succeeding Prop. that shall be passed over in Silence, having sufficently displayed the same heretofore, what I intend to treat of hereafter, is the Method of taking and protracting the Bearings in the Field, with the Manner of deducing a Plan therefrom.

To draw the Plan.

Chuse any Point (⊙1) for your first Station; apply the Edge of a Parallel Ruler to the Center ⊙ and the Point 1, and having extended the other Edge to ⊙1,
draw

draw the Line 11 = 370, which will give the Corner *A*: In like Manner find the other Corners *B, I, D*, together with ⊙2, which being joined, finishes the Field *A B I D*. After the same Method construct the other Fields *B E F I, D I H K, I F G H*, and you have done.

The FIELD BOOK.

REMARKS	N°	Dist	REMARKS
		⊙1	In *ABID*
The open	1	370	Field
	2	380	*BEFI*
	⊙2	580	
	3	403	*DIHK*.
Sir Will. Jones's	4	440	Ground.
		⊙2	In *BEFI*.
	2		
John Simpson's	5	400	Ground.
	6	460	*IFGH*
	7	———	
BEFI closes at	3		
Return to		⊙1	In *ABID*.
	⊙3	600	
		⊙3	In *DIHK*.
	7	———	*IFGH*.
	⊙1	630	
South	8	432	Field
John Spencer's	9	400	Ground.
DIHK closes at	4	———	
		⊙4	In *IFGH*.
Edward Johnstone's	6	———	Ground.
South	10	380	Field
IFGH closes at	8	———	

Prop

Sect. I. *by the* PLAIN TABLE. 455

PROP. IV.

To take the Plot of a Field A B C D E F, *by going round the same.* (FIG 60)

Set up your Plain Table at the first Station in the Field, move the fiducial Edge of the Index on the Center ⊙, and take an Observation at the Mark placed at the 2d Station, then will the same fiducial Edge cut the Circle O P Q R in the Point 1 Then remove your Instrument to the 2d Station, and placing the Edge of the Index on ⊙ and the Point 1, take a Back-Sight to the 1st (or last) Station, then directing the Index on the Center ⊙ to the 3d (or next) Station, the Edge thereof will cross the Circle in the Point 2 In like Manner the Instrument being planted at every Station, a Back-Sight taken to the last preceeding One, and the Index directed forward to the next succeeding Station, will give the protracted Points 3, 4, 5, 6.

The FIELD-BOOK.

REMARKS	O	⊙L	O	REMARKS
		⊙1		In *A B C D E F*
	70	0		
	50	250		
	85	550		
		⊙2		In Ditto
	84	0		
Corner	65	440		
		⊙3		In Ditto
		0		
	60	465		

The FIELD-BOOK

REMARKS	◯	⊙L	◯	REMARKS
		⊙4		In Ditto
	72	0		
	58	365		
	80	750		
		⊙5		In Ditto
	40	0		
	68	302		
	60	680		
		⊙6		In Ditto
	58	0		
	50	355		
	67	663	to ⊙1	Clofe Ditto

To draw the Plan

Chufe any Point ⊙1, to denote the firft Station. Lay the Edge of a Parallel Ruler on the Center ⊙ and the Point 1, and extend the other Edge 'till it touch ⊙1, and draw by the Side thereof the Line 1 2 = 550, then apply the Ruler to ⊙ and the Mark 2, and extend the other Edge to ⊙2, and draw thereby the Line 2 3 = 440; again, lay the Edge of the Ruler to ⊙ and the Point 3, and the other Edge being extended to ⊙3, draw the Line 3 4 = 465, after the fame Method lay down the remaining Stations, and the Traverfe is delineated. As for drawing the Hedges, that fhall be left for the Learner's Exercife.

PROP.

Sect. I   *by the* PLAIN TABLE   457

Prop. V.

To take the Plot of several Fields A, B, C, D, *by Circulation*   Fig 61

From the projecting Point ⊙ (by Prop IV) project the Stations in *A*, into the Points 1, 2, 3, 4, then the Instrument being planted at the 2d Station, from the same projecting Point ⊙ project that Station (the 2d in *A*) into the Point 2^2 (2^2 denoting the Instrument being planted a second Time at that Station) which is done thus Lay the Index to ⊙ and the Point 2, and take a Back-Sight to the first Station (that being the Station immediately preceding that you are at in the Field-Book), then on the Center ⊙ take a Fore-Observation at the next succeeding Station, and the Index will cut the Circle in the Point 2· Thus project every other remaining Station.

The FIELD-BOOK.

REMARKS	⊙	⊙L	⊙	REMARKS
		⊙1		In Field *A*
	53	0		
	80	290		
Corner	85	610		
	60	695		
		⊙2		In Ditto
	70	0		
	65	560		
		⊙3		In Ditto.
	60	0		
	75	368		
	55	680		

458   *The* NEW ART *of* SURVEYING

The FIELD-BOOK.

REMARKS	0	⊙L	0	REMARKS.
		⊙4		In Ditto
	50	0		
	48	440		to⊙1. Close here *A*.
Return to		⊙2		In *A*.
		0		
Corner	60	80		into *B*.
	50	402		
		⊙5		In *B*.
	50	0		
	60	340		
	50	650		
		⊙6		In Ditto.
	50	0		
Ag Hedge	51	500		
		560		bye ⊙ for closing *C*,
Closes at Cor. of *A*	50	620	×	the Hedge,
		682		to ⊙3 in *A*.
Ret to		⊙4		In *A*.
		0		
		60	70	
		into *C*		
		380	60	
		682	68	
		⊙7		In *C*
		0	40	
		300	60	
		720	50	
		⊙8		In Ditto.
		0	70	
		400	24	
		780	63	Close *C*.
		Cross Hedge		
		820		bye ⊙ at 560 l 6, 4.

The

Sect. II *by the* PLAIN TABLE.   459

The FIELD-BOOK.

REMARKS.	O	⊙L	O	REMARKS.
Ret. to	☾8 0 60 into 220 554		50 D. 50 40	In Ditto Corner.
	☾9 0 250		40 38	In D.
	⊙10 0 64 530 into 570		50 64 B to ⊙6 in B	In Ditto Close D at Cor. B.

To draw the Plan.

The Bearings being protracted in the Circle O P Q R, the Plan may readily be drawn by Prop. XVI. B. VIII. to which I refer the Reader.

SECT. II.

The Method of ascertaining the just Measure of any Angle in Degrees, Minutes, Seconds, &c.

Prop. VI.

To find the exact Measure of any Angle B A C, *that is, to ascertain the just Quantity thereof to a Minute, Second, &c* Fig. 62.

Mr Martin, in his New Art of Surveying by the Goniometer, has given the Method of measuring

ing an Angle to great Exactness by an Instrument called A Goniometer, which is performed by measuring the Angle many Times over, and afterwards taking a Mean of the Whole; which Mean is the just Measurement of the Angle. But this is much more conveniently performed by a Theodolite, when an Instrument of that Kind is ready at Hand, but as these are Instruments of great Value, and consequently rarely met with, I shall by Means of a Plain-Table only and a Sheet of Paper placed thereon, perform the Work of measuring an Angle with as great Correctness (and Double the Expedition) as by an Instrument of superior Value. However I shall in the first Place shew the Performance hereof by the Theodolite, and then proceed to the Use of the Plain-Table.

I. *By the Theodolite.*

Fix your Theodolite at A, set the Index to 360 on the Limb, direct the Telescope to B, and fasten the Limb, then discharging the Index, direct the Telescope to C, and fasten the Index, so is the Arch c 1 = the Angle once measured. Then turn back the Telescope to the Mark B, and fastening the Limb, direct the Telescope to C, and the Angle is twice measured, as denoted by the Arches c 1, 1 2, for c 1 + 1 2 = the Angle twice measured. Again, the Index being fixed to the Limb, bring back the Telescope to B, and fasten the Instrument, then direct the Telescope to C, and the Angle is thrice measured, as is represented by the Arches c 1, 1 2, 2 3; therefore c 1 + 1 2 + 2 3 = the Angle thrice measured; for the Arches c 1, 1 2, 2 3 are each = the Measure

of

of the Angle BAC, and equal to one another Fig 62, 63, 64, 65, 66, 67.

In like Manner proceed to quadruple it, quintuple it, and laſtly ſextuple it. Now it is evident, that the Index in all this Time has paſſed over the Circumference of a Circle and the overplus Arch $c\ 6 = 14° \ 15'$, which added to 360°, the Sum 374° 15′ is ſix Times the true Quantity of the Angle.

The overplus Arch $c\ 6$ being known, the true Meaſure of the Angle BAC is $= \frac{360° + 14° \ 15'}{6} =$ 62° 22′ 30″ = the Mean of ſix Obſervations.

Note, You may meaſure the Angle as many Times over as you pleaſe, only obſerve to divide the whole Sum or Total of the Degrees, &c by a Number equal to the Times the Angle hath been meaſured, and the Quote will be the Mean of them all This Method of meaſuring an Angle is undoubtedly the moſt accurate, and much more ſo than Occaſion requires in Practical Surveying, except in ſome particular Caſes, and therefore may be practiſed more for Curioſity than real Service.

II. *By the Plain-Table.* (Fig 68)

The Plain-Table being covered with Paper, draw thereon with a Chord of 60° the Circle $O\ P\ Q\ R$, and draw the Radius AD. Plant the Table at A, lay the Index on AD, and move the Table 'till you obſerve the Mark B, faſten the Table in this Direction, and bring the Index (the ſame moving on the Center A) to the Mark C, and the Edge thereof will cut the Circle in 1, ſo is the Arch D, 1 = the Angle once meaſured. Unſcrew the Table,

and

and holding the Index in the fame Pofition, move the fame 'till you obferve the Mark B, and faften the Inftrument; then move the Index forward to C, and the Edge thereof will cut the Circle in the Point 2, and the Angle is twice meafured, for the Arch D 1 is = the Arch 1 2, and therefore D 1 + 1 2 = D 2 = the Angle twice meafured, after the fame Method triple it, quadruple it, quintuple it, and fextuple it, for the Arches D 1, 1 2, 2 3, 3 4, 4 5, 5 6 put together are equal to the Angle fix Times meafured.

It is evident from the Figure, that the Index has paffed over the Circumference of the Circle and the overplus Arch D 6 (as before with the Theodolite), and therefore D 6 meafured and added to 360°, and that Sum divided by 6, will give the true Quantity of the Angle $B A C = 62° \ 22' \ 30''$, the fame as before

But the beft and moft expeditious Method of meafuring the Angle is thus Plant the Inftrument at A, (Fig 69) lay the Index on the Radius $A D$, and meafure the $\angle B A C$ once over, whofe Quantity is = the Arch D 1 Take D 1 in your Compaffes, and lay it on the Circumference of the Circle fix Times (the Angle being required to be meafured fix Times over) from D to 1, from 1 to 2, from 2 to 3, from 3 to 4, from 4 to 5, and from 5 to 6, which gives the overplus Arch D 6 as before, which being meafured and added to 360°, gives the true Meafure of the Angle $B A C = 62° \ 22' \ 30''$, the fame as before by the other Methods.

A

A TABLE

OF THE

LOGARITHMS,

OF ALL

NUMBERS,

From 1 to 10000.

A TABLE, &c.

Number 1 to 100, and their Log. with Indices.

1	0 000000	26	1·414973	51	1 707570	76	1 880814
2	0 301030	27	1 431364	52	1 716003	77	1 886491
3	0 477121	28	1 447158	53	1 724276	78	1 892095
4	0·602060	29	1·462398	54	1·732394	79	1 897627
5	0 698970	30	1·477121	55	1 740363	80	1 903090
6	0 778151	31	1 491362	56	1 748188	81	1·908485
7	0·845098	32	1 505150	57	1 755875	82	1 913814
8	0 903090	33	1 518514	58	1 763428	83	1 919078
9	0 954243	34	1 531479	59	1 770852	84	1 924279
10	1·000000	35	1 544068	60	1 778151	85	1·929419
11	1 041393	36	1 556303	61	1 785330	86	1 934499
12	1 079181	37	1·568202	62	1 792392	87	1 939519
13	1 113943	38	1·579784	63	1·799341	88	1 944483
14	1 146128	39	1 591065	64	1 806180	89	1 949390
15	1·176091	40	1·602060	65	1·812913	90	1·954243
16	1 204120	41	1·612784	66	1 819544	91	1 959041
17	1 230449	42	1·623249	67	1 826075	92	1·963788
18	1 255273	43	1 633469	68	1 832509	93	1 968483
19	1 278754	44	1 643453	69	1·838849	94	1·973128
20	1 301030	45	1 653213	70	1 845098	95	1 977724
21	1 322219	46	1 662758	71	1 851258	96	1 982271
22	1 342423	47	1 672098	72	1 857333	97	1·986772
23	1 361728	48	1 681241	73	1 863323	98	1 991226
24	1 380211	49	1 690196	74	1·869232	99	1 995635
25	1 397940	50	1 698970	75	1 875061	100	2 000000

A TABLE of

N°	0	1	2	3	4	5	6	7	8	9
100	000000	0434	0868	1301	1734	2166	2598	3030	3461	3891
101	4321	4751	5181	5609	6038	6466	6894	7321	7748	8174
102	8600	9026	9451	9876	0300	0724	1147	1570	1993	2415
103	012837	3259	3680	4100	4521	4940	5360	5779	6197	6616
104	7033	7451	7868	8284	8701	9116	9532	9947	0361	0776
105	021189	1603	2016	2428	2841	3253	3664	4075	4486	4896
106	5306	5715	6125	6533	6942	7350	7757	8164	8571	8978
107	9384	9790	0195	0600	1004	1409	1812	2216	2619	3021
108	033424	3826	4227	4629	5029	5430	5830	6230	6629	7028
109	7427	7825	8223	8620	9017	9414	9811	0207	0602	0998
110	041393	1787	2182	2576	2969	3362	3755	4148	4540	4932
111	5323	5714	6105	6495	6885	7275	7664	8053	8442	8830
112	9218	9606	9993	0380	0766	1153	1538	1924	2309	2694
113	053078	3463	3846	4230	4613	4996	5378	5761	6142	6524
114	6905	7286	7666	8046	8426	8806	9185	9563	9942	0320
115	060698	1075	1453	1829	2206	2582	2958	3333	3709	4083
116	4458	4832	5206	5580	5953	6326	6699	7071	7443	7815
117	8186	8557	8928	9298	9668	0038	0407	0777	1145	1514
118	071882	2250	2618	2985	3352	3718	4085	4451	4816	5182
119	5547	5912	6276	6640	7004	7368	7731	8094	8457	8819
120	9181	9543	9905	0266	0627	0987	1347	1707	2067	2426
121	082785	3144	3503	3861	4219	4576	4934	5291	5647	6004
122	6360	6716	7071	7427	7781	8136	8491	8845	9198	9552
123	9905	0258	0611	0963	1315	1667	2019	2370	2721	3071
124	093422	3772	4122	4471	4820	5169	5518	5867	6215	6562
125	6910	7257	7604	7951	8298	8644	8990	9335	9681	0026
126	100371	0715	1059	1403	1747	2091	2434	2777	3119	3462
127	3804	4146	4487	4828	5169	5510	5851	6191	6531	6871
128	7210	7549	7888	8227	8565	8903	9241	9579	9916	0253
129	110590	0926	1263	1599	1934	2270	2605	2940	3275	3609
130	3943	4277	4611	4944	5278	5611	5943	6276	6608	6940
131	7271	7603	7934	8265	8595	8926	9256	9586	9915	0245
132	120574	0903	1232	1560	1888	2216	2544	2871	3198	3525
133	3852	4178	4504	4830	5156	5481	5807	6131	6456	6781
134	7105	7429	7753	8076	8399	8722	9045	9368	9690	0012

LOGARITHMS.

N.	0	1	2	3	4	5	6	7	8	9
135	130334	0655	0977	1298	1619	1939	2260	2580	2900	3220
136	3539	3858	4177	4496	4814	5133	5451	5769	6086	6403
137	6721	7038	7354	7671	7987	8303	8618	8934	9249	9564
138	9879	0194	0508	0822	1136	1450	1763	2077	2390	2702
139	143015	3327	3639	3951	4263	4574	4885	5196	5507	5818
140	6128	6438	6748	7058	7367	7676	7985	8294	8603	8911
141	9219	9527	9835	0142	0449	0756	1063	1370	1676	1982
142	152288	2594	2900	3205	3510	3815	4120	4424	4728	5032
143	5336	5640	5943	6246	6549	6852	7154	7457	7759	8061
144	8363	8664	8965	9266	9567	9868	0168	0469	0769	1068
145	161368	1667	1967	2266	2564	2863	3161	3460	3758	4055
146	4353	4650	4947	5244	5541	5838	6134	6430	6726	7022
147	7317	7613	7908	8203	8498	8792	9086	9381	9674	9968
148	170262	0555	0848	1141	1434	1727	2019	2311	2603	2895
149	3186	3478	3769	4060	4351	4641	4932	5222	5512	5802
150	176091	6381	6670	6959	7248	7537	7825	8113	8401	8689
151	8977	9265	9552	9839	0126	0413	0699	0986	1272	1558
152	181844	2129	2415	2700	2985	3270	3555	3839	4123	4408
153	4691	4975	5259	5542	5825	6108	6391	6674	6956	7239
154	7521	7803	8084	8366	8647	8929	9210	9490	9771	0051
155	190332	0612	0892	1172	1451	1730	2010	2289	2568	2846
156	3125	3403	3681	3959	4237	4514	4792	5069	5346	5623
157	5900	6176	6453	6729	7005	7281	7556	7832	8107	8382
158	8657	8932	9207	9481	9755	0029	0303	0577	0851	1124
159	201397	1670	1943	2216	2488	2761	3033	3305	3577	3849
160	4120	4391	4663	4934	5204	5475	5746	6016	6286	6556
161	6826	7096	7365	7634	7904	8173	8441	8710	8979	9247
162	9515	9783	0051	0319	0586	0853	1121	1388	1654	1921
163	212188	2454	2720	2986	3252	3518	3783	4049	4314	4579
164	4844	5109	5373	5638	5902	6166	6430	6694	6957	7221
165	7484	7747	8010	8273	8536	8798	9060	9323	9585	9846
166	220108	0370	0631	0892	1153	1414	1675	1936	2196	2456
167	2717	2976	3236	3496	3756	4015	4274	4533	4792	5051
168	5309	5568	5826	6084	6342	6600	6858	7115	7372	7630
169	7887	8144	8400	8657	8913	9170	9426	9682	9938	0193

A Table of

N°	0	1	2	3	4	5	6	7	8	9
170	230449	0704	0960	1215	1470	1724	1979	2234	2488	2742
171	2996	3250	3504	3757	4011	4264	4517	4770	5023	5276
172	5528	5781	6033	6285	6537	6789	7041	7292	7544	7795
173	8046	8297	8548	8799	9049	9300	9550	9800	0050	0300
174	240549	0799	1048	1297	1547	1795	2044	2293	2541	2790
175	3038	3286	3534	3782	4030	4277	4525	4772	5019	5266
176	5513	5759	6006	6252	6499	6745	6991	7237	7482	7728
177	7973	8219	8464	8709	8954	9198	9443	9687	9932	0176
178	250420	0664	0908	1151	1395	1638	1882	2125	2368	2610
179	2853	3096	3338	3580	3822	4065	4306	4548	4790	5031
180	5273	5514	5755	5996	6237	6477	6718	6958	7198	7439
181	7679	7919	8158	8398	8637	8877	9116	9355	9594	9833
182	260071	0310	0548	0787	1025	1263	1501	1739	1976	2214
183	2451	2688	2926	3163	3399	3636	3873	4109	4346	4582
184	4818	5054	5290	5525	5761	5996	6232	6467	6702	6937
185	7172	7406	7641	7875	8110	8344	8578	8812	9046	9279
186	9513	9746	9980	0213	0446	0679	0912	1144	1377	1609
187	271842	2074	2306	2538	2770	3001	3233	3464	3696	3927
188	4158	4389	4620	4850	5081	5311	5542	5772	6002	6232
189	6462	6692	6921	7151	7380	7609	7838	8067	8296	8525
190	8754	8982	9211	9439	9667	9895	0123	0351	0578	0806
191	281033	1261	1488	1715	1942	2169	2396	2622	2849	3075
192	3301	3527	3753	3979	4205	4431	4656	4882	5107	5332
193	5557	5782	6007	6232	6457	6681	6905	7130	7354	7578
194	7802	8026	8249	8473	8696	8920	9143	9366	9589	9812
195	290035	0257	0480	0702	0925	1147	1369	1591	1813	2034
196	2256	2478	2699	2920	3142	3363	3584	3804	4025	4246
197	4466	4687	4907	5127	5347	5567	5787	6007	6226	6446
198	6665	6885	7104	7323	7542	7761	7979	8198	8416	8635
199	8853	9071	9289	9507	9725	9943	0161	0378	0596	0813
200	301030	1247	1464	1681	1898	2114	2331	2547	2764	2980
201	3196	3412	3628	3844	4060	4275	4491	4706	4921	5136
202	5351	5566	5781	5996	6211	6425	6639	6854	7068	7282
203	7496	7710	7924	8137	8351	8564	8778	8991	9204	9417
204	9630	9843	0056	0268	0481	0693	0906	1118	1330	1542

LOGARITHMS.

N°	0	1	2	3	4	5	6	7	8	9
205	311754	1966	2177	2389	2600	2812	3023	3234	3445	3656
206	3867	4078	4289	4499	4710	4920	5130	5341	5551	5761
207	5970	6180	6390	6599	6809	7018	7227	7437	7646	7855
208	8063	8272	8481	8689	8898	9106	9314	9522	9731	9938
209	320146	0354	0562	0769	0977	1184	1391	1598	1806	2012
210	2219	2426	2633	2839	3046	3252	3458	3665	3871	4077
211	4283	4488	4694	4900	5105	5310	5516	5721	5926	6131
212	6336	6541	6745	6950	7155	7359	7563	7768	7972	8176
213	8380	8583	8787	8991	9194	9398	9601	9805	0008	0211
214	330414	0617	0820	1022	1225	1427	1630	1832	2034	2236
215	2439	2640	2842	3044	3246	3447	3649	3850	4051	4253
216	4454	4655	4856	5057	5257	5458	5659	5859	6059	6260
217	6460	6660	6860	7060	7260	7459	7659	7858	8058	8257
218	8457	8656	8855	9054	9253	9451	9650	9849	0047	0246
219	340444	0642	0841	1039	1237	1435	1632	1830	2028	2225
220	2423	2620	2817	3015	3212	3409	3606	3802	3999	4196
221	4392	4589	4785	4981	5178	5374	5570	5766	5962	6157
222	6353	6549	6744	6940	7135	7330	7525	7720	7915	8110
223	8305	8500	8694	8889	9083	9278	9472	9666	9860	0054
224	350248	0442	0636	0829	1023	1216	1410	1603	1796	1990
225	2183	2376	2568	2761	2954	3147	3339	3532	3724	3916
226	4108	4301	4493	4685	4876	5068	5260	5452	5643	5835
227	6026	6217	6408	6599	6791	6981	7172	7363	7554	7744
228	7935	8125	8316	8506	8696	8886	9076	9266	9456	9646
229	9836	0025	0215	0404	0593	0783	0972	1161	1350	1539
230	361728	1917	2105	2294	2483	2671	2859	3048	3236	3424
231	3612	3800	3988	4176	4363	4551	4739	4926	5113	5301
232	5488	5675	5862	6049	6236	6423	6610	6796	6983	7170
233	7356	7542	7729	7915	8101	8287	8473	8659	8845	9030
234	9216	9401	9587	9772	9958	0143	0328	0513	0698	0883
235	371068	1253	1437	1622	1807	1991	2175	2360	2544	2728
236	2912	3096	3280	3464	3648	3831	4015	4198	4382	4565
237	4748	4932	5115	5298	5481	5664	5846	6029	6212	6394
238	6577	6759	6942	7124	7306	7488	7670	7852	8034	8216
239	8398	8580	8761	8943	9124	9306	9487	9668	9849	0030

N°.	0	1	2	3	4	5	6	7	8	9
240	380211	0392	0573	0754	0935	1115	1296	1476	1657	1837
241	2017	2197	2377	2557	2737	2917	3097	3277	3456	3636
242	3815	3995	4174	4353	4533	4712	4891	5070	5249	5428
243	5606	5785	5964	6142	6321	6499	6677	6856	7033	7212
244	7390	7568	7746	7924	8101	8279	8457	8634	8811	8989
245	9166	9343	9521	9698	9875	0052	0228	0405	0582	0759
246	390935	1112	1288	1464	1641	1817	1993	2169	2345	2521
247	2697	2873	3049	3224	3400	3575	3751	3926	4101	4277
248	4452	4627	4802	4977	5152	5326	5501	5676	5850	6025
249	6199	6374	6548	6722	6896	7071	7245	7419	7592	7766
250	397940	8114	8287	8461	8634	8808	8981	9154	9328	9501
251	9674	9847	0020	0193	0365	0538	0711	0883	1056	1228
252	401401	1573	1745	1917	2089	2261	2433	2605	2777	2949
253	3121	3292	3464	3635	3807	3978	4149	4321	4492	4663
254	4834	5005	5176	5346	5517	5688	5858	6029	6199	6370
255	6540	6711	6881	7051	7221	7391	7561	7731	7901	8070
256	8240	8410	8579	8749	8918	9087	9257	9426	9595	9764
257	9933	0102	0271	0440	0609	0777	0946	1114	1283	1451
258	411620	1788	1956	2124	2293	2461	2629	2796	2964	3132
259	3300	3467	3635	3803	3970	4137	4305	4472	4639	4806
260	4973	5140	5307	5474	5641	5808	5974	6141	6308	6474
261	6641	6807	6973	7139	7306	7472	7638	7804	7970	8136
262	8301	8467	8633	8798	8964	9129	9295	9460	9625	9791
263	9956	0121	0286	0451	0616	0781	0945	1110	1275	1439
264	421604	1768	1933	2097	2261	2426	2590	2754	2918	3082
265	3246	3410	3574	3737	3901	4065	4228	4392	4555	4718
266	4882	5045	5208	5371	5534	5697	5860	6023	6186	6349
267	6511	6674	6837	6999	7161	7324	7486	7648	7811	7973
268	8135	8297	8459	8621	8783	8944	9106	9268	9429	9591
269	9752	9914	0075	0236	0398	0559	0720	0881	1042	1203
270	431364	1525	1685	1846	2007	2167	2328	2488	2649	2809
271	2969	3130	3290	3450	3610	3770	3930	4090	4250	4409
272	4569	4729	4888	5048	5207	5367	5526	5685	5844	6004
273	6163	6322	6481	6640	6799	6957	7116	7275	7433	7592
274	7751	7909	8068	8226	8384	8542	8701	8859	9017	9175

LOGARITHMS.

N°	0	1	2	3	4	5	6	7	8	9
275	9333	9491	9648	9806	9964	0122	0279	0437	0594	0752
276	440909	1066	1224	1381	1538	1695	1852	2009	2166	2323
277	2480	2637	2793	2950	3107	3263	3420	3576	3732	3889
278	4045	4201	4357	4513	4669	4825	4981	5137	5293	5449
279	5604	5760	5915	6071	6226	6382	6537	6693	6848	7003
280	7158	7313	7468	7623	7778	7933	8088	8242	8397	8552
281	8706	8861	9015	9170	9324	9478	9633	9787	9941	0095
282	450249	0403	0557	0711	0865	1019	1172	1326	1479	1633
283	1786	1940	2093	2247	2400	2553	2706	2859	3012	3165
284	3318	3471	3624	3777	3930	4082	4235	4388	4540	4692
285	4845	4997	5150	5302	5454	5606	5758	5910	6062	6214
286	6366	6518	6670	6821	6973	7125	7276	7428	7579	7731
287	7882	8033	8184	8336	8487	8638	8789	8940	9091	9242
288	9393	9543	9694	9845	9995	0146	0296	0447	0597	0748
289	460898	1048	1198	1348	1499	1649	1799	1949	2098	2248
290	2398	2548	2697	2847	2997	3146	3296	3445	3594	3744
291	3893	4042	4191	4341	4490	4639	4788	4936	5085	5234
292	5383	5532	5680	5829	5977	6126	6274	6423	6571	6719
293	6868	7016	7164	7312	7460	7608	7756	7904	8052	8200
294	8347	8495	8643	8790	8938	9085	9233	9380	9528	9675
295	9822	9969	0116	0263	0411	0558	0704	0851	0998	1145
296	471292	1438	1585	1732	1878	2025	2171	2318	2464	2610
297	2756	2903	3049	3195	3341	3487	3633	3779	3925	4071
298	4216	4362	4508	4653	4799	4944	5090	5235	5381	5526
299	5671	5816	5962	6107	6252	6397	6542	6687	6832	6977
300	477121	7266	7411	7555	7700	7845	7989	8133	8278	8422
301	8567	8711	8855	8999	9143	9287	9431	9575	9719	9863
302	480007	0151	0295	0438	0582	0725	0869	1012	1156	1299
303	1443	1586	1729	1872	2016	2159	2302	2445	2588	2731
304	2874	3016	3159	3302	3445	3587	3730	3873	4015	4157
305	4300	4442	4585	4727	4869	5011	5153	5295	5438	5580
306	5721	5863	6005	6147	6289	6431	6572	6714	6855	6997
307	7138	7280	7421	7563	7704	7845	7986	8128	8269	8410
308	8551	8692	8833	8974	9111	9255	9396	9537	9677	9818
309	9959	0099	0240	0380	0520	0661	0801	0941	1081	1222

3 P

A Table of

N°	0	1	2	3	4	5	6	7	8	9
310	491362	1502	1642	1782	1922	2062	2202	2341	2481	2621
311	2760	2900	3040	3179	3319	3458	3597	3737	3876	4015
312	4155	4294	4433	4572	4711	4850	4989	5128	5267	5406
313	5544	5683	5822	5960	6099	6238	6376	6515	6653	6791
314	6930	7068	7206	7344	7483	7621	7759	7897	8035	8173
315	8311	8448	8586	8724	8862	8999	9137	9275	9412	9550
316	9687	9825	9762	0099	0237	0374	0511	0648	0785	0922
317	501059	1196	1333	1470	1607	1744	1881	2017	2154	2291
318	2427	2564	2700	2837	2973	3109	3246	3382	3518	3655
319	3791	3927	4063	4199	4335	4471	4607	4743	4879	5014
320	5150	5286	5421	5557	5693	5828	5964	6099	6234	6370
321	6505	6640	6776	6911	7046	7181	7316	7451	7586	7721
322	7856	7991	8126	8260	8395	8530	8664	8799	8934	9068
323	9203	9337	9471	9606	9740	9874	0009	0143	0277	0411
324	510545	0679	0813	0947	1081	1215	1349	1482	1616	1750
325	1883	2017	2151	2284	2418	2551	2684	2818	2951	3084
326	3218	3351	3484	3617	3750	3883	4016	4149	4282	4415
327	4548	4681	4813	4946	5079	5211	5344	5476	5609	5711
328	5874	6006	6139	6271	6403	6535	6668	6800	6932	7064
329	7196	7328	7460	7592	7724	7855	7987	8119	8251	8382
330	8514	8646	8777	8909	9040	9172	9303	9434	9566	9697
331	9828	9959	0090	0221	0353	0484	0615	0746	0876	1007
332	521138	1269	1400	1530	1661	1792	1922	2053	2183	2314
333	2444	2575	2705	2835	2966	3096	3226	3356	3486	3616
334	3747	3877	4006	4136	4266	4396	4526	4656	4785	4915
335	5045	5174	5304	5434	5563	5693	5822	5951	6081	6210
336	6339	6469	6598	6727	6856	6985	7114	7243	7372	7501
337	7630	7759	7888	8016	8145	8274	8402	8531	8660	8788
338	8917	9045	9174	9302	9430	9559	9687	9815	9943	0072
339	530200	0328	0456	0584	0712	0840	0968	1096	1223	1351
340	1479	1607	1734	1862	1990	2117	2245	2372	2500	2627
341	2754	2882	3009	3136	3264	3391	3518	3645	3772	3899
342	4026	4153	4280	4407	4534	4661	4787	4914	5041	5168
343	5294	5421	5547	5674	5800	5927	6053	6180	6306	6432
344	6558	6685	6811	6937	7063	7189	7315	7441	7567	7693

LOGARITHMS. 473

N°	0	1	2	3	4	5	6	7	8	9
345	7819	7945	8071	8197	8322	8448	8574	8699	8825	8951
346	9076	9202	9327	9453	9578	9703	9829	9954	0079	0204
347	540330	0455	0580	0705	0830	0955	1080	1205	1330	1454
348	1579	1704	1829	1954	2078	2203	2327	2452	2577	2701
349	2825	2950	3074	3199	3323	3447	3571	3696	3820	3944
350	544068	4192	4316	4440	4564	4688	4812	4936	5060	5183
351	5307	5431	5555	5678	5802	5925	6049	6172	6296	6419
352	6543	6666	6789	6913	7036	7159	7282	7406	7529	7652
353	7775	7898	8021	8144	8267	8389	8512	8635	8758	8881
354	9003	9126	9249	9371	9494	9616	9739	9861	9984	0106
355	550228	0351	0473	0595	0717	0840	0962	1084	1206	1328
356	1450	1572	1694	1816	1938	2060	2181	2303	2425	2547
357	2668	2790	2912	3033	3155	3276	3398	3519	3640	3762
358	3883	4004	4126	4247	4368	4489	4610	4731	4852	4974
359	5094	5215	5336	5457	5578	5699	5820	5940	6061	6182
360	6303	6423	6544	6664	6785	6905	7026	7146	7267	7387
361	7507	7628	7748	7868	7988	8108	8228	8349	8469	8589
362	8709	8829	8948	9068	9188	9308	9428	9548	9667	9787
363	9907	0026	0146	0265	0385	0504	0624	0743	0863	0982
364	561101	1221	1340	1459	1578	1698	1817	1936	2055	2174
365	2293	2412	2531	2650	2769	2887	3006	3125	3244	3362
366	3481	3600	3718	3837	3956	4074	4193	4311	4429	4548
367	4666	4784	4903	5021	5139	5257	5376	5494	5612	5730
368	5848	5966	6084	6202	6320	6438	6555	6673	6791	6909
369	7026	7144	7262	7379	7497	7614	7732	7850	7967	8084
370	8202	8319	8436	8554	8671	8788	8905	9023	9140	9257
371	9374	9491	9608	9725	9842	9959	0076	0193	0309	0426
372	570543	0660	0776	0893	1010	1126	1243	1359	1476	1592
373	1709	1825	1942	2058	2174	2291	2407	2523	2639	2756
374	2872	2988	3104	3220	3336	3452	3568	3684	3800	3915
375	4031	4147	4263	4379	4494	4610	4726	4841	4957	5072
376	5188	5303	5419	5534	5650	5765	5880	5996	6111	6226
377	6341	6457	6572	6687	6802	6917	7032	7147	7262	7377
378	7492	7607	7722	7836	7951	8066	8181	8295	8410	8525
379	8639	8754	8868	8983	9097	9212	9326	9441	9555	9669

3 P 2

A TABLE of

N°	0	1	2	3	4	5	6	7	8	9
380	9784	9898	0012	0126	0241	0355	0469	0583	0697	0811
381	580925	1039	1153	1267	1381	1495	1608	1722	1836	1950
382	2063	2177	2291	2404	2518	2631	2745	2859	2972	3085
383	3199	3312	3426	3539	3652	3765	3879	3992	4105	4218
384	4531	4444	4557	4670	4783	4896	5009	5122	5235	5348
385	5461	5574	5686	5799	5912	6024	6137	6250	6362	6475
386	6587	6700	6812	6925	7037	7150	7262	7374	7487	7599
387	7711	7823	7935	8048	8160	8272	8384	8496	8608	8720
388	8832	8944	9056	9167	9279	9391	9503	9615	9726	9838
389	9950	0061	0173	0284	0396	0508	0619	0730	0842	0953
390	591065	1176	1287	1399	1510	1621	1732	1843	1955	2066
391	2177	2288	2399	2510	2621	2732	2843	2954	3064	3175
392	3286	3397	3508	3618	3729	3840	3950	4061	4172	4282
393	4393	4503	4614	4724	4834	4945	5055	5165	5276	5386
394	5496	5606	5717	5827	5937	6047	6157	6267	6377	6487
395	6597	6707	6817	6927	7037	7147	7256	7366	7476	7586
396	7695	7805	7915	8024	8134	8243	8353	8462	8572	8681
397	8791	8900	9009	9119	9228	9337	9446	9556	9665	9774
398	9883	9992	0101	0210	0319	0428	0537	0646	0755	0864
399	600973	1082	1191	1299	1408	1517	1626	1734	1843	1951
400	602060	2169	2277	2386	2494	2603	2711	2819	2928	3036
401	3144	3253	3361	3469	3577	3686	3794	3902	4010	4118
402	4226	4334	4442	4550	4658	4766	4874	4982	5090	5197
403	5305	5413	5521	5628	5736	5844	5951	6059	6166	6274
404	6381	6489	6596	6704	6811	6919	7026	7133	7241	7348
405	7455	7562	7669	7777	7884	7991	8098	8205	8312	8419
406	8526	8633	8740	8847	8954	9061	9167	9274	9381	9488
407	9594	9701	9808	9914	0021	0128	0234	0341	0447	0554
408	610660	0767	0873	0979	1086	1192	1298	1405	1511	1617
409	1723	1830	1936	2042	2148	2254	2360	2466	2572	2677
410	2784	2890	2996	3102	3207	3313	3419	3525	3630	3736
411	3842	3948	4053	4159	4264	4370	4475	4581	4686	4792
412	4897	5003	5108	5213	5319	5424	5529	5635	5740	5845
413	5950	6055	6160	6265	6371	6476	6581	6686	6791	6895
414	7000	7105	7210	7315	7420	7525	7629	7734	7839	7943

LOGARITHMS. 475

N°	0	1	2	3	4	5	6	7	8	9
415	8048	8153	8257	8362	8467	8571	8676	8780	8885	8989
416	9093	9198	9302	9406	9511	9615	9719	9824	9928	0032
417	620136	0240	0344	0448	0552	0657	0761	0865	0968	1072
418	1176	1280	1384	1488	1592	1696	1799	1903	2007	2110
419	2214	2318	2421	2525	2628	2732	2836	2939	3042	3146
420	3249	3353	3456	3559	3663	3766	3869	3973	4076	4179
421	4282	4385	4488	4592	4695	4798	4901	5004	5107	5210
422	5313	5415	5518	5621	5724	5827	5930	6032	6135	6238
423	6340	6443	6546	6648	6751	6853	6956	7059	7161	7263
424	7366	7468	7571	7673	7775	7878	7980	8082	8185	8287
425	8389	8491	8593	8695	8798	8900	9002	9104	9206	9308
426	9410	9512	9613	9715	9817	9919	0021	0123	0224	0326
427	630428	0530	0631	0733	0835	0936	1038	1139	1241	1342
428	1444	1545	1647	1748	1850	1951	2052	2154	2255	2356
429	2457	2559	2660	2761	2862	2963	3064	3165	3266	3367
430	3469	3569	3670	3771	3872	3973	4074	4175	4276	4377
431	4477	4578	4679	4780	4880	4981	5081	5182	5283	5383
432	5484	5584	5685	5785	5886	5986	6087	6187	6287	6388
433	6488	6588	6688	6789	6889	6989	7089	7189	7290	7390
434	7490	7590	7690	7790	7890	7990	8090	8190	8290	8389
435	8489	8589	8689	8789	8858	8988	9088	9188	9287	9387
436	9487	9586	9686	9785	9885	9984	0084	0183	0283	0382
437	640481	0581	0680	0780	0879	0978	1077	1177	1276	1375
438	1474	1573	1672	1772	1871	1970	2069	2168	2267	2366
439	2465	2563	2662	2761	2860	2959	3058	3157	3255	3354
440	3453	3551	3650	3749	3847	3946	4045	4143	4242	4340
441	4439	4537	4636	4734	4832	4931	5029	5127	5226	5324
442	5422	5521	5619	5717	5815	5913	6011	6110	6208	6306
443	6404	6502	6600	6698	6796	6894	6992	7089	7187	7285
444	7383	7481	7579	7676	7774	7872	7970	8067	8165	8262
445	8360	8458	8555	8653	8750	8848	8945	9043	9140	9238
446	9335	9432	9530	9627	9724	9822	9919	0016	0113	0210
447	650308	0405	0502	0599	0696	0793	0890	0987	1084	1181
448	1278	1375	1472	1569	1666	1762	1859	1956	2053	2150
449	2246	2343	2440	2536	2633	2730	2826	2923	3020	3116

A Table of

N°.	0	1	2	3	4	5	6	7	8	9
450	653213	3309	3406	3502	3598	3695	3791	3888	3984	4080
451	4177	4273	4369	4465	4562	4658	4754	4850	4946	5042
452	5138	5235	5331	5427	5523	5619	5715	5811	5906	6002
453	6098	6194	6290	6386	6482	6577	6673	6769	6865	6960
454	7056	7152	7247	7343	7438	7534	7629	7725	7821	7916
455	8011	8107	8202	8298	8393	8488	8584	8679	8774	8870
456	8965	9060	9155	9251	9346	9441	9536	9631	9726	9821
457	9916	0011	0106	0201	0296	0391	0486	0581	0676	0771
458	660866	0960	1055	1150	1245	1339	1434	1529	1623	1718
459	1813	1907	2002	2096	2191	2286	2380	2475	2569	2663
460	2758	2852	2947	3041	3135	3230	3324	3418	3513	3607
461	3701	3795	3889	3984	4078	4172	4266	4360	4454	4548
462	4642	4736	4830	4924	5018	5112	5206	5300	5393	5487
463	5581	5675	5769	5862	5956	6050	6143	6237	6331	6424
464	6518	6612	6705	6799	6892	6986	7079	7173	7266	7360
465	7453	7546	7640	7733	7826	7920	8013	8106	8200	8293
466	8386	8479	8572	8665	8759	8852	8945	9038	9131	9224
467	9317	9410	9503	9596	9689	9782	9875	9967	0060	0153
468	670246	0339	0431	0524	0617	0710	0802	0895	0988	1080
469	1173	1265	1358	1451	1543	1636	1728	1821	1913	2005
470	2098	2190	2283	2375	2467	2560	2652	2744	2837	2929
471	3021	3113	3205	3297	3390	3482	3574	3666	3758	3850
472	3942	4034	4126	4218	4310	4402	4494	4586	4678	4769
473	4861	4953	5045	5137	5228	5320	5412	5503	5595	5687
474	5778	5870	5962	6053	6145	6236	6328	6419	6511	6602
475	6694	6785	6876	6968	7059	7151	7242	7333	7424	7516
476	7607	7698	7789	7881	7972	8063	8154	8245	8336	8427
477	8518	8609	8700	8791	8882	8973	9064	9155	9246	9337
478	9428	9519	9610	9700	9791	9882	9973	0063	0154	0245
479	680336	0426	0517	0607	0698	0789	0879	0970	1060	1151
480	1241	1332	1422	1513	1603	1693	1784	1874	1965	2055
481	2145	2235	2326	2416	2506	2596	2687	2777	2867	2957
482	3047	3137	3227	3317	3407	3497	3587	3677	3767	3857
483	3947	4037	4127	4217	4307	4397	4486	4576	4666	4756
484	4845	4935	5025	5115	5204	5294	5383	5473	5563	5652

LOGARITHMS. 477

N°.	0	1	2	3	4	5	6	7	8	9
485	5742	5831	5921	6010	6100	6189	6279	6368	6458	6547
486	6636	6726	6815	6904	6994	7083	7172	7261	7351	7440
487	7529	7618	7707	7796	7886	7975	8064	8153	8242	8331
488	8420	8509	8598	8687	8776	8865	8954	9042	9131	9220
489	9309	9398	9486	9575	9664	9753	9841	9930	0019	0107
490	690196	0285	0373	0462	0551	0639	0728	0816	0905	0993
491	1082	1170	1258	1347	1435	1524	1612	1700	1789	1877
492	1965	2053	2142	2230	2318	2406	2494	2583	2671	2759
493	2847	2935	3023	3111	3199	3287	3375	3463	3551	3639
494	3727	3815	3903	3991	4079	4166	4254	4342	4430	4518
495	4605	4693	4781	4868	4956	5044	5131	5219	5307	5394
496	5482	5569	5657	5744	5832	5919	6007	6094	6182	6269
497	6356	6444	6531	6619	6706	6793	6880	6968	7055	7142
498	7229	7317	7404	7491	7578	7665	7752	7839	7926	8014
499	8101	8188	8275	8362	8449	8536	8622	8709	8796	8883
500	698970	9057	9144	9231	9317	9404	9491	9578	9664	9751
501	9838	9924	0011	0098	0184	0271	0358	0444	0531	0617
502	700704	0790	0877	0963	1050	1136	1223	1309	1395	1482
503	1568	1654	1741	1827	1913	2000	2086	2172	2258	2344
504	2431	2517	2603	2689	2775	2861	2947	3033	3119	3205
505	3291	3377	3463	3549	3635	3721	3807	3893	3979	4065
506	4151	4236	4322	4408	4494	4579	4665	4751	4837	4922
507	5008	5094	5179	5265	5351	5436	5522	5607	5693	5778
508	5864	5949	6035	6120	6206	6291	6376	6462	6547	6633
509	6718	6803	6888	6974	7059	7144	7229	7315	7400	7485
510	7570	7655	7741	7826	7911	7996	8081	8166	8251	8336
511	8421	8506	8591	8676	8761	8846	8931	9015	9100	9185
512	9270	9355	9440	9524	9609	9694	9779	9863	9948	0033
513	710117	0202	0287	0371	0456	0540	0625	0710	0794	0879
514	0963	1048	1132	1217	1301	1385	1470	1554	1639	1723
515	1807	1892	1976	2060	2144	2229	2313	2397	2481	2566
516	2650	2734	2818	2902	2986	3070	3154	3239	3323	3407
517	3491	3575	3659	3743	3826	3910	3994	4078	4162	4246
518	4330	4414	4497	4581	4665	4749	4833	4916	5000	5084
519	5167	5251	5335	5418	5502	5586	5669	5753	5836	5920

N°.	0	1	2	3	4	5	6	7	8	9
520	6002	6087	6170	6254	6337	6421	6504	6588	6671	6754
521	6838	6921	7004	7038	7171	7254	7338	7421	7504	7587
522	7671	7754	7837	7920	8003	8086	8169	8253	8336	8419
523	8502	8585	8668	8751	8834	8917	9000	9083	9166	9248
524	9331	9414	9497	9580	9663	9746	9828	9911	9994	0077
525	720159	0242	0325	0407	0490	0573	0655	0738	0821	0903
526	0986	1068	1151	1233	1316	1398	1481	1563	1646	1728
527	1811	1893	1975	2058	2140	2223	2305	2387	2469	2552
528	2634	2716	2798	2881	2963	3045	3127	3209	3291	3374
529	3456	3538	3620	3702	3784	3866	3948	4030	4112	4194
530	4276	4358	4440	4522	4604	4685	4767	4849	4931	5013
531	5095	5176	5258	5340	5422	5503	5585	5667	5748	5830
532	5912	5993	6075	6157	6238	6320	6401	6483	6564	6646
533	6727	6809	6890	6972	7053	7134	7216	7297	7379	7460
534	7541	7623	7704	7785	7866	7948	8029	8110	8191	8273
535	8354	8435	8516	8597	8678	8760	8841	8922	9003	9084
536	9165	9246	9327	9408	9489	9570	9651	9732	9813	9893
537	9974	0055	0136	0217	0298	0379	0459	0540	0621	0702
538	730782	0863	0944	1024	1105	1186	1266	1347	1428	1508
539	1589	1669	1750	1830	1911	1991	2072	2152	2233	2313
540	2394	2474	2555	2635	2715	2776	2876	2956	3037	3117
541	3197	3278	3358	3438	3518	3599	3679	3759	3839	3919
542	3999	4079	4160	4240	4320	4400	4480	4560	4640	4720
543	4800	4880	4960	5040	5120	5200	5279	5359	5439	5519
544	5599	5679	5759	5838	5918	5998	6078	6157	6237	6317
545	6397	6476	6556	6636	6715	6795	6874	6954	7034	7113
546	7193	7272	7352	7431	7511	7590	7670	7749	7829	7908
547	7987	8067	8146	8225	8305	8384	8463	8543	8622	8701
548	8781	8860	8939	9018	9097	9177	9256	9335	9414	9493
549	9572	9651	9731	9810	9889	9968	0047	0126	0205	0284
550	740363	0442	0521	0600	0678	0757	0836	0915	0994	1073
551	1152	1230	1309	1388	1467	1546	1624	1703	1782	1860
552	1939	2018	2096	2175	2254	2332	2411	2490	2568	2647
553	2725	2804	2882	2961	3039	3118	3196	3275	3353	3431
554	3510	3588	3667	3745	3823	3902	3980	4058	4137	4215

LOGARITHMS.

No	0	1	2	3	4	5	6	7	8	9
555	744293	4371	4450	4528	4606	4684	4762	4840	4919	4997
556	5075	5153	5231	5309	5387	5465	5543	5621	5699	5777
557	5855	5933	6011	6089	6167	6245	6323	6401	6479	6556
558	6634	6712	6790	6868	6945	7023	7101	7179	7256	7334
559	7412	7490	7567	7645	7723	7800	7878	7955	8033	8111
560	8188	8266	8343	8421	8498	8576	8653	8731	8808	8885
561	8963	9040	9118	9595	9272	9350	9427	9504	9552	9659
562	9736	9814	9891	9968	0045	0123	0200	0277	0354	0431
563	750508	0586	0663	0740	0817	0894	0971	1048	1125	1202
564	1279	1356	1433	1510	1587	1664	1741	1818	1895	1972
565	2048	2125	2202	2279	2356	2433	2509	2586	2663	2740
566	2816	2893	2970	3047	3123	3200	3277	3353	3430	3507
567	3583	3660	3736	3813	3889	3966	4042	4119	4195	4272
568	4348	4425	4501	4578	4654	4731	4807	4883	4960	5036
569	5112	5189	5265	5341	5418	5494	5570	5646	5722	5798
570	5875	5951	6027	6103	6180	6256	6332	6408	6484	6560
571	6636	6712	6788	6864	6940	7016	7092	7168	7244	7320
572	7396	7472	7548	7624	7700	7775	7851	7927	8003	8079
573	8155	8230	8306	8382	8458	8533	8609	8685	8761	8836
574	8912	8988	9063	9139	9214	9290	9366	9441	9517	9592
375	9668	9743	9819	9894	9970	0045	0121	0196	0272	0347
576	760423	0498	0573	0649	0724	0799	0875	0950	1025	1101
577	1176	1251	1326	1402	1477	1552	1627	1702	1778	1853
578	1928	2003	2078	2153	2228	2303	2378	2454	2529	2604
579	2679	2754	2829	2904	2979	3053	3128	3203	3278	3353
580	3428	3503	3578	3653	3727	3802	3877	3952	4027	4101
581	4176	4251	4326	4400	4475	4550	4624	4699	4774	4848
582	4923	4998	5072	5147	5221	5296	5371	5445	5520	5594
583	5669	5743	5818	5892	5966	6041	6115	6190	6264	6338
584	6413	6487	6562	6636	6710	6785	6859	6933	7007	7082
585	7156	7230	7304	7379	7453	7527	7601	7675	7749	7823
586	7898	7972	8046	8120	8194	8268	8342	8416	8490	8564
587	8638	8712	8786	8860	8934	9008	9082	9156	9230	9304
588	9377	9451	9525	9599	9673	9747	9820	9894	9968	0042
589	770115	0189	0263	0336	0410	0484	0558	0631	0705	0778

3 Q

A Table of

N°	0	1	2	3	4	5	6	7	8	9
590	770852	0926	0999	1072	1146	1220	1293	1367	1441	1514
591	1588	1661	1734	1808	1881	1955	2028	2102	2175	2248
592	2322	2395	2468	2542	2615	2688	2762	2835	2908	2981
593	3055	3128	3201	3274	3348	3421	3494	3567	3640	3713
594	3786	3860	3933	4006	4079	4152	4225	4298	4371	4444
595	4517	1590	4663	4736	4809	4882	4955	5028	5101	5173
596	5246	5319	5392	5465	5538	5610	5683	5756	5829	5902
597	5974	6047	6120	6193	6265	6338	6411	6483	6556	6629
598	6701	6774	6846	6919	6992	7064	7137	7209	7282	7354
599	7427	7490	7572	7644	7717	7789	7862	7934	8007	8079
600	8151	8224	8296	8368	8441	8513	8585	8658	8730	8802
601	8875	8947	9019	9091	9163	9236	9308	9380	9452	9524
602	9597	9669	9741	9813	9885	9957	0029	0101	0173	0245
603	780317	0389	0461	0533	0605	0677	0749	0821	0893	0965
604	1037	1109	1181	1253	1325	1396	1468	1540	1612	1684
605	1755	1827	1899	1971	2042	2114	2186	2258	2329	2401
606	2473	2544	2616	2688	2759	2831	2902	2974	3046	3117
607	3189	3260	3332	3403	3475	3546	3618	3689	3761	3832
608	3904	3975	4046	4118	4189	4261	4332	4403	4475	4546
609	4617	4689	4760	4831	4902	4974	5045	5116	5187	5259
610	5330	5401	5472	5543	5615	5686	5757	5828	5899	5970
611	6041	6112	6183	6254	6325	6397	6468	6539	6610	6680
612	6751	6822	6893	6964	7035	7106	7177	7248	7319	7390
613	7461	7531	7602	7673	7744	7815	7885	7956	8027	8098
614	8168	8239	8310	8381	8451	8522	8593	8663	8734	8805
615	8875	8946	9016	9087	9158	9228	9299	9369	9440	9510
616	9581	9651	9722	9792	9863	9933	0004	0074	0144	0215
617	90285	0356	0426	0496	0567	0637	0707	0778	0848	0918
618	0989	1059	1129	1199	1270	1340	1410	1480	1550	1621
619	1691	1761	1831	1901	1971	2041	2111	2182	2252	2322
620	2392	2462	2532	2602	2672	2742	2812	2882	2952	3022
621	3092	3162	3231	3301	3371	3441	3511	3581	3651	3721
622	3790	3860	3930	4000	4070	4139	4209	4279	4349	4418
623	4488	4558	4627	4697	4767	4837	4906	4976	5045	5115
624	5185	5254	5324	5393	5463	5532	5602	5672	5741	5811

LOGARITHMS.

N°	0	1	2	3	4	5	6	7	8	9
625	795880	5950	6019	6088	6158	6227	6297	6366	6436	6505
626	6574	6644	6713	6782	6852	6921	6990	7060	7129	7198
627	7268	7337	7406	7475	7545	7614	7683	7752	7821	7891
628	7960	8029	8098	8167	8236	8305	8374	8444	8513	8582
629	8651	8720	8789	8858	8927	8996	9065	9134	9203	9272
630	9341	9410	9478	9547	9616	9685	9754	9823	9892	9961
631	800029	0098	0167	0236	0305	0373	0442	0511	0580	0648
632	0717	0786	0855	0923	0992	1061	1129	1198	1267	1335
633	1404	1472	1541	1610	1678	1747	1815	1884	1952	2021
634	2089	2158	2226	2295	2363	2432	2500	2569	2637	2705
634	2774	2842	2911	2979	3047	3116	3184	3252	3321	3389
636	3457	3525	3594	3662	3730	3798	3867	2935	4003	4071
637	4139	4208	4276	4344	4412	4480	4548	4616	4685	4753
638	4821	4889	4957	5025	5093	5161	5229	5297	5365	5433
639	5501	5569	5637	5705	5773	5841	5909	5976	6044	6112
640	6180	6248	6316	6384	6451	6519	6587	6655	6723	6790
641	6858	6926	6994	7061	7129	7197	7264	7332	7400	7467
642	7535	7603	7670	7738	7806	7873	7941	8008	8076	8143
643	8211	8279	8346	8414	8481	8549	8616	8684	8751	8818
644	8886	8953	9021	9088	9156	9223	9290	9358	9425	9492
645	9560	9627	9694	9762	9829	9896	9964	0031	0098	0165
646	810233	0300	0367	0434	0501	0569	0636	0703	0770	0837
647	0904	0971	1039	1106	1173	1240	1307	1374	1441	1508
648	1575	1642	1709	1776	1843	1910	1977	2044	2111	2178
649	2245	2312	2379	2445	2512	2579	2646	2713	2780	2847
650	2913	2980	3047	3114	3181	3247	3314	3381	3448	3514
651	3581	3648	3714	3781	3848	3914	3981	4048	4114	4181
652	4248	4314	4381	4447	4514	4581	4647	4714	4780	4847
653	4913	4980	5046	5113	5179	5246	5312	5379	5445	5511
654	5578	5644	5711	5777	5843	5910	5976	6042	6109	6175
655	6241	6308	6374	6440	6506	6573	6639	6705	6771	6838
656	6904	6970	7036	7102	7169	7235	7301	7367	7433	7499
657	7565	7632	7698	7764	7830	7896	7962	8028	8094	8160
658	8226	8292	8358	8424	8490	8556	8622	8688	8754	8820
659	8885	8951	9017	9083	9149	9215	9281	9347	9412	9478

3 Q 2

N°.	0	1	2	3	4	5	6	7	8	9
660	819544	9610	9676	9741	9807	9873	9939	0004	0070	0136
661	820202	0267	0333	0399	0464	0530	0596	0661	0727	0792
662	0858	0924	0989	1055	1120	1186	1251	1317	1383	1448
663	1514	1579	1645	1710	1776	1841	1906	1972	2037	2103
664	2168	2234	2299	2364	2430	2495	2560	2626	2691	2756
665	2822	2887	2952	3018	3083	3148	3213	3279	3344	3409
666	3474	3539	3605	3670	3735	3800	3865	3931	3996	4061
667	4126	4191	4256	4321	4386	4451	4516	4581	4646	4711
668	4777	4842	4907	4972	5030	5101	5166	5231	5296	5361
669	5426	5491	5556	5621	5686	5751	5815	5880	5945	6010
670	6075	6140	6204	6269	6334	6399	6464	6528	6593	6658
671	6723	6787	6852	6917	6981	7046	7111	7175	7240	7305
672	7369	7434	7499	7563	7628	7692	7757	7821	7886	7951
673	8015	8080	8144	8209	8273	8338	8402	8467	8531	8596
674	8660	8724	8789	8853	8918	8982	9046	9111	9175	9239
675	9304	9368	9432	9497	9561	9625	9690	9754	9818	9882
676	9947	0011	0075	0139	0204	0268	0332	0396	0460	0525
677	830589	0653	0717	0781	0845	0909	0973	1038	1102	1166
678	1230	1294	1358	1422	1486	1550	1614	1678	1742	1806
679	1870	1934	1998	2062	2126	2190	2253	2317	2381	2445
680	2509	2573	2637	2701	2764	2828	2892	2956	3020	3083
681	3147	3211	3275	3338	3402	3466	3530	3593	3657	3721
682	3784	3848	3912	3975	4039	4103	4166	4230	4294	4357
683	4421	4484	4548	4611	4675	4739	4802	4866	4929	4993
684	5056	5120	5183	5247	5310	5374	5437	5500	5564	5627
685	5691	5754	5817	5881	5944	6008	6071	6134	6198	6261
686	6324	6387	6451	6514	6577	6641	6704	6767	6830	6894
687	6957	7020	7083	7146	7210	7273	7336	7399	7462	7525
688	7588	7652	7715	7778	7841	7904	7967	8030	8093	8156
689	8219	8282	8345	8408	8471	8534	8597	8660	8723	8786
690	8849	8912	8975	9038	9101	9164	9227	9290	9352	9415
691	9478	9541	9604	9667	9709	9792	9855	9918	9981	0043
692	840106	0169	0232	0294	0357	0420	0483	0545	0608	0671
693	0733	0796	0859	0921	0984	1047	1109	1172	1234	1297
694	1360	1422	1485	1547	1610	1672	1735	1797	1860	1922

LOGARITHMS.

N°	0	1	2	3	4	5	6	7	8	9
695	841985	2047	2110	2172	2235	2297	2360	2422	2484	2547
696	2609	2672	2734	2796	2859	2921	2984	3046	3108	3171
697	3233	3295	3357	3420	3482	3544	3607	3669	3731	3793
698	3855	3918	3980	4042	4104	4166	4229	4291	4353	4415
699	4477	4539	4601	4664	4726	4788	4850	4912	4974	5036
700	5098	5160	5222	5284	5346	5408	5470	5532	5594	5656
701	5718	5780	5842	5904	5966	6028	6090	6152	6213	6275
702	6337	6399	6461	6523	6585	6646	6708	6770	6832	6894
703	6955	7017	7079	7141	7202	7264	7326	7388	7449	7511
704	7573	7634	7696	7758	7819	7881	7943	8004	8066	8128
705	8189	8251	8312	8374	8436	8497	8559	8620	8682	8743
706	8805	8866	8928	8989	9051	9112	9174	9235	9297	9358
707	9419	9481	9542	9604	9665	9726	9788	9849	9911	9972
708	850033	0095	0156	0217	0279	0340	0401	0462	0524	0585
709	0646	0708	0769	0830	0891	0952	1014	1075	1136	1197
710	1258	1320	1381	1442	1503	1564	1625	1686	1747	1809
711	1870	1931	1992	2053	2114	2175	2236	2297	2358	2419
712	2480	2541	2602	2663	2724	2785	2846	2907	2968	3029
713	3090	3150	3211	3272	3333	3394	3455	3516	3577	3637
714	3698	3759	3820	3881	3941	4002	4063	4124	4185	4245
715	4306	4367	4428	4488	4549	4610	4670	4731	4792	4852
716	4913	4974	5034	5095	5156	5216	5277	5337	5398	5459
717	5519	5580	5640	5701	5761	5822	5882	5913	6004	6064
718	6124	6185	6245	6306	6366	6427	6487	6548	6608	6669
719	6729	6789	6850	6910	6970	7031	7091	7152	7212	7272
720	7333	7393	7453	7513	7574	7634	7694	7755	7815	7875
721	7935	7996	8056	8116	8176	8236	8297	8357	8417	8477
722	8537	8597	8658	8718	8778	8838	8898	8958	9018	9078
723	9138	9198	9258	9319	9379	9439	9499	9559	9619	9679
724	9739	9799	9859	9919	9978	0038	0098	0158	0218	0278
724	860338	0398	0458	0518	0578	0637	0697	0757	0817	0877
726	0937	0996	1056	1116	1176	1236	1295	1355	1415	1475
727	1534	1594	1654	1714	1773	1833	1893	1952	2012	2072
728	2131	2191	2251	2310	2370	2430	2489	2519	2608	2668
729	2728	2787	2847	2906	2966	3025	3085	3144	3204	3263

A Table of

N°	0	1	2	3	4	5	6	7	8	9
730	863323	3382	3442	3501	3561	3620	3680	3739	3799	3858
731	3917	3977	4036	4096	4155	4214	4274	4333	4392	4452
732	4511	4570	4630	4689	4748	4808	4867	4926	4986	5045
733	5104	5163	5223	5282	5341	5400	5459	5519	5578	5637
734	5696	5755	5814	5874	5933	5992	6051	6110	6169	6228
735	6287	6346	6406	6465	6524	6583	6642	6701	6760	6819
736	6878	6937	6996	7055	7114	7173	7232	7291	7350	7409
737	7468	7526	7585	7644	7703	7762	7821	7880	7939	7998
738	8056	8115	8174	8233	8292	8351	8409	8468	8527	8586
739	8644	8703	8762	8821	8879	8938	8997	9056	9114	9173
740	9232	9290	9349	9408	9466	9525	9584	9642	9701	9760
741	9818	9877	9935	9994	0053	0111	0170	0228	0287	0345
742	870404	0462	0521	0579	0630	0697	0755	0813	0872	0930
743	0989	1047	1106	1164	1223	1281	1339	1398	1456	1515
744	1573	1631	1690	1748	1806	1865	1923	1981	2040	2098
745	2156	2215	2273	2331	2389	2448	2506	2564	2622	2681
746	2739	2797	2855	2913	2972	3030	3088	3146	3204	3263
747	3321	3379	3437	3495	3553	3611	3669	3727	3786	3844
748	3902	3960	4018	4076	4134	4192	4250	4308	4366	4424
749	4482	4540	4598	4656	4714	4772	4830	4888	4945	5003
750	5061	5119	5177	5235	5293	5351	5409	5466	5524	5582
751	5640	5698	5756	5813	5871	5929	5987	6045	6102	6160
752	6218	6276	6333	6391	6449	6507	6564	6622	6680	6737
753	6795	6853	6910	6968	7026	7083	7141	7199	7256	7314
754	7371	7429	7487	7544	7602	7659	7717	7774	7832	7889
755	7947	8005	8062	8120	8177	8235	8292	8349	8407	8464
756	8522	8579	8637	8694	8752	8809	8866	8924	8981	9039
757	9096	9153	9211	9268	9325	9383	9440	9497	9555	9612
758	9669	9727	9784	9841	9898	9956	0013	0070	0127	0185
759	880242	0299	0356	0413	0471	0528	0585	0642	0699	0756
760	0814	0871	0928	0985	1042	1099	1156	1213	1271	1328
761	1385	1442	1499	1556	1613	1670	1727	1784	1841	1898
762	1955	2012	2069	2126	2183	2240	2297	2354	2411	2468
763	2525	2582	2638	2695	2752	2809	2866	2923	2980	3037
764	3093	3150	3207	3264	3321	3378	3434	3491	3548	3605

LOGARITHMS.

N°	0	1	2	3	4	5	6	7	8	9
765	883661	3718	3775	3832	3889	3945	4002	4059	4115	4172
766	4229	4286	4342	4399	4456	4512	4569	4626	4682	4739
767	4795	4852	4909	4965	5022	5078	5135	5192	5248	5305
768	5361	5418	5474	5531	5587	5644	5700	5757	5813	5870
769	5926	5983	6039	6096	6152	6209	6265	6322	6378	6434
770	6491	6547	6604	6660	6716	6773	6829	6885	6942	6998
771	7054	7111	7167	7223	7280	7336	7392	7449	7505	7561
772	7617	7674	7730	7786	7842	7899	7955	8011	8067	8123
773	8180	8236	8292	8348	8404	8460	8517	8573	8629	8685
774	8741	8797	8853	8909	8965	9021	9078	9134	9190	9246
775	9302	9358	9414	9470	9526	9582	9638	9694	9750	9806
776	9862	9918	9974	0030	0086	0142	0197	0253	0309	0365
777	890421	0477	0533	0589	0645	0700	0756	0812	0868	0924
778	0980	1035	1091	1147	1203	1259	1314	1370	1426	1482
779	1538	1593	1649	1705	1760	1816	1872	1928	1983	2039
780	2095	2150	2206	2262	2317	2373	2429	2484	2540	2595
781	2651	2707	2762	2818	2873	2929	2985	3040	3096	3151
782	3207	3262	3318	3373	3429	3484	3540	3595	3651	3706
783	3762	3817	3873	3928	3984	4039	4094	4150	4205	4261
784	4316	4372	4427	4482	4538	4593	4648	4704	4759	4814
785	4870	4925	4980	5036	5091	5146	5202	5257	5312	5367
786	5423	5478	5533	5588	5644	5699	5754	5809	5864	5920
787	5975	6030	6085	6140	6195	6251	6306	6361	6416	6471
788	6526	6581	6636	6692	6747	6802	6857	6912	6967	7022
789	7077	7132	7187	7242	7297	7352	7407	7462	7517	7572
790	7627	7682	7737	7792	7847	7902	7957	8012	8067	8122
791	8177	8231	8286	8341	8396	8451	8506	8561	8616	8670
792	8725	8780	8835	8890	8945	8999	9055	9109	9164	9218
793	9273	9328	9383	9438	9492	9547	9602	9656	9711	9766
794	9821	9875	9930	9985	0039	0094	0149	0203	0258	0313
795	900367	0422	0476	0531	0586	0640	0695	0749	0804	0859
796	0913	0968	1022	1077	1131	1186	1240	1295	1349	1404
797	1458	1513	1567	1622	1676	1731	1785	1840	1894	1949
798	2003	2057	2112	2166	2221	2275	2329	2384	2438	2492
799	2547	2601	2656	2710	2764	2819	2873	2927	2981	3036

A Table of

N°	0	1	2	3	4	5	6	7	8	9
800	903090	3144	3199	3253	3307	3361	3416	3470	3524	3578
801	3633	3687	3741	3795	3849	3904	3958	4012	4066	4120
802	4174	4229	4283	4337	4391	4445	4499	4553	4607	4662
803	4716	4770	4824	4878	4932	4986	5040	5094	5148	5202
804	5256	5310	5364	5418	5472	5526	5580	5634	5688	5742
805	5796	5850	5904	5958	6012	6066	6120	6173	6227	6281
806	6335	6389	6443	6497	6551	6604	6658	6712	6766	6820
807	6874	6927	6981	7035	7089	7143	7196	7250	7304	7358
808	7411	7465	7519	7573	7626	7680	7734	7787	7841	7895
809	7949	8002	8056	8110	8163	8217	8271	8324	8378	8431
810	8485	8539	8592	8646	8699	8753	8807	8860	8914	8967
811	9021	9074	9128	9182	9235	9289	9342	9396	9449	9503
812	9556	9610	9663	9717	9770	9823	9877	9930	9984	0037
813	910091	0144	0197	0251	0304	0358	0411	0464	0518	0571
814	0624	0678	0731	0784	0838	0891	0944	0998	1051	1104
815	1158	1211	1264	1317	1371	1424	1477	1531	1584	1637
816	1690	1743	1797	1850	1903	1956	2009	2063	2116	2169
817	2222	2275	2328	2382	2435	2488	2541	2594	2647	2700
818	2753	2806	2860	2913	2966	3019	3072	3125	3178	3231
819	3284	3337	3390	3443	3496	3549	3602	3655	3708	3761
820	3814	3867	3920	3973	4026	4079	4132	4184	4237	4290
821	4343	4396	4449	4502	4555	4608	4660	4713	4766	4819
822	4872	4925	4978	5030	5083	5136	5189	5242	5294	5347
823	5400	5453	5505	5558	5611	5664	5716	5769	5822	5875
824	5927	5980	6033	6085	6138	6191	6243	6296	6349	6401
825	6454	6507	6559	6612	6665	6717	6770	6822	6875	6928
826	6980	7033	7085	7138	7190	7243	7295	7348	7401	7453
827	7506	7558	7611	7663	7716	7768	7821	7873	7925	7978
828	8030	8083	8135	8188	8240	8293	8345	8397	8450	8502
829	8555	8607	8659	8712	8764	8816	8869	8921	8973	9026
830	9078	9130	9183	9235	9287	9340	9392	9444	9497	9549
831	9601	9653	9706	9758	9810	9862	9915	9967	0019	0071
832	920123	0176	0228	0280	0332	0384	0436	0489	0541	0593
833	0645	0697	0749	0801	0854	0906	0958	1010	1062	1114
834	1166	1218	1270	1322	1374	1426	1478	1530	1582	1635

LOGARITHMS.

N°	0	1	2	3	4	5	6	7	8	9
835	921687	1739	1791	1843	1895	1947	1998	2050	2102	2154
836	2206	2258	2310	2362	2414	2466	2518	2570	2622	2674
837	2726	2777	2829	2881	2933	2985	3037	3089	3140	3192
838	3244	3296	3348	3400	3451	3503	3555	3607	3658	3710
839	3762	3814	3866	3917	3969	4021	4072	4124	4176	4228
840	4279	4331	4383	4434	4486	4538	4589	4641	4693	4744
841	4796	4848	4899	4951	5003	5054	5106	5157	5209	5261
842	5312	5364	5415	5467	5518	5570	5622	5673	5725	5776
843	5828	5879	5931	5982	6034	6085	6137	6188	6240	6291
844	6342	6394	6445	6497	6548	6600	6651	6703	6754	6805
845	6857	6908	6960	7011	7062	7114	7165	7216	7268	7319
846	7370	7422	7473	7524	7576	7627	7678	7730	7781	7832
847	7883	7935	7986	8037	8089	8140	8191	8242	8293	8345
848	8396	8447	8498	8550	8601	8652	8703	8754	8805	8857
849	8908	8959	9010	9061	9112	9163	9215	9266	9317	9368
850	9419	9470	9521	9572	9623	9674	9725	9776	9828	9879
851	9930	9981	0032	0083	0134	0185	0236	0287	0338	0389
852	930440	0491	0542	0593	0643	0694	0745	0796	0847	0898
853	0949	1000	1051	1102	1153	1204	1254	1305	1356	1407
854	1458	1509	1560	1610	1661	1712	1763	1814	1865	1915
855	1966	2017	2068	2119	2169	2220	2271	2322	2372	2423
856	2474	2525	2575	2626	2677	2727	2778	2829	2880	2930
857	2981	3032	3082	3133	3184	3234	3285	3335	3386	3437
858	3487	3538	3589	3639	3690	3740	3791	3842	3892	3943
859	3993	4044	4094	4145	4195	4246	4296	4347	4397	4448
860	4499	4549	4599	4650	4700	4751	4801	4852	4902	4953
861	5003	5054	5104	5154	5205	5255	5306	5356	5407	5457
862	5507	5558	5608	5658	5709	5759	5810	5860	5910	5961
863	6011	6061	6111	6162	6212	6262	6313	6363	6113	6164
864	6514	6564	6614	6665	6715	6765	6815	6866	6916	6966
865	7016	7066	7117	7167	7217	7267	7317	7367	7418	7468
866	7518	7568	7618	7668	7718	7769	7819	7869	7919	7969
867	8019	8069	8119	8169	8219	8270	8320	8370	8420	8470
868	8520	8570	8620	8670	8720	8770	8820	8870	8920	8970
869	9020	9070	9120	9170	9220	9270	9320	9370	9419	9469

3 R

A Table of

N°	0	1	2	3	4	5	6	7	8	9
870	939519	9569	9619	9669	9719	9769	9819	9869	9918	9968
871	940018	0068	0118	0168	0218	0267	0317	0367	0417	0467
872	0517	0566	0616	0666	0716	0765	0815	0865	0915	0965
873	1014	1064	1114	1164	1213	1263	1313	1362	1412	1462
874	1511	1561	1611	1661	1710	1760	1810	1859	1909	1958
875	2008	2058	2107	2157	2207	2256	2306	2355	2405	2455
876	2504	2554	2603	2653	2702	2752	2802	2851	2901	2950
877	3000	3049	3099	3148	3198	3247	3297	3346	3396	3445
878	3495	3544	3593	3643	3692	3742	3791	3841	3890	3940
879	3989	4038	4088	4137	4187	4236	4285	4335	4384	4433
880	4483	4532	4581	4631	4680	4729	4779	4828	4877	4927
881	4976	5025	5075	5124	5173	5222	5272	5321	5370	5419
882	5469	5518	5567	5616	5666	5715	5764	5813	5862	5912
883	5961	6010	6059	6108	6157	6207	6256	6305	6354	6403
884	6452	6501	6551	6600	6649	6698	6747	6796	6845	6894
885	6943	6992	7041	7091	7140	7189	7238	7287	7336	7385
886	7434	7483	7532	7581	7630	7679	7728	7777	7826	7875
887	7924	7973	8022	8071	8119	8168	8217	8266	8315	8364
888	8413	8462	8511	8560	8609	8657	8706	8755	8804	8853
889	8902	8951	9000	9048	9097	9146	9195	9244	9292	9341
890	9390	9439	9488	9536	9585	9634	9683	9732	9780	9829
891	9878	9926	9975	0024	0073	0121	0170	0219	0267	0316
892	950365	0414	0462	0511	0560	0608	0657	0706	0754	0803
893	0852	0900	0949	0997	1046	1095	1143	1192	1240	1289
894	1338	1386	1435	1483	1532	1580	1629	1677	1726	1775
895	1823	1872	1920	1969	2017	2066	2114	2163	2211	2260
896	2308	2357	2405	2453	2502	2550	2599	2647	2696	2744
897	2792	2841	2889	2938	2986	3035	3083	3131	3180	3228
898	3276	3325	3373	3421	3470	3518	3566	3615	3663	3711
899	3760	3808	3856	3905	3953	4001	4049	4098	4146	4194
900	4243	4291	4339	4387	4436	4484	4532	4580	4628	4677
901	4725	4773	4821	4869	4918	4966	5014	5062	5110	5158
902	5207	5255	5303	5351	5399	5447	5495	5543	5592	5640
903	5688	5736	5784	5832	5880	5928	5976	6024	6072	6120
904	6168	6217	6265	6313	6361	6409	6457	6505	6553	6601

LOGARITHMS.

N°	0	1	2	3	4	5	6	7	8	9
905	956649	6697	6745	6793	6841	6889	6937	6984	7032	7080
906	7128	7176	7224	7272	7320	7368	7416	7464	7512	7559
907	7607	7655	7703	7751	7799	7847	7895	7942	7990	8038
908	8086	8134	8182	8229	8277	8325	8373	8421	8468	8516
909	8564	8612	8659	8707	8755	8803	8851	8898	8946	8994
910	9041	9089	9137	9185	9232	9280	9328	9375	9423	9471
911	9518	9566	9614	9661	9709	9757	9804	9852	9900	9947
912	9995	0043	0090	0138	0185	0233	0281	0328	0376	0423
913	960471	0518	0566	0614	0661	0709	0756	0804	0851	0899
914	0946	0994	1041	1089	1136	1184	1231	1279	1326	1374
915	1421	1469	1516	1564	1611	1658	1706	1753	1801	1848
916	1896	1943	1990	2038	2085	2133	2180	2227	2275	2322
917	2369	2417	2464	2511	2559	2606	2653	2701	2748	2795
918	2843	2890	2937	2985	3032	3079	3126	3174	3221	3268
919	3316	3363	3410	3457	3505	3552	3599	3646	3693	3741
920	3788	3835	3882	3929	3977	4024	4071	4118	4165	4213
921	4260	4307	4354	4401	4448	4495	4543	4590	4637	4684
922	4731	4778	4825	4872	4919	4966	5014	5061	5108	5155
923	5202	5249	5296	5343	5390	5437	5484	5531	5578	5625
924	5672	5719	5766	5813	5860	5907	5954	6001	6048	6095
925	6142	6189	6236	6283	6330	6376	6423	6470	6517	6564
926	6611	6658	6705	6752	6799	6845	6892	6939	6986	7033
927	7080	7127	7173	7220	7267	7314	7361	7408	7454	7501
928	7548	7595	7642	7688	7735	7782	7829	7875	7922	7969
929	8016	8063	8109	8156	8203	8249	8296	8343	8390	8436
930	8483	8530	8576	8623	8670	8716	8763	8810	8856	8903
931	8950	8996	9043	9090	9136	9183	9230	9276	9323	9369
932	9416	9463	9509	9556	9602	9649	9695	9742	9789	9835
933	9882	9928	9975	0021	0068	0114	0161	0207	0254	0300
934	970347	0393	0440	0486	0533	0579	0626	0672	0719	0765
935	0812	0858	0905	0951	0997	1044	1090	1137	1183	1229
936	1276	1322	1369	1415	1461	1508	1554	1601	1647	1693
937	1740	1786	1832	1879	1925	1971	2018	2064	2110	2157
938	2203	2249	2295	2342	2388	2434	2481	2527	2573	2619
939	2666	2712	2758	2804	2851	2897	2943	2989	3035	3082

3 R 2

490   *A* Table *of*

Nº	0	1	2	3	4	5	6	7	8	9
940	973128	3174	3220	3266	3313	3359	3405	3451	3497	3544
941	3590	3636	3682	3728	3774	3820	3866	3913	3959	4005
942	4051	4097	4143	4189	4235	4281	4327	4374	4420	4466
943	4512	4558	4604	4650	4697	4742	4788	4834	4880	4926
944	4972	5018	5064	5110	5156	5202	5248	5294	5340	5386
945	5432	5478	5524	5570	5616	5662	5708	5753	5799	5845
946	5891	5937	5983	6029	6075	6121	6167	6212	6258	6304
947	6350	6396	6442	6488	6533	6579	6625	6671	6717	6763
948	6808	6854	6900	6946	6992	7037	7083	7129	7175	7220
949	7266	7312	7358	7404	7449	7495	7541	7586	7632	7678
950	7724	7769	7815	7861	7906	7952	7998	8044	8089	8135
951	8181	8226	8272	8318	8363	8409	8454	8500	8546	8591
952	8637	8683	8728	8774	8819	8865	8911	8956	9002	9047
953	9093	9139	9184	9230	9275	9321	9366	9412	9457	9503
954	9518	9594	9639	9685	9730	9776	9821	9867	9912	9958
955	980003	0049	0094	0140	0185	0231	0276	0321	0367	0413
956	0458	0503	0549	0594	0640	0685	0730	0776	0821	0867
957	0912	0957	1003	1048	1093	1139	1184	1230	1275	1320
958	1366	1411	1456	1502	1547	1592	1637	1683	1728	1773
959	1819	1864	1909	1954	2000	2045	2090	2136	2181	2226
960	2271	2317	2362	2407	2452	2497	2543	2588	2633	2678
961	2723	2769	2814	2859	2904	2949	2995	3040	3085	3130
962	3175	3220	3265	3311	3356	3401	3446	3491	3536	3581
963	3626	3671	3717	3762	3807	3852	3897	3942	3987	4032
964	4077	4122	4167	4212	4257	4302	4347	4392	4437	4482
965	4527	4572	4617	4662	4707	4752	4797	4842	4887	4932
966	4977	5022	5067	5112	5157	5202	5247	5292	5337	5382
967	5427	5471	5516	5561	5606	5651	5696	5741	5786	5831
968	5875	5920	5965	6010	6055	6100	6145	6189	6234	6279
969	6324	6369	6413	6458	6503	6548	6593	6637	6682	6727
970	6772	6817	6861	6906	6951	6996	7040	7085	7130	7175
971	7219	7264	7309	7353	7398	7443	7488	7532	7577	7622
972	7666	7711	7756	7800	7845	7890	7934	7979	8024	8068
973	8113	8158	8202	8247	8291	8336	8381	8425	8470	8514
974	8559	8604	8648	8693	8737	8782	8826	8871	8916	8960

LOGARITHMS.

N.	0	1	2	3	4	5	6	7	8	9
975	989005	9049	9094	9138	9183	9227	9272	9316	9361	9405
976	9450	9494	9539	9583	9628	9672	9717	9761	9806	9850
977	9895	9939	9984	0028	0072	0117	0161	0206	0250	0294
978	990339	0383	0428	0472	0516	0561	0605	0650	0694	0738
979	0783	0827	0871	0916	0960	1004	1049	1093	1137	1182
980	1226	1270	1315	1359	1403	1448	1492	1536	1581	1625
981	1669	1713	1758	1802	1846	1890	1935	1979	2023	2067
982	2112	2156	2200	2244	2288	2333	2377	2421	2465	2509
983	2554	2598	2642	2686	2730	2774	2819	2863	2907	2951
984	2995	3039	3083	3128	3172	3216	3260	3304	3348	3392
985	3436	3480	3524	3569	3613	3657	3701	3745	3789	3833
986	3877	3921	3965	4009	4053	4097	4141	4185	4229	4273
987	4317	4361	4405	4449	4493	4537	4581	4625	4669	4713
988	4757	4801	4845	4889	4933	4977	5021	5065	5109	5152
989	5196	5240	5284	5328	5372	5416	5460	5504	5547	5591
990	5635	5679	5723	5767	5811	5855	5898	5942	5986	6030
991	6074	6118	6161	6205	6249	6293	6337	6380	6424	6468
992	6512	6555	6599	6643	6687	6731	6774	6818	6862	6906
993	6949	6993	7037	7080	7124	7168	7212	7255	7299	7343
994	7386	7430	7474	7517	7561	7605	7648	7692	7736	7779
995	7823	7867	7910	7954	7998	8041	8085	8129	8172	8216
996	8259	8303	8347	8390	8434	8477	8521	8565	8608	8652
997	8695	8739	8782	8826	8869	8913	8956	9000	9044	9087
998	9131	9174	9218	9261	9305	9348	9392	9435	9479	9522
999	9566	9609	9652	9696	9739	9783	9826	9870	9913	9957

A TABLE

OF

LOGARITHMIC SINES

AND

TANGENTS

TO EVERY

DEGREE and MINUTE

OF THE

QUADRANT.

A Table of

0 Degrees.

M	Sines	Co-sines	Tangents	Co-tang	
0	0 000000	10 000000	0 000000	Infinite	60
1	6 463726	10 000000	6 463726	13 536274	59
2	6 764756	9 999999	6 764756	13 235244	58
3	6 940847	9 999999	6 940848	13 059153	57
4	7 065786	9 999999	7 065786	12 934214	56
5	7 162696	9 999999	7 162696	12 837304	55
6	7 241877	9 999999	7 241878	12 758122	54
7	7 308824	9 999999	7 308825	12 691175	53
8	7 366816	9 999999	7 366817	12 633183	52
9	7 417968	9 999999	7 417970	12 582030	51
10	7 463726	9 999998	7 463727	12 536273	50
11	7 505118	9 999998	7 505120	12 494880	49
12	7 542907	9 999997	7 542909	12 457091	48
13	7 577068	9 999997	7 577072	12 422329	47
14	7 609853	9 999996	7 609857	12 390143	46
15	7 639816	9 999996	7 639820	12 360180	45
16	7 667845	9 999995	7 667849	12 332151	44
17	7 694173	9 999995	7 694179	12 305821	43
18	7 718997	9 999994	7 719003	12 280997	42
19	7 742478	9 999993	7 742484	12 257516	41
20	7 764754	9 999993	7 764761	12 235239	40
21	7 785943	9 999992	7 785951	12 214049	39
22	7 806146	9 999991	7 806155	12 193845	38
23	7 825451	9 999990	7 825460	12 174540	37
24	7 843934	9 999989	7 843944	12 156056	36
25	7 861662	9 999989	7 861674	12 138326	35
26	7 878695	9 999988	7 878708	12 121292	34
27	7 895085	9 999987	7 895099	12 104901	33
28	7 910879	9 999986	7 910894	12 089106	32
29	7 926119	9 999985	7 926134	12 073866	31
30	7 940842	9 999984	7 940858	12 059142	30
	Co-sines	Sines	Co-tang.	Tangents	M

89 Degrees.

Sines and Tangents

0 Degrees

M	Sines	Co-sines	Tangents	Co-tang	
30	7 940842	9 999984	7 940858	12 059142	30
31	7·955082	9 999982	7·955100	12 044900	29
32	7 968870	9 999981	7 968889	12 031111	28
33	7 982233	9 999980	7 982253	12 017747	27
34	7 995198	9 999979	7 995219	12 004781	26
35	8 007787	9 999978	8 007809	11 992191	25
36	8 020021	9 999976	8 020045	11 979956	24
37	8 031920	9 999975	8 031945	11 968055	23
38	8 043501	9 999974	8 043527	11 956473	22
39	8 054781	9 999972	8 054809	11 945191	21
40	8 065776	9 999971	8 065806	11 934194	20
41	8 076500	9 999969	8 076531	11 923469	19
42	8 086965	9 999968	8 086997	11 913003	18
43	8 097183	9 999966	8 097217	11·902783	17
44	8 107167	9 999964	8 107203	11 892798	16
45	8 116926	9 999963	8 116963	11 883037	15
46	8 126471	9 999961	8 126510	11·873490	14
47	8 135810	9 999959	8 135851	11 864149	13
48	8 144953	9 999958	8 144996	11 855004	12
49	8 153908	9 999956	8 153952	11 846048	11
50	8 162681	9 999954	8 162727	11·837273	10
51	8 171280	9 999952	8 171328	11·828672	9
52	8·179713	9 999950	8 179763	11 820237	8
53	8·187985	9 999948	8·188036	11 811964	7
54	8 196102	9 999946	8 196156	11 803844	6
55	8 204070	9·999944	8 204126	11 795874	5
56	8·211895	9·999942	8 211953	11·788047	4
57	8 219581	9 999940	8 219641	11 780359	3
58	8 227134	9 999938	8 227195	11·772805	2
59	8·234557	9 999936	8 234621	11 765379	1
60	8 241855	9 999934	8·241922	11 758079	0
	Co-sines	Sines	Co-tang	Tangents	M

89 Degrees.

3 S

A Table of
1 Degree

M	Sines	Co-sines	Tangents	Co-tang	
0	8 241855	9 999934	8 241922	11 758079	60
1	8 249033	9 999932	8 249102	11 750899	59
2	8 256094	9 999929	8 256165	11 743835	58
3	8 263042	9 999927	8 263115	11 736885	57
4	8 269881	9 999925	8 269956	11 730044	56
5	8 276614	9 999922	8 276691	11 723309	55
6	8 283243	9 999920	8 283323	11 716677	54
7	8 289773	9 999918	8 289856	11 710144	53
8	8 296207	9 999915	8 296292	11 703708	52
9	8 302546	9 999913	8 302634	11 697367	51
10	8 308794	9 999910	8 308884	11 691116	50
11	8 314954	9 999907	8 315046	11 684954	49
12	8 321027	9 999905	8 321122	11 678878	48
13	8 327016	9 999902	8 327114	11 672886	47
14	8 332924	9 999899	8 333025	11 666975	46
15	8 338753	9 999897	8 338856	11 661144	45
16	8 344504	9 999894	8 344611	11 655390	44
17	8 350181	9 999891	8 350290	11 649711	43
18	8 355784	9 999888	8 355895	11 644105	42
19	8 361315	9 999885	8 361430	11·638570	41
20	8 366777	9 999882	8 366895	11 633106	40
21	8 372171	9 999879	8 372292	11 627709	39
22	8 377499	9 999876	8 377622	11 622378	38
23	8 382762	9 999873	8 382889	11·617111	37
24	8 387962	9 999870	8 388092	11 611908	36
25	8 393101	9 999867	8 393234	11 606766	35
26	8 398179	9 999864	8 398315	11 601685	34
27	8 403199	9 999861	8 403338	11 596662	33
28	8 408161	9 999858	8 408304	11 591696	32
29	8 413068	9 999854	8 413213	11 586787	31
30	8 417919	9·999851	8 418068	11 581932	30
	Co-sines	Sines	Co-tang	Tangents	M

89 Degrees.

SINES and TANGENTS

1 Degree

M	Sines	Co-sines	Tangents	Co-tang	
30	8 417919	9 999851	8 418068	11 581922	30
31	8 422717	848	8 422869	11 577131	29
32	7462	845	7618	2382	28
33	8 432156	841	8 432315	11 567685	27
34	6800	838	6962	3038	26
35	8 441394	834	8 441560	11 558440	25
36	5941	831	6110	3890	24
37	8 450440	827	8 450613	11 549387	23
38	4893	824	5070	4930	22
39	9301	820	9481	0519	21
40	8 463665	816	8 463849	11 536151	20
41	7985	813	8173	1828	19
42	8 472263	809	8 472454	11 527546	18
43	6498	805	6693	3307	17
44	8 480693	801	8 480892	11 519108	16
45	4848	797	5051	4950	15
46	8963	794	9170	0830	14
47	8 493040	790	8 493250	11 506750	13
48	7078	786	7293	2707	12
49	8 501080	782	8 501298	11 498702	11
50	5045	778	5267	4733	10
51	8974	774	9200	0800	9
52	8 512867	770	8 513098	11 486902	8
53	6726	765	6961	3039	7
54	8 520551	761	8 520790	11 479210	6
55	4343	757	4586	5414	5
56	8102	753	8349	1651	4
57	8 531828	748	8 532080	11 467920	3
58	5523	744	5779	4221	2
59	9186	740	9447	0553	1
60	8 542819	735	8 543084	11 456916	0
	Co-sines	Sines	Co-tang.	Tangents	M

88 Degrees

2 Degrees

M	Sines	Co-sines	Tangents	Co-tang.	
0	8 542819	9 999735	8 543084	11 456916	60
1	6422	731	6691	3309	59
2	9995	727	8 550268	11 449732	58
3	8 553539	722	3817	6183	57
4	7054	717	7336	2664	56
5	8 560540	713	8 560828	11·439172	55
6	3999	708	4291	5709	54
7	7431	704	7728	2273	53
8	8 570836	699	8 571137	11 428863	52
9	4214	694	4520	5480	51
10	7566	689	7877	2123	50
11	8 580892	685	8 581208	11 418792	49
12	4193	680	4514	5486	48
13	7469	675	7795	2206	47
14	8 590721	670	8 591051	11 408949	46
15	3948	665	4283	5717	45
16	7152	660	7492	2508	44
17	8 600332	655	8 600677	11 399323	43
18	3489	650	3839	6161	42
19	6623	645	6978	3022	41
20	9734	640	8 610094	11 389906	40
21	8 612824	635	3189	6811	39
22	5891	629	6262	3738	38
23	8937	624	9313	0687	37
24	8 621962	619	8 622343	11·377657	36
25	4965	614	5352	4648	35
26	7948	608	8340	1660	34
27	8 630911	603	8·631308	11 368692	33
28	3854	597	4256	5744	32
29	6776	592	7185	2816	31
30	9680	587	8 640093	11 359907	30
	Co-sines	Sines	Co-tang	Tangents	M

87 Degrees

Sines and Tangents.

2 Degrees

M	Sines	Co-sines	Tangents	Co-tang	
30	8 639680	9 999587	8 640093	11 359907	30
31	8 642563	581	2983	7018	29
32	5428	575	5853	4147	28
33	8274	570	8704	1296	27
34	8 651102	564	8 651538	11 348463	26
35	3911	558	4352	5648	25
36	6702	553	7149	2851	24
37	9475	547	9928	0072	23
38	8·662230	541	8 662689	11·338463	22
39	4968	535	5433	4567	21
40	7689	530	8160	1840	20
41	8 670393	524	8·670870	11·329130	19
42	3080	518	3563	6437	18
43	5751	512	6239	3761	17
44	8405	506	8900	1100	16
45	8 681043	500	8 681544	11 318456	15
46	3665	494	4172	5828	14
47	6272	487	6784	3216	13
48	8863	481	9381	0619	12
49	8 691438	475	8 691963	11·308037	11
50	3998	469	4529	5471	10
51	6543	463	7081	2919	9
52	9073	456	9617	0383	8
53	8 701589	450	8 702139	11·297861	7
54	4090	444	4647	5354	6
55	6577	437	7140	2861	5
56	9049	431	9619	0382	4
57	8 711508	424	8 712083	11·287917	3
58	3952	418	4535	5466	2
59	6383	411	6972	3028	1
60	8800	404	9396	0604	0
	Co-sines	Sines	Co-tang	Tangents	M

87 Degrees.

A Table of
3 Degrees

M	Sines	Co-sines	Tangents	Co-tang	
0	8 718800	9 999404	8 719396	11 280604	60
1	8 721204	398	8 721806	11 278194	59
2	3595	391	4204	5797	58
3	5972	384	6588	3412	57
4	8337	378	8959	1041	56
5	8 730688	371	8 731317	11 268683	55
6	3027	364	3663	6337	54
7	5354	357	5996	4004	53
8	7668	350	8317	1683	52
9	9969	343	8·740626	11·259374	51
10	8 742259	336	2922	7078	50
11	4536	329	5207	4793	49
12	6802	322	7479	2521	48
13	9055	315	9740	0260	47
14	8 751297	308	8 751989	11 248011	46
15	3528	301	4227	5773	45
16	5747	294	6453	3547	44
17	7955	287	8668	1332	43
18	8 760151	279	8 760872	11 239128	42
19	2337	272	3065	6935	41
20	4511	265	5247	4754	40
21	6675	257	7418	2583	39
22	8828	250	9578	0422	38
23	8 770970	242	8 771727	11 228273	37
24	3101	235	3867	6134	36
25	5223	227	5995	4005	35
26	7333	220	8114	1886	34
27	9434	212	8 780222	11 219778	33
28	8·781525	205	2320	7680	32
29	3605	197	4408	5592	31
30	5675	189	6486	3514	30
	Co-sines	Sines	Co-tang	Tangents	M

86 Degrees.

Sines and Tangents.

3 Degrees

M	Sines	Co-sines	Tangents	Co-tang	
30	8 785675	9 999189	8 786486	11 213514	30
31	7736	182	8554	1446	29
32	9787	174	8 790613	11 209387	28
33	8 791828	166	2662	7338	27
34	3859	158	4701	5299	26
35	5881	150	6731	3269	25
36	7894	142	8752	1248	24
37	9897	134	8 800763	11 199237	23
38	8 801892	126	2765	7235	22
39	3876	118	4758	5242	21
40	5852	110	6742	3258	20
41	7819	102	8717	1283	19
42	9777	094	8 810683	11 189317	18
43	8 811726	086	2641	7359	17
44	3667	077	4589	5411	16
45	5599	069	6529	3471	15
46	7522	061	8461	1539	14
47	9436	053	8 820384	11 179616	13
48	8 821343	044	2298	7702	12
49	3240	036	4205	5795	11
50	5130	027	6103	3897	10
51	7011	019	7992	2008	9
52	8884	010	9874	0126	8
53	8 830750	002	8 831748	11 168252	7
54	2607	9 998993	6313	6387	6
55	4456	985	5471	4529	5
56	6297	976	7321	2679	4
57	8130	967	9163	0837	3
58	9956	958	8 840998	11 159002	2
59	8 841774	950	2825	7176	1
60	3585	941	4644	5356	0
	Co-sines	Sines	Co-tang	Tangents	M

86 Degrees.

A Table of

4 Degrees

M	Sines	Co-sines	Tangents	Co-tang	
0	8·843585	9·998941	8·844644	11·155356	60
1	5387	932	6455	3545	59
2	7183	923	8260	1740	58
3	8971	914	8·850057	11·149943	57
4	8·850751	905	1846	8154	56
5	2525	896	3628	6372	55
6	4291	887	5403	4597	54
7	6049	878	7171	2829	53
8	7801	869	8932	1068	52
9	9546	860	8·860686	11·139314	51
10	8·861283	851	2433	7567	50
11	3014	841	4173	5828	49
12	4738	832	5906	4095	48
13	6455	823	7632	2368	47
14	8165	814	9351	0649	46
15	9868	804	8·871064	11·128936	45
16	8·871565	795	2770	7230	44
17	3255	785	4469	5531	43
18	4938	776	6162	3838	42
19	6615	766	7849	2151	41
20	8285	757	9529	0471	40
21	9949	747	8·881202	11·118798	39
22	8·881607	738	2869	7131	38
23	3258	728	4530	5470	37
24	4903	718	6185	3815	36
25	6542	708	7833	2106	35
26	8174	699	9476	0524	34
27	9801	689	8·891112	11·108888	33
28	8·891421	679	2742	7258	32
29	3035	669	4366	5634	31
30	4643	659	5984	4016	30
	Co-sines	Sines	Tangents	Tangents	

85 Degrees.

4 Degrees

M	Sines	Co-sines	Tangents	Co-tang	
30	8·894643	9 998659	8·895984	11·104016	30
31	6246	649	7596	2404	29
32	7842	639	9203	0797	28
33	9432	629	8 900803	11·099197	27
34	8 901017	619	2398	7602	26
35	2596	609	3987	6013	25
36	4169	599	5570	4430	24
37	5736	589	7147	2853	23
38	7298	578	8719	1281	22
39	8854	568	8 910285	11 089715	21
40	8 910404	558	1846	8154	20
41	1949	548	3401	6599	19
42	3488	537	4951	5049	18
43	5022	527	6495	3505	17
44	6550	516	8034	1966	16
45	8073	506	9568	0433	15
46	9591	495	8 921096	11 078904	14
47	8 921103	485	2619	7381	13
48	2611	474	4136	5864	12
49	4112	464	5649	4351	11
50	5609	453	7156	2844	10
51	7100	442	8658	1342	9
52	8587	432	8 930155	11·069845	8
53	8 930068	421	1647	8353	7
54	1544	410	3134	6866	6
55	3015	399	4616	5384	5
56	4481	388	6093	3907	4
57	5942	377	7565	2435	3
58	7398	366	9032	0968	2
59	8850	355	8 940494	11·059506	1
60	8 940296	344	1952	8048	0
	Co-sines	Sines	Co-tang	Tangents	M

85 Degrees.

5 Degrees

M	Sines	Co-sines	Tangents	Co-tang	
0	8 940296	9 998344	8 941952	11 059648	60
1	1738	333	3404	6596	59
2	3174	322	4852	5148	58
3	4606	311	6295	3705	57
4	6034	300	7734	2266	56
5	7456	289	9168	0832	55
6	8874	277	8·950597	11·049403	54
7	8 950287	266	2021	7979	53
8	1696	255	3441	6559	52
9	3100	243	4856	5144	51
10	4499	232	6267	3733	50
11	5894	220	7674	2327	49
12	7284	209	9075	0925	48
13	8670	197	8·960473	11 039527	47
14	8·960052	186	1866	8134	46
15	1429	174	3255	6746	45
16	2801	163	4639	5361	44
17	4170	151	6019	3981	43
18	5534	139	7394	2606	42
19	6893	128	8766	1234	41
20	8249	116	8 970133	11·029867	40
21	9600	104	1496	8504	39
22	8·970947	092	2855	7145	38
23	2290	080	4209	5791	37
24	3628	068	5500	4440	36
25	4962	056	6906	3094	35
26	6293	044	8248	1752	34
27	7619	032	9587	0414	33
28	8941	020	8·980921	11·019079	32
29	8 980259	008	2251	7749	31
30	1573	9·997996	3577	6423	30
	Co-sines	Sines	Co-tang.	Tangents	M

84 Degrees.

Sines and Tangents.

5 Degrees

M	Sines	Co-sines	Tangents	Co tang.	
30	8·981573	9 997996	8·983577	11 016423	30
31	2883	984	4899	5101	29
32	4189	972	6217	3783	28
33	5491	959	7532	2468	27
34	6789	947	8842	1158	26
35	8083	935	8 990149	11·009851	25
36	9374	922	1451	8549	24
37	0660	910	2750	7250	23
38	8 991943	898	4045	5955	22
39	3222	885	5337	4663	21
40	4497	873	6624	3376	20
41	5768	860	7908	2092	19
42	7036	847	9188	0812	18
43	8299	835	9·000465	10 999535	17
44	9560	822	1738	8263	16
45	9 000816	809	3007	6993	15
46	2069	797	4272	5728	14
47	3318	784	5534	4466	13
48	4563	771	6792	3208	12
49	5805	758	8047	1953	11
50	7044	745	9298	0702	10
51	8278	732	9·010546	10 989454	9
52	9510	719	1790	8210	8
53	9 010737	706	3031	6969	7
54	1962	693	4268	5732	6
55	3182	680	5502	4498	5
56	4400	667	6733	3268	4
57	5614	654	7959	2041	3
58	6824	641	9183	0817	2
59	8031	628	9·020403	10·979597	1
60	9235	614	1620	8380	0
	Co-fines	Sines	Co-tang.	Tangents	M

84 Degrees.

A Table of
6 Degrees

M	Sines	Co-sines	Tangents	Co-tang	
0	9 019235	9 997614	9 021620	10 978380	60
1	9 020435	601	2834	7166	59
2	1632	588	4044	5956	58
3	2825	574	5251	4749	57
4	4016	561	6455	3545	56
5	5203	548	7655	2345	55
6	6387	534	8852	1148	54
7	7567	521	9 030046	10 969954	53
8	8744	507	1237	8763	52
9	9918	493	2425	7575	51
10	9 031089	480	3609	6391	50
11	2257	466	4791	5209	49
12	3421	452	5969	4031	48
13	4583	439	7144	2856	47
14	5741	425	8316	1684	46
15	6896	411	9485	0515	45
16	8048	397	9 040651	10 959349	44
17	9197	383	1813	8187	43
18	9 040342	369	2973	7027	42
19	1485	355	4130	5870	41
20	2625	341	5283	4716	40
21	3762	327	6434	3566	39
22	4895	313	7582	2418	38
23	6026	299	8727	1273	37
24	7154	285	9869	0131	36
25	8279	271	9 051008	10 948992	35
26	9401	257	2144	7856	34
27	9 050519	242	3277	6723	33
28	1635	228	4407	5593	32
29	2749	214	5535	4465	31
30	3859	199	6660	3341	30
	Co-sines	Sines	Co-tang	Tangents	M

83 Degrees

Sines and Tangents.

6 Degrees

M	Sines	Co-sines	Tangents	Co-tang.	
30	9 053859	9 997199	9 056660	10·943341	30
31	4966	185	7781	2219	29
32	6071	170	8900	1100	28
33	7172	156	9 060016	10 939984	27
34	8271	141	1130	8870	26
35	9367	127	2240	7760	25
36	9 660460	112	3348	6652	24
37	1551	098	4453	5547	23
38	2639	083	5556	4444	22
39	3724	068	6655	3345	21
40	4806	054	7752	2248	20
41	5885	039	8847	1154	19
42	6962	024	9938	0062	18
43	8036	009	9·071027	10 928973	17
44	9107	9 996994	2113	7887	16
45	9 070176	979	3197	6803	15
46	1242	964	4278	5722	14
47	2306	949	5356	4644	13
48	3366	934	6432	3568	12
49	4424	919	7505	2495	11
50	5480	904	8576	1424	10
51	6533	889	9644	0356	9
52	7583	874	9 080710	10 919290	8
53	8631	858	1773	8227	7
54	9676	843	2833	7167	6
55	9·080719	828	3891	6109	5
56	1759	813	4947	5053	4
57	2797	797	6000	4000	3
58	3832	782	7050	2950	2
59	4864	766	8098	1902	1
60	5895	751	9144	0856	0
	Co-sines	Sines	Co-tang.	Tangents	M

83 Degrees.

7 Degrees

M	Sines	Co-sines	Tangents	Co-tang.	
0	9 085895	9 996751	9 089144	10 910856	60
1	6922	735	9 090187	10 909813	59
2	7947	720	1228	8772	58
3	8970	704	2266	7734	57
4	9990	688	3302	6698	56
5	9 091008	673	4336	5665	55
6	2024	657	5367	4633	54
7	3037	641	6396	3605	53
8	4947	625	7422	2578	52
9	5056	610	8446	1554	51
10	6062	594	9468	0532	50
11	7065	578	9·100487	10·899513	49
12	8066	562	1504	8496	48
13	9065	546	2519	7480	47
14	9·100062	530	3532	6468	46
15	1056	514	4542	5458	45
16	2048	498	5550	4450	44
17	3037	482	6556	3444	43
18	4025	466	7559	2441	42
19	5010	449	8560	1440	41
20	5992	433	9559	0441	40
21	6973	417	9 110556	10·889444	39
22	7951	400	1551	8449	38
23	8927	384	2543	7457	37
24	9901	368	3533	6467	36
25	9 110873	351	4521	5479	35
26	1842	335	5507	4493	34
27	2809	318	6491	3509	33
28	3774	302	7472	2528	32
29	4737	285	8452	1548	31
30	5698	269	9429	0571	30
	Co-sines	Sines	Co-tang.	Tangents	M

82 Degrees.

Sines and Tangents.

7 Degrees

M	Sines	Co-sines	Tangents	Co-tang	
30	9·115698	9·996269	9·119429	10·880571	30
31	6656	252	9·120404	10·879596	29
32	7613	235	1377	8623	28
33	8567	219	2348	7652	27
34	9519	202	3317	6683	26
35	9·120469	185	4284	5716	25
36	1417	168	5249	4751	24
37	2362	151	6211	3789	23
38	3306	134	7172	2828	22
39	4248	117	8130	1870	21
40	5187	100	9087	0913	20
41	6125	083	9·130041	10·869959	19
42	7060	066	0994	9006	18
43	7993	049	1944	8056	17
44	8925	032	2893	7107	16
45	9854	015	3839	6161	15
46	9·130781	9·995998	4784	5217	14
47	1706	980	5726	4274	13
48	2630	963	6667	3334	12
49	3551	946	7605	2395	11
50	4470	928	8542	1458	10
51	5388	911	9476	0524	9
52	6303	894	9·140409	10·859591	8
53	7216	876	1340	8660	7
54	8128	859	2269	7731	6
55	9037	841	3196	6804	5
56	9945	824	4121	5879	4
57	9·140850	806	5044	4956	3
58	1754	788	5966	4035	2
59	2656	771	6885	3115	1
60	3555	753	7803	2198	0
	Co-sines	Sines	Co-tang.	Tangents	M

82 Degrees

8 Degrees

M	Sines	Co-sines	Tangents	Co-tang	
0	9 143555	9 995753	9·147803	10 852198	60
1	4453	735	8718	1282	59
2	5349	717	9632	0368	58
3	6244	699	9·150544	10 849456	57
4	7136	682	1454	8546	56
5	8026	664	2363	7637	55
6	8915	646	3269	6731	54
7	9802	628	4172	5826	53
8	9·150686	610	5077	4923	52
9	1569	592	5978	4022	51
10	2451	573	6877	3123	50
11	3330	555	7775	2225	49
12	4208	537	8671	1329	48
13	5083	519	9565	0435	47
14	5957	501	9 160457	10 839543	46
15	6830	482	1347	8653	45
16	7700	464	2236	7764	44
17	8569	446	3123	6877	43
18	9435	427	4008	5992	42
19	9 160301	409	4892	5108	41
20	1164	390	5774	4226	40
21	2025	372	6654	3346	39
22	2885	353	7532	2468	38
23	3743	335	8409	1591	37
24	4600	316	9284	0716	36
25	5454	297	9 170157	10 829843	35
26	6307	279	1029	8971	34
27	7159	260	1899	8101	33
28	8008	241	2767	7233	32
29	8856	222	3634	6306	31
30	9702	203	4499	5501	30
	Co-sines	Sines	Co tang	Tangents	

81 Degrees.

SINES and TANGENTS

8 Degrees

M	Sines	Co-sines	Tangents	Co-tang.	
30	9 169702	9 995203	9 174499	10 825501	30
31	9 170547	184	5362	4638	29
32	1389	165	6224	3776	28
33	2231	146	7084	2916	27
34	3070	127	7943	2058	26
35	3908	108	8799	1201	25
36	4744	089	9655	0345	24
37	5578	070	9 180508	10 819492	23
38	6411	051	1360	8640	22
39	7243	032	2211	7789	21
40	8072	013	3060	6941	20
41	8900	9 994993	3907	6093	19
42	9727	974	4753	5248	18
43	9·180551	955	5597	4403	17
44	1374	935	6439	3561	16
45	2196	916	7280	2720	15
46	3016	896	8120	1880	14
47	3834	877	8958	1043	13
48	4651	857	9794	0206	12
49	5467	838	9 190629	10 809371	11
50	6280	818	1462	8538	10
51	7092	799	2294	7706	9
52	7903	779	3124	6876	8
53	8712	759	3953	6047	7
54	9520	739	4780	5220	6
55	9·190325	720	5606	4394	5
56	1130	700	6430	3570	4
57	1933	680	7253	2747	3
58	2734	660	8074	1926	2
59	3534	640	8894	1106	1
60	4332	620	9713	0288	0
	Co-sines	Sines	Co-tang	Tangents	M

81 Degrees.

3 U

A Table of

9 Degrees

M	Sines	Co-sines	Tangents	Co-tang	
0	9 194332	9 994620	9 199713	10 800288	60
1	5129	600	9 200529	10,799471	59
2	5925	580	1345	8655	58
3	6719	560	2156	7841	57
4	7511	540	2971	7029	56
5	8302	519	3783	6218	55
6	9091	499	4592	5408	54
7	9879	479	5400	4600	53
8	9 200666	459	6207	3793	52
9	1451	438	7013	2987	51
10	2235	418	7817	2184	50
11	3017	398	8619	1381	49
12	3797	377	9420	0580	48
13	4577	357	9 210220	10 789780	47
14	5355	336	1018	8982	46
15	6131	315	1815	8185	45
16	6906	295	2611	7389	44
17	7680	274	3405	6595	43
18	8452	254	4198	5802	42
19	9222	233	4989	5011	41
20	9992	212	5780	4221	40
21	9 210760	191	6568	3432	39
22	1526	171	7356	2644	38
23	2291	150	8142	1858	37
24	3055	129	8926	1074	36
25	3818	108	9710	0290	35
26	4579	087	9 220492	10·779508	34
27	5338	066	1272	8728	33
28	6097	045	2052	7948	32
29	6854	024	2830	7170	31
30	7609	003	3607	6394	30
	Co-sines	Sines	Co-tang	Tangents	

80 Degrees.

SINES and TANGENTS.

9 Degrees

M	Sines	Co-sines	Tangents	Co-tang.	
30	9 217609	9 994003	9 223607	10 776394	30
31	8364	9 993982	4382	5618	29
32	9116	960	5156	4844	28
33	9868	939	5929	4071	27
34	9·220618	918	6700	3300	26
35	1367	897	7471	2529	25
36	2115	875	8240	1761	24
37	2861	854	9007	0993	23
38	3606	832	9774	0227	22
39	4350	811	9 230539	10 769461	21
40	5092	789	1302	8698	20
41	5833	768	2065	7935	19
42	6573	746	2826	7174	18
43	7311	725	3586	6414	17
44	8048	703	4345	5655	16
45	8784	681	5103	4897	15
46	9519	660	5859	4141	14
47	9 230252	638	6614	3386	13
48	0984	616	7368	2632	12
49	1715	594	8120	1880	11
50	2444	572	8872	1128	10
51	3172	550	9622	0378	9
52	3899	529	9 240371	10 759629	8
53	4625	507	1119	8882	7
54	5349	484	1865	8135	6
55	6073	462	2610	7390	5
56	6795	440	3354	6646	4
57	7515	418	4097	5903	3
58	8235	396	4839	5161	2
59	8953	374	5579	4421	1
60	9670	352	6319	3681	0
	Co-sines	Sines	Co-ting	Tangents	M

80 Degrees

A Table of
10 Degrees

M	Sines	Co-sines	Tangents	Co-tang.	
0	9.239670	9.993352	9.246319	10.753681	60
1	9.240386	329	7057	2943	59
2	1101	307	7794	2206	58
3	1814	285	8530	1470	57
4	2526	262	9264	0736	56
5	3237	240	9998	0002	55
6	3947	217	9.250730	10.749270	54
7	4656	195	1461	8539	53
8	5363	172	2191	7809	52
9	6070	149	2920	7080	51
10	6775	127	3648	6352	50
11	7478	104	4374	5626	49
12	8181	081	5100	4900	48
13	8883	059	5824	4176	47
14	9583	036	6547	3453	46
15	9.250288	013	7269	2731	45
16	0980	9.992990	7990	2010	44
17	1677	967	8710	1290	43
18	2373	944	9429	0572	42
19	3068	921	9.260146	10.739854	41
20	3761	898	0863	9138	40
21	4453	875	1578	8422	39
22	5144	852	2292	7708	38
23	5834	829	3005	6995	37
24	6523	806	3717	6283	36
25	7211	783	4428	5572	35
26	7898	760	5138	4862	34
27	8583	736	5847	4153	33
28	9268	713	6555	3445	32
29	9951	690	7261	2739	31
30	9.260633	666	7967	2033	30
	Co-sines	Sines	Co-tang.	Tangents	M

79 Degrees.

Sines and Tangents.

10 Degrees

M	Sines	Co-sines	Tangents	Co-tang.	
30	9·260633	9·992666	9 267967	10 732033	30
31	1314	643	8671	1329	29
32	1994	619	9375	0625	28
33	2673	596	9 270077	10 729923	27
34	3351	572	0779	9221	26
35	4027	549	1479	8521	25
36	4703	525	2178	7822	24
37	5378	501	2876	7124	23
38	6051	478	3573	6427	22
39	6723	454	4269	5731	21
40	7395	430	4964	5036	20
41	8065	406	5658	4342	19
42	8734	382	6351	3649	18
43	9402	359	7043	2957	17
44	9·270069	335	7734	2266	16
45	0735	311	8424	1576	15
46	1400	287	9113	0887	14
47	2064	263	9801	0199	13
48	2726	239	9 280408	10 719512	12
49	3388	214	1174	8826	11
50	4049	190	1859	8142	10
51	4708	166	2542	7458	9
52	5367	142	3325	6775	8
53	6025	118	3907	6093	7
54	6681	093	4588	5412	6
55	7337	069	5268	4732	5
56	7991	045	5947	4053	4
57	8645	020	6625	3376	3
58	9297	9 991996	7301	2699	2
59	9948	971	7977	2023	1
60	9 280599	947	8652	1348	0
	Co-sines	Sines	Co-tang	Tangent	M

79 Degrees.

11 Degrees

M	Sines	Co-sines	Tangents	Co-tang	
0	9 280599	9 991947	9 288652	10 711348	60
1	1248	922	9326	0674	59
2	1897	897	9999	0001	58
3	2544	873	9 290671	10 709329	57
4	3191	848	1342	8658	56
5	3836	823	2013	7987	55
6	4480	799	2682	7318	54
7	5124	774	3350	6650	53
8	5766	749	4017	5983	52
9	6408	724	4684	5316	51
10	7048	699	5349	4651	50
11	7688	674	6013	3987	49
12	8326	649	6677	3323	48
13	8964	624	7340	2661	47
14	9600	599	8001	1999	46
15	9 290236	574	8662	1338	45
16	0870	549	9322	0678	44
17	1504	524	9980	0020	43
18	2137	498	9 300638	10 699362	42
19	2769	473	1295	8705	41
20	3399	448	1951	8049	40
21	4029	423	2607	7393	39
22	4658	397	3261	6739	38
23	5286	372	3914	6086	37
24	5913	346	4567	5433	36
25	6539	321	5218	4782	35
26	7164	295	5869	4131	34
27	7788	270	6519	3481	33
28	8412	244	7168	2833	32
29	9034	218	7816	2185	31
30	9655	193	8463	1537	30
	Co-sines	Sines	Co-tang.	Tangents	M

78 Degrees.

Sines *and* Tangents.

11 Degrees

M	Sines	Co-sines	Tangents	Co-tang.	
30	9 299655	9 991193	9 308463	10 691537	30
31	9·300276	167	9109	0891	29
32	0895	141	9754	0246	28
33	1514	115	9 310399	10 689602	27
34	2132	090	1042	8958	26
35	2749	064	1685	8315	25
36	3364	038	2327	7673	24
37	3979	012	2968	7033	23
38	4593	9 990786	3608	6392	22
39	5207	960	4247	5753	21
40	5819	934	4885	5115	20
41	6430	908	5522	4477	19
42	7041	882	6159	3841	18
43	7650	855	6795	3205	17
44	8259	829	7430	2570	16
45	8867	803	8064	1936	15
46	9474	777	8697	1303	14
47	9·310080	750	9330	0671	13
48	0685	724	9961	0039	12
49	1289	697	9 320592	10 679408	11
50	1893	671	1222	8778	10
51	2495	645	1851	8149	9
52	3097	618	2479	7521	8
53	3698	591	3106	6894	7
54	4298	565	3733	6267	6
55	4897	538	4358	5642	5
56	5495	512	4983	5017	4
57	6092	485	5607	4393	3
58	6689	458	6231	3770	2
59	7284	431	6853	3147	1
60	7879	404	7475	2526	0
	Co-sines	Sines	Co-tang	Tangents	M

78 Degrees.

12 Degrees.

M	Sines	Co-sines	Tangents	Co-tang	
0	9 317879	9 990404	9 327475	10 672526	60
1	8473	378	8095	1905	59
2	9066	351	8715	1285	58
3	9658	324	9335	0666	57
4	9 320250	297	9953	0047	56
5	0840	270	9·330570	10 669430	55
6	1430	243	1187	8813	54
7	2019	216	1803	8197	53
8	2607	188	2418	7582	52
9	3194	161	3033	6967	51
10	3780	134	3646	6354	50
11	4366	107	4259	5741	49
12	4951	079	4871	5129	48
13	5534	052	5482	4518	47
14	6117	025	6093	3907	46
15	6700	9 989997	6702	3298	45
16	7281	970	7311	2689	44
17	7862	942	7919	2081	43
18	8442	915	8527	1473	42
19	9021	887	9133	0867	41
20	9599	860	9739	0261	40
21	9 330176	832	9 340344	10 659626	39
22	0753	804	0948	9052	38
23	1329	777	1552	8448	37
24	1904	749	2155	7845	36
25	2478	721	2757	7243	35
26	3051	693	3358	6642	34
27	3624	665	3958	6042	33
28	4196	637	4558	5442	32
29	4767	610	5157	4843	31
30	5337	582	5755	4245	30
	Co-sines	Sines	Co-tang.	Tangents	M

77 Degrees

Sines *and* Tangents.

12 Degrees

M	Sines	Co-sines	Tangents	Co-tang	
30	9 335337	9 989582	9 345755	10 654245	30
31	5906	554	6353	3647	29
32	6475	525	6949	3051	28
33	7043	497	7545	2455	27
34	7610	469	8141	1859	26
35	8176	441	8735	1265	25
36	8742	413	9329	0671	24
37	9307	385	9922	0078	23
38	9871	356	9 350514	10 649486	22
39	9 340434	328	1106	8894	21
40	0996	300	1697	8303	20
41	1558	271	2287	7713	19
42	2119	243	2876	7124	18
43	2679	214	3465	6535	17
44	3239	186	4053	5947	16
45	3797	157	4640	5360	15
46	4355	129	5227	4773	14
47	4912	100	5813	4187	13
48	5469	071	6398	3602	12
49	6025	042	6982	3018	11
50	6579	014	7566	2431	10
51	7134	9 988985	8149	1851	9
52	7687	956	8731	1269	8
53	8240	927	9313	0687	7
54	8792	898	9894	0107	6
55	9343	869	9 360474	10 639526	5
56	9893	840	1053	8947	4
57	9 350443	811	1632	8368	3
58	0992	782	2210	7790	2
59	1541	753	2787	7213	1
60	2088	724	3364	6636	0
	Co-sines	Sines	Co-tang	Tangents	M

77 Degrees.

3 X

13 Degrees

M	Sines	Co-sines	Tangents	Co-tang	
0	9 352088	9 988724	9 363364	10 636636	60
1	2635	695	3940	6060	59
2	3181	666	4516	5485	58
3	3726	636	5090	4910	57
4	4271	607	5664	4336	56
5	4815	578	6237	3763	55
6	5358	548	6810	3190	54
7	5901	519	7382	2618	53
8	6443	489	7953	2047	52
9	6984	460	8524	1476	51
10	7524	430	9094	0906	50
11	8064	401	9663	0337	49
12	8603	371	9 370232	10·629769	48
13	9141	342	0799	9201	47
14	9679	312	1367	8633	46
15	9 360215	282	1933	8067	45
16	0752	252	2499	7501	44
17	1287	223	3065	6936	43
18	1822	193	3629	6371	42
19	2356	163	4193	5807	41
20	2889	133	4756	5244	40
21	3422	103	5319	4681	39
22	3954	073	5881	4119	38
23	4485	043	6442	3558	37
24	5016	013	7003	2997	36
25	5546	9 987983	7563	2437	35
26	6075	953	8123	1878	34
27	6604	922	8681	1319	33
28	7132	892	9239	0761	32
29	7659	862	9797	0203	31
30	8185	832	9 380354	10 619646	30
	Co-sines	Sines	Co-tang	Tangents	M

76 Degrees.

SINES and TANGENTS

13 Degrees

M	Sines	Co-sines	Tangents	Co-t ing	
30	9 368185	9 987832	9 380354	10 619646	30
31	8711	801	0910	9090	29
32	9236	771	1466	8535	28
33	9761	740	2021	7980	27
34	9 370285	710	2575	7425	26
35	0808	679	3129	6872	25
36	1330	649	3682	6318	24
37	1852	618	4234	5766	23
38	2374	588	4786	5214	22
39	2894	557	5337	4663	21
40	3414	526	5888	4112	20
41	3933	496	6438	3562	19
42	4452	465	6987	3013	18
43	4970	434	7536	2464	17
44	5487	403	8084	1916	16
45	6003	372	8631	1369	15
46	6519	341	7178	0822	14
47	7035	310	9724	0276	13
48	7549	279	9 390270	10 609730	12
49	8063	248	0815	9185	11
50	8577	217	1360	8641	10
51	9089	186	1903	8097	9
52	9602	155	2447	7553	8
53	9 380113	124	2989	7011	7
54	0624	092	3531	6469	6
55	1134	061	4073	5927	5
56	1643	030	4614	5386	4
57	2152	9 986998	5154	4846	3
58	2661	967	5694	4307	2
59	3168	936	6233	3767	1
60	3675	904	6771	3229	0
	Co-sines	Sines	Co-t ing	Tangents	M

76 Degrees.

14 Degrees

M	Sines	Co-fines	Tangents	Co-tang	
0	9 383675	9 986904	9 396771	10 603229	60
1	4182	873	7309	2691	59
2	4687	841	7846	2154	58
3	5192	809	8383	1617	57
4	5697	778	8919	1081	56
5	6201	746	9455	0545	55
6	6704	714	9990	0010	54
7	7207	683	9 400524	10 599476	53
8	7709	651	1058	8942	52
9	8210	619	1591	8409	51
10	8711	587	2124	7876	50
11	9211	555	2656	7344	49
12	9711	523	3187	6813	48
13	9 390210	491	3718	6282	47
14	0708	459	4249	5751	46
15	1206	427	4778	5222	45
16	1703	395	5308	4692	44
17	2199	363	5836	4164	43
18	2695	331	6364	3636	42
19	3191	299	6892	3108	41
20	3685	266	7419	2581	40
21	4179	234	7945	2055	39
22	4673	202	8471	1529	38
23	5166	169	8997	1004	37
24	5658	137	9521	0479	36
25	6150	105	9 410045	10 589955	35
26	6641	072	0569	9431	34
27	7132	039	1092	8908	33
28	7622	007	1615	8385	32
29	8111	9 985974	2137	7863	31
30	8600	942	2658	7342	30
	Co-fines	Sines	Co-tang	Tangents	M

75 Degrees.

A Table of
14 Degrees.

M	Sines	Co-fines	Tangents	Co-tang.	
30	9 398600	9 985942	9 412658	10 587342	30
31	9088	909	3179	6821	29
32	9575	876	3699	6301	28
33	9·400063	843	4219	5781	27
34	0549	811	4738	5262	26
35	1035	778	5257	4743	25
36	1520	745	5775	4225	24
37	2005	712	6293	3707	23
38	2489	679	6810	3190	22
39	2972	646	7327	2674	21
40	3455	613	7843	2158	20
41	3938	580	8358	1642	19
42	4420	547	8873	1127	18
43	4901	514	9387	0613	17
44	5382	480	9901	0099	16
45	5862	447	9 420415	10 579585	15
46	6341	414	0928	9073	14
47	6820	381	1440	8560	13
48	7299	347	1952	8049	12
49	7777	314	2463	7537	11
50	8254	280	2974	7027	10
51	8731	247	3484	6516	9
52	9207	213	3994	6007	8
53	9682	180	4503	5497	7
54	9 410158	146	5011	4989	6
55	0632	113	5519	4481	5
56	1106	079	6027	3973	4
57	1579	045	6534	3466	3
58	2052	011	7041	2959	2
59	2525	9·984978	7547	2453	1
60	2996	944	8053	1948	0
	Co-fines	Sines	Co-tang.	Tangents	M

75 Degrees

A Table of
15 Degrees

M	Sines	Co-sines	Tangents	Co-tang	
0	9 412996	9 984944	9 428053	10 571948	60
1	9 413167	910	558	443	59
2	338	876	9 429062	10 570938	58
3	9 414403	842	566	434	57
4	578	808	9 430070	10 569930	56
5	9 415347	774	573	427	55
6	515	740	9 431075	10 568925	54
7	9 416283	706	577	423	53
8	751	672	9 432079	10 567921	52
9	9 417217	638	580	420	51
10	684	603	9 433080	10 566920	50
11	9 418150	569	581	420	49
12	615	535	9 434080	10 565920	48
13	9 419080	500	579	421	47
14	544	466	9 435078	10 564922	46
15	9·420007	432	576	424	45
16	470	397	9 436073	10 563927	44
17	933	363	570	430	43
18	9 421395	328	9 437067	10 562933	42
19	857	294	563	437	41
20	9 422318	259	9 438059	10 561941	40
21	778	224	554	446	39
22	9 423238	190	9·439049	10 560952	38
23	697	155	543	457	37
24	9 424156	120	9 440036	10 559964	36
25	615	085	530	471	35
26	9 425073	050	9 441022	10 558978	34
27	530	015	515	486	33
28	987	9 983981	9 442006	10 557994	32
29	9 426443	946	498	502	31
30	899	911	988	012	30
	Co-sines	Sines	Co-tang	Tangents	M

74 Degrees.

Sines and Tangents. 525

15 Degrees

M	Sines	Co-sines	Tangents	Co-tang	
30	9 426899	9 983911	9 442988	10 557012	30
31	9 427354	876	9·443479	10 556521	29
32	809	840	969	032	28
33	9 428263	805	9·444458	10 555542	27
34	717	770	947	053	26
35	9 429170	735	9·445435	10 554565	25
36	623	700	923	077	24
37	9 430073	664	9 446411	10 553589	23
38	527	629	898	102	22
39	978	574	9 447384	10 552616	21
40	9 431429	558	870	130	20
41	879	523	9 448356	10·551644	19
42	9 432329	487	841	159	18
43	778	452	9 449326	10 550674	17
44	9 433226	416	810	190	16
45	675	381	9 450294	10 549706	15
46	9 434122	345	777	223	14
47	569	309	9·451260	10 548740	13
48	9 435016	274	743	257	12
49	462	238	9 452225	10·547775	11
50	908	202	706	294	10
51	9 436353	166	9 453187	10 546813	9
52	798	130	668	332	8
53	9 437242	094	9 454148	10 545852	7
54	686	058	628	372	6
55	9·438129	022	9 455107	10 544893	5
56	572	9 982986	586	414	4
57	9 439014	950	9 456064	10 543936	3
58	456	914	542	458	2
59	897	878	9·457019	10 542981	1
60	9 440338	842	496	504	0
	Co-sines	Sines	Co-tang	Tangents	M

74 Degrees.

A Table of
16 Degrees

M	Sines	Co-sines	Tangents	Co-tang	
0	9 440338	9 982842	9 457496	10 542504	60
1	778	805	973	027	59
2	9 441218	769	9 458449	10·541551	58
3	658	733	925	075	57
4	9 442097	696	9 459400	10 540600	56
5	535	660	875	125	55
6	973	624	9 460349	10 539651	54
7	9·443410	587	823	177	53
8	847	551	9 461297	10 538703	52
9	9 444284	514	770	230	51
10	720	477	9 462242	10 537758	50
11	9 445155	441	715	286	49
12	590	404	9 463186	10 536814	48
13	9·446025	367	658	342	47
14	459	331	9 464129	10 535872	46
15	893	294	599	401	45
16	9·447326	257	9 465069	10 534931	44
17	759	220	539	461	43
18	9 448191	183	9 466008	10 533992	42
19	623	146	477	524	41
20	9·449054	109	945	055	40
21	485	072	9 467413	10·532587	39
22	915	035	880	120	38
23	9 450345	9 981998	9·468347	10 531653	37
24	775	961	814	186	36
25	9 451204	924	9 469280	10 530720	35
26	632	886	746	254	34
27	9·452060	849	9 470211	10·529789	33
28	488	812	676	324	32
29	915	774	9 471141	10 528859	31
30	9 453342	737	605	395	30
	Co-sines	Sines	Co-tang.	Tangents	M

73 Degrees

SINES and TANGENTS

16 Degrees

M	Sines	Co-fines	Tangents	Co-t ing	
30	9 453342	9·981737	9 471605	10 528395	30
31	768	700	9 472069	10·527932	29
32	9·454194	662	532	468	28
33	619	625	995	005	27
34	9 455044	587	9·473457	10 526543	26
35	469	549	919	081	25
36	893	512	9 474381	10 525619	24
37	9 456316	474	842	158	23
38	739	436	9 475303	10 524697	22
39	9·457162	399	763	237	21
40	584	361	9 476223	10 523777	20
41	9 458006	323	683	317	19
42	427	285	9 477142	10 522858	18
43	848	247	601	399	17
44	9 459268	209	9 478059	10 521941	16
45	688	171	517	483	15
46	9·460108	133	975	025	14
47	527	095	9 479432	10 520568	13
48	946	057	889	111	12
49	9·461364	019	9·480345	10 519655	11
50	782	9 980981	801	199	10
51	9 462199	942	9 481257	10 518743	9
52	616	904	712	288	8
53	9·463032	866	9 482167	10 517833	7
54	448	827	621	379	6
55	864	789	9 483075	10 516925	5
56	9 464279	751	529	471	4
57	694	712	982	018	3
58	9 465108	674	9 484435	10 515565	2
59	522	635	887	113	1
60	935	596	9 485339	10 514661	0
	Co-fines	Sines	Co-t ing	Tangents	M

73 Degrees.

3 Y

17 Degrees

M	Sines	Co-fines	Tangents	Co-tang.	
0	9 465935	9 980596	9·485339	10 514661	60
1	9·466348	558	791	209	59
2	761	519	9 486242	10 513758	58
3	9 467173	480	693	307	57
4	585	442	9 487143	10 512857	56
5	996	403	593	407	55
6	9 468407	364	9·488043	10 511957	54
7	817	325	492	508	53
8	9 469227	286	941	059	52
9	637	247	9 489390	10·510610	51
10	9 470046	208	838	162	50
11	455	169	9 490286	10·509714	49
12	863	130	733	267	48
13	9 471271	091	9 491180	10 508820	47
14	679	052	627	373	46
15	9 472086	012	9 492073	10 507927	45
16	492	9 979973	519	481	44
17	899	934	965	035	43
18	9 473304	895	9 493410	10·506590	42
19	710	855	855	146	41
20	9 474115	816	9 494300	10·505701	40
21	519	776	743	257	39
22	923	737	9 495187	10 504814	38
23	9 475327	697	630	370	37
24	730	658	9 496073	10 503927	36
25	9 476133	618	515	485	35
26	536	579	957	043	34
27	938	539	9·497399	10 502601	33
28	9 477340	499	841	159	32
29	741	459	9 498282	10 501718	31
30	9 478142	420	722	278	30
	Co-fines	Sines	Co-t ing.	Tangents	M

72 Degrees

Sines and Tangents.

17 Degrees

M	Sines	Co-sines	Tangents	Co-tang	
30	9 478142	9 979420	9 498722	10 501278	30
31	542	380	9 499163	10 500837	29
32	942	340	603	397	28
33	9·479342	300	9 500042	10 499958	27
34	741	260	481	519	26
35	9·480140	220	920	080	25
36	539	180	9 501359	10·498641	24
37	937	140	797	203	23
38	9 481334	100	9 502235	10 497765	22
39	732	059	672	328	21
40	9 482128	019	9 503109	10 496891	20
41	525	9 978979	546	454	19
42	921	939	982	018	18
43	9·483317	898	9 504418	10 495582	17
44	712	858	854	146	16
45	9 484107	818	9 505289	10 494711	15
46	501	777	724	276	14
47	895	737	9 506159	10·493841	13
48	9 485289	696	593	407	12
49	682	655	9 507027	10 492973	11
50	9 486075	615	460	540	10
51	467	574	893	107	9
52	860	533	9 508326	10 491674	8
53	9·487251	493	759	241	7
54	643	452	9 509191	10·490809	6
55	9 488034	411	622	378	5
56	424	370	9 510054	10 489946	4
57	814	329	485	515	3
58	9·489204	288	916	084	2
59	593	247	9 511346	10 488654	1
60	982	206	776	224	0
	Co-fines	Sines	Co-t ing	Tangents	M

72 Degrees.

A Table of

18 Degrees.

M	Sines	Co-sines	Tangents	Co-tang.	
0	9.489982	9.978206	9.511776	10.488224	60
1	9.490371	165	9.512206	10.487794	59
2	759	124	635	365	58
3	9.491147	083	9.513064	10.486936	57
4	535	042	493	507	56
5	922	001	921	079	55
6	9.492308	9.977959	9.514349	10.485651	54
7	695	918	777	223	53
8	9.493081	877	9.515204	10.484796	52
9	466	835	631	369	51
10	851	794	9.516058	10.483943	50
11	9.494236	752	484	516	49
12	621	711	910	090	48
13	9.495005	669	9.517335	10.482665	47
14	388	628	761	239	46
15	772	586	9.518186	10.481815	45
16	9.496155	544	610	390	44
17	537	503	9.519034	10.480966	43
18	919	461	458	542	42
19	9.497301	419	882	118	41
20	682	377	9.520305	10.479695	40
21	9.498064	335	728	272	39
22	444	293	9.521151	10.478849	38
23	825	252	573	437	37
24	9.499205	210	995	005	36
25	584	167	9.522417	10.477583	35
26	963	125	838	162	34
27	9.500342	083	9.523259	10.476741	33
28	721	041	680	321	32
29	9.501099	9.976999	9.524100	10.475900	31
30	476	957	520	480	30
	Co-sines	Sines	Co-tang	Tangents	M

71 Degrees.

SINES *and* TANGENTS. 531

18 Degrees

M	Sines	Co-sines	Tangents	Co-tang	
30	9 501476	9 976957	9·524520	10 475480	30
31	854	914	940	061	29
32	9 502231	872	9 525359	10 474641	28
33	608	830	778	222	27
34	984	787	9 526197	10·473803	26
35	9 503360	745	615	385	25
36	735	702	9 527033	10 472967	24
37	9 504111	660	451	549	23
38	485	617	868	132	22
39	860	575	9 528285	10·471715	21
40	9·505234	532	702	298	20
41	608	489	9 529119	10·470881	19
42	981	446	535	465	18
43	9 506354	404	951	050	17
44	727	361	9 530366	10·469634	16
45	9 507099	318	781	219	15
46	471	275	9 531196	10 468804	14
47	843	232	611	389	13
48	9 508214	189	9 532025	10·467975	12
49	585	146	439	561	11
50	956	103	853	147	10
51	9·509326	060	9 533266	10 466734	9
52	696	017	679	321	8
53	9·510065	9·975974	9 534092	10 465908	7
54	434	930	504	496	6
55	803	887	916	083	5
56	9 511172	844	9 535328	10 464672	4
57	540	800	739	261	3
58	907	757	9 536151	10·463850	2
59	9 512275	713	561	439	1
60	642	670	972	028	0
	Co-sines	Sines	Co-tang.	Tangents	M

71 Degrees.

A Table of
19 Degrees

M	Sines	Co-sines	Tangents	Co-tang.	
0	9 512642	9 975670	9·536972	10 463028	60
1	9 513009	627	9 537382	10 462618	59
2	375	583	792	208	58
3	741	539	9 538202	10·461798	57
4	9 514107	496	611	389	56
5	472	452	9 539020	10·460980	55
6	837	408	429	571	54
7	9 515202	365	837	163	53
8	566	321	9 540245	10·459755	52
9	930	277	653	347	51
10	9 516294	233	9·541061	10·458939	50
11	657	189	468	532	49
12	9 517020	145	875	125	48
13	382	101	9 542281	10·457719	47
14	745	057	688	312	46
15	9 518107	013	9 543094	10 456906	45
16	468	9 974969	499	501	44
17	830	925	905	095	43
18	9 519190	880	9 544310	10 455690	42
19	551	836	715	285	41
20	911	792	9 545119	10 454881	40
21	9 520271	748	524	476	39
22	631	703	928	072	38
23	990	659	9 546331	10 453669	37
24	9 521349	614	735	265	36
25	707	570	9 547138	10 452862	35
26	9 522066	525	511	460	34
27	424	481	943	057	33
28	781	436	9 548345	10 451655	32
29	9 523138	391	747	253	31
30	495	347	9 549149	10·450851	30
	Co-sines	Sines	Co-tang	Tangents	M

70 Degrees

Sines and Tangents.

19 Degrees

M	Sines	Co-sines	Tangents	Co-tang.	
30	9 523495	9 974347	9 549149	10 450851	30
31	852	302	550	450	29
32	9·524208	257	951	049	28
33	564	212	9·550352	10 449648	27
34	920	167	752	248	26
35	9 525275	122	9·551153	10 448848	25
36	630	077	552	448	24
37	984	032	952	048	23
38	9·526339	9 973987	9 552351	10 447649	22
39	693	942	750	250	21
40	9 527046	897	9 553149	10 446851	20
41	400	852	548	452	19
42	753	807	946	054	18
43	9 528105	762	9 554344	10 445656	17
44	458	716	742	259	16
45	810	671	9·555139	10 444861	15
46	9 529161	626	536	464	14
47	513	580	933	067	13
48	864	535	9 556329	10·443671	12
49	9 530215	489	726	275	11
50	565	444	9·557121	10·442879	10
51	915	398	517	483	9
52	9·531265	352	913	088	8
53	614	307	9·558308	10 441692	7
54	964	261	703	298	6
55	9 532312	215	9 559097	10 440903	5
56	661	169	491	509	4
57	9·533009	124	885	115	3
58	357	078	9 560279	10 439721	2
59	704	032	673	327	1
60	9 534052	9 972986	9 561066	931	0
	Co-sines	Sines	Co-tang	Tangents	M

70 Degrees

A Table of
20 Degrees

M	Sines	Co-sines	Tangents	Co-tang	
0	9 534052	9 972986	9 561066	10 438934	60
1	399	940	459	541	59
2	745	894	852	149	58
3	9 535092	848	9 562244	10 437756	57
4	438	802	636	364	56
5	783	755	9 563028	10 436972	55
6	9·536129	709	419	581	54
7	474	663	811	189	53
8	818	617	9·564202	10 435798	52
9	9·537163	570	593	408	51
10	507	524	983	017	50
11	851	478	9 565373	10 434627	49
12	9 538194	431	763	237	48
13	538	385	9 566153	10 433847	47
14	880	338	542	458	46
15	9 539223	291	932	068	45
16	565	245	9 567321	10·432680	44
17	907	198	709	291	43
18	9 540249	151	9 568098	10 431903	42
19	590	105	486	514	41
20	931	058	874	127	40
21	9 541272	011	9 569261	10 430739	39
22	613	9·971964	648	352	38
23	953	917	9·570036	10 429965	37
24	9 542293	870	422	578	36
25	632	823	809	191	35
26	971	776	9 571195	10·428805	34
27	9 543310	729	581	419	33
28	649	682	967	033	32
29	987	635	9 572352	10 427648	31
30	9 544325	588	738	262	30
	Co-fines	Sines	Co-tang.	Tangents	M

69 Degrees.

SINES and TANGENTS.

20 Degrees

M	Sines	Co-sines	Tangents	Co-tang.	
30	9·544325	9·971588	9 572738	10 427262	30
31	663	540	9·573123	10 426877	29
32	9·545001	493	507	493	28
33	338	446	892	108	27
34	675	398	9·574276	10·424724	26
35	9·546011	351	660	340	25
36	347	304	9 575044	10·429956	24
37	683	256	427	573	23
38	9·547019	208	810	190	22
39	354	161	9·576193	10·423807	21
40	689	113	576	424	20
41	9·548024	066	959	042	19
42	359	018	9 577341	10 422659	18
43	693	9·970970	723	277	17
44	9·549027	922	9·578104	10·421896	16
45	360	874	486	514	15
46	694	827	867	133	14
47	9·550027	779	9 579284	10 420752	13
48	359	731	629	371	12
49	692	683	9·580009	10·419991	11
50	9 551024	635	389	611	10
51	356	587	769	231	9
52	687	538	9·581149	10·418851	8
53	9·552018	490	528	472	7
54	349	442	907	093	6
55	680	394	9·582286	10 417714	5
56	9·553011	345	665	335	4
57	341	297	9 583044	10·416957	3
58	670	249	422	578	2
59	9·554000	200	800	200	1
60	329	152	9·584177	10·415823	0
	Co-fines	Sines	Co-tang.	Tangents	M

69 Degrees.

3 Z

A Table of

21 Degrees

M	Sines	Co-sines	Tangents	Co-tang	
0	9 554329	9 970152	9 584177	10 415823	30
1	658	103	555	445	29
2	987	055	932	068	28
3	9 555315	006	9 585309	10 414691	27
4	643	9 969957	686	314	26
5	971	909	9·586062	10 413938	25
6	9 556299	860	439	561	24
7	626	811	815	185	23
8	953	762	9·587190	10 412810	22
9	9 557280	714	566	434	21
10	606	665	941	059	20
11	932	616	9·588316	10 411684	19
12	9 558258	567	691	309	18
13	584	518	9 589066	10 410934	17
14	909	469	440	560	16
15	9 559234	420	814	186	15
16	559	370	9·590188	10 409812	14
17	883	321	562	438	13
18	9 560207	272	935	065	12
19	531	223	9·591308	10·408692	11
20	855	173	681	319	10
21	9 561178	124	9·592054	10 407946	9
22	501	075	426	574	8
23	824	025	799	202	7
24	9·562146	9 968976	9 593171	10·406830	6
25	469	926	542	458	5
26	790	877	914	086	4
27	9·563112	827	9·594285	10·405715	3
28	434	777	656	344	2
29	755	728	9·595027	10 404973	1
30	9 564075	678	398	603	0
	Co-sines	Sines	Co-tang.	Tangents	M

68 Degrees.

SINES and TANGENTS.

21 Degrees

M	Sines	Co-sines	Tangents	Co-tang.	
30	9 564075	9 968678	9 595398	10 404603	30
31	396	628	768	232	29
32	716	578	9 596138	10 403862	28
33	9 565036	528	508	492	27
34	356	479	878	122	26
35	676	429	9 597247	10 402753	25
36	995	379	616	384	24
37	9 566314	329	985	015	23
38	632	278	9 598354	10 401646	22
39	951	228	723	278	21
40	9 567269	178	9 599091	10 400909	20
41	587	128	459	541	19
42	904	078	827	173	18
43	9 568222	027	9 600191	10 399806	17
44	539	9 967977	562	438	16
45	856	927	929	071	15
46	9 569172	876	9 601296	10 398704	14
47	488	826	663	338	13
48	804	775	9 602029	10 397971	12
49	9 570120	725	395	605	11
50	436	674	761	239	10
51	751	624	9 603127	10 396873	9
52	9 571066	573	493	507	8
53	380	522	858	142	7
54	695	471	9 604223	10 395777	6
55	9 572009	421	588	412	5
56	323	370	953	047	4
57	636	319	9 605317	10 394683	3
58	950	268	682	318	2
59	9 573263	217	9 606046	10 393954	1
60	575	166	410	590	0
	Co-fines	Sines	Co-tang	Tangents	M

68 Degrees.

A Table of
22 Degrees

M	Sines	Co-sines	Tangents	Co-tang.	
0	9·573575	9·967166	9 606410	10·393590	60
1	888	115	773	227	59
2	9 574200	064	9·607137	10·392863	58
3	512	013	500	500	57
4	824	9 966961	863	137	56
5	9 575136	910	9 608225	10 391775	55
6	447	859	588	412	54
7	758	808	950	050	53
8	9 576069	756	9 609312	10·390688	52
9	379	705	674	326	51
10	689	653	9·610036	10 389964	50
11	999	602	397	603	49
12	9 577309	550	759	241	48
13	618	499	9 611120	10·388880	47
14	928	447	480	520	46
15	9·578236	395	841	159	45
16	545	344	9·612201	10 387799	44
17	854	292	562	439	43
18	9·579162	240	921	079	42
19	470	188	9·613281	10 386719	41
20	777	137	641	359	40
21	9·580085	085	9 614000	000	39
22	392	033	359	10·385641	38
23	699	9 965981	718	282	37
24	9·581005	929	9·615077	10·384923	36
25	312	876	435	565	35
26	618	824	793	207	34
27	924	772	9 616151	10·383849	33
28	9·582229	720	509	491	32
29	535	668	867	133	31
30	840	615	9·617224	382776	30
	Co-sines	Sines	Co-tang.	Tangents	M

17 Degrees

SINES and TANGENTS.

22 Degrees

M	Sines	Co-sines	Tangents	Co-tang	
30	9·582840	9 965615	9·617224	10·382776	30
31	9·583145	563	582	419	29
32	449	511	939	062	28
33	754	458	9·618295	10·381705	27
34	9 584058	406	652	348	26
35	362	353	9 619008	10 380992	25
36	665	301	365	636	24
37	969	248	721	280	23
38	9·585272	195	9·620076	10 379924	22
39	575	143	432	568	21
40	877	090	787	213	20
41	9 586180	037	9 621142	10 378858	19
42	482	9 964984	497	503	18
43	784	931	852	148	17
44	9 587085	879	9·622207	10·377793	16
45	387	826	561	439	15
46	688	773	915	085	14
47	989	720	9 623269	10 376731	13
48	9 588289	667	623	377	12
49	590	613	976	024	11
50	890	560	9·624330	10 375670	10
51	9·589190	507	683	317	9
52	489	454	9 625036	19 374964	8
53	789	400	388	612	7
54	9 590088	347	741	259	6
55	387	294	9 626093	10 373907	5
56	686	240	445	555	4
57	984	187	797	203	3
58	9 591282	133	9·627149	10 372852	2
59	580	080	501	499	1
60	878	026	852	148	0
	Co-sines	Sines	Co-tang.	Tangents	M

67 Degrees.

A Table of

23 Degrees.

M	Sines	Co-sines	Tangents	Co-tang.	
0	9 591878	9 964026	9 627852	10 372148	60
1	9·592176	9·963972	9 628203	10 371797	59
2	473	919	554	446	58
3	770	865	905	095	57
4	9·593067	811	9 629255	10·370745	56
5	363	757	606	394	55
6	659	704	956	044	54
7	956	650	9 630306	10 369694	53
8	9·594251	596	656	344	52
9	547	542	9 631005	10·368995	51
10	842	488	355	646	50
11	9 595137	434	704	296	49
12	432	380	9 632053	10 367947	48
13	727	325	402	599	47
14	9·596021	271	750	250	46
15	315	217	9 633099	10 366902	45
16	609	163	447	553	44
17	903	108	795	205	43
18	9 597197	054	9·634143	10·365857	42
19	490	9 962999	490	510	41
20	783	945	838	162	40
21	9 598075	890	9 635185	10·364815	39
22	368	836	532	468	38
23	660	781	879	121	37
24	952	727	9 636226	10 363774	36
25	9·599244	672	572	428	35
26	536	617	919	082	34
27	837	562	9 637265	10 362735	33
28	9·600118	508	611	389	32
29	409	453	956	044	31
30	700	398	9·638302	10·361698	30
	Co-sines	Sines	Co-tang.	Tangents	M

66 Degrees.

SINES and TANGENTS.

23 Degrees

M	Sines	Co-sines	Tangents	Co-tang	
30	9 600700	9·962398	9·638302	10·361698	30
31	990	343	647	353	29
32	9 661280	288	993	008	28
33	570	233	9·639338	10·360663	27
34	860	178	682	318	26
35	9·602150	123	9·640027	10 359973	25
36	439	067	371	629	24
37	728	012	716	284	23
38	9·603017	9·961957	9 641060	10·358940	22
39	305	902	404	596	21
40	594	846	747	253	20
41	882	791	9·642091	10 357909	19
42	9 604170	736	434	566	18
43	457	680	777	223	17
44	745	625	9 643120	10·356880	16
45	9 605032	569	463	537	15
46	319	513	806	194	14
47	606	458	9·644148	10 355852	13
48	892	402	490	510	12
49	9·606179	346	832	168	11
50	465	290	9·645174	10 354826	10
51	751	235	516	484	9
52	9·607036	179	858	143	8
53	322	123	9 646199	10·353801	7
54	607	067	540	460	6
55	892	011	881	119	5
56	9·608177	9 960955	9·647222	10 352778	4
57	461	899	562	438	3
58	745	843	903	097	2
59	9·609029	786	9 648243	10 351757	1
60	313	730	583	417	0
	Co-sines	Sines	Co-tang	Tangents	M

66 Degrees.

A Table of

24 Degrees.

M	Sines	Co-fines	Tangents	Co-tang.	
0	9.609313	9.960730	9.648583	10.351417	60
1	597	674	923	077	59
2	880	618	9.649263	10.350737	58
3	9.610164	561	602	398	57
4	447	505	942	058	56
5	729	448	9.650281	10.349719	55
6	9.611012	392	620	380	54
7	294	335	959	041	53
8	576	279	9.651297	10.348703	52
9	858	222	636	364	51
10	9.612140	166	974	026	50
11	421	109	9.652312	10.347687	49
12	702	052	650	350	48
13	983	9.959995	988	012	47
14	9.613264	938	9.653326	10.346674	46
15	545	882	663	337	45
16	825	825	9.654000	000	44
17	9.614105	768	338	10.345663	43
18	385	711	674	326	42
19	665	654	9.655011	10.344989	41
20	944	596	348	652	40
21	9.615223	539	684	316	39
22	502	482	9.656020	10.343980	38
23	781	425	356	644	37
24	9.616060	368	692	308	36
25	338	310	9.657028	10.342972	35
26	616	253	364	636	34
27	894	195	699	301	33
28	9.617172	138	9.658034	10.341966	32
29	450	081	369	631	31
30	727	023	704	296	30
	Co-fines	Sines	Co-tang.	Tangents	M

65 Degrees.

SINES and TANGENTS.

24 Degrees

M	Sines	Co-sines	Tangents	Co-tang	
30	9·617727	9 959023	9 658704	10 341296	30
31	9 618004	9 958965	9·659039	10 340961	29
32	281	908	373	627	28
33	558	850	708	292	27
34	834	792	9·660042	10·339958	26
35	9 619110	735	376	624	25
36	386	677	710	290	24
37	662	619	9 661043	10 338957	23
38	938	561	377	623	22
39	9·620213	503	710	290	21
40	488	445	9 662043	10 337957	20
41	763	387	377	624	19
42	9 621038	329	709	291	18
43	313	271	9·663042	10 336958	17
44	587	213	375	626	16
45	861	154	707	293	15
46	9 622135	096	9·664039	10·335961	14
47	409	038	371	629	13
48	682	9·957979	703	297	12
49	956	921	9 665035	10 334965	11
50	9·623229	863	366	634	10
51	502	804	698	303	9
52	774	746	9 666029	10 333971	8
53	9 624047	687	360	640	7
54	319	628	691	309	6
55	591	570	9 667021	10 332979	5
56	863	511	352	648	4
57	9·625135	452	682	318	3
58	406	393	9 668013	10 331987	2
59	677	335	343	657	1
60	948	276	673	328	0
	Co-sine	Sines	Co-tang	Tangent	M

65 Degrees.

4 A

25 Degrees.

M	Sines	Co-sines	Tangents	Co-tang.	
0	9 625948	9 957276	9 668673	10 331328	60
1	9 626219	217	9 669002	10 330998	59
2	490	158	332	668	58
3	760	099	661	339	57
4	9 627030	040	991	009	56
5	300	9 956981	9 670320	10 329680	55
6	570	922	649	351	54
7	840	862	977	023	53
8	9 628109	803	9 671306	10 328694	52
9	378	744	635	366	51
10	647	684	963	037	50
11	916	625	9 672291	10 327709	49
12	9 629185	566	619	381	48
13	453	506	947	053	47
14	721	447	9 673275	10 326726	46
15	989	387	602	398	45
16	9 630257	327	929	071	44
17	524	268	9 674257	10 325743	43
18	792	208	584	416	42
19	9 631059	148	911	090	41
20	326	089	9 675237	10 324763	40
21	593	029	564	436	39
22	859	9 955969	890	110	38
23	9 632126	909	9 676217	10 323784	37
24	392	849	543	457	36
25	658	789	869	131	35
26	923	729	9 677194	10 322806	34
27	9 633189	669	520	480	33
28	454	609	846	154	32
29	719	549	9 678171	10 321829	31
30	984	408	496	504	30
	Co-sines	Sines	Co-tang	Tangents	M

64 Degrees.

Sines and Tangents.

25 Degrees

M	Sines	Co-sines	Tangents	Co-tang	
30	9·633984	9 955488	9·678496	10 321504	30
31	9 634249	428	821	179	29
32	514	368	9 679146	10 320854	28
33	778	307	471	529	27
34	9 635042	247	795	205	26
35	306	186	9 680120	10 319880	25
36	570	126	441	550	24
37	834	065	768	232	23
38	9 636097	005	9 681092	10 318908	22
39	360	9 954944	416	584	21
40	623	883	740	260	20
41	886	823	9·682063	10 317937	19
42	9 637148	762	387	614	18
43	411	701	710	290	17
44	673	640	9 683033	10 316967	16
45	935	579	356	644	15
46	9 638197	518	679	322	14
47	459	457	9 684001	10 315999	13
48	720	396	324	676	12
49	981	335	646	354	11
50	9 639242	274	968	032	10
51	503	213	9 685290	10 314710	9
52	764	152	612	388	8
53	9 640024	090	934	066	7
54	284	029	9 686255	10 313745	6
55	545	9 953968	577	423	5
56	804	906	898	102	4
57	9 641064	845	9 687219	10·312781	3
58	324	783	540	460	2
59	583	722	861	139	1
60	842	660	9 688182	10 311818	0
	Co-sines	Sines	Co-tang	Tangents	M

64 Degrees.

26 Degrees

M	Sines	Co-fines	Tangents	Co-tang	
0	9 641842	9 953660	9 688182	10 311818	60
1	9 642101	599	502	498	59
2	360	537	823	177	58
3	618	475	9 689143	10 310857	57
4	877	413	463	537	56
5	9 643135	352	783	217	55
6	393	290	9 690103	10 309897	54
7	650	228	423	577	53
8	908	166	742	258	52
9	9 644165	104	9 961062	10 308938	51
10	423	042	381	619	50
11	680	9 952980	700	300	49
12	937	918	9 692019	10 307981	48
13	9 645193	855	338	662	47
14	450	793	657	344	46
15	706	731	975	025	45
16	962	669	9 693293	10 306707	44
17	9 646218	606	612	388	43
18	474	544	930	070	42
19	729	481	9 694248	10 305752	41
20	984	419	566	434	40
21	9 647240	356	883	117	39
22	495	294	9 695201	10 304799	38
23	749	231	518	482	37
24	9 648004	168	836	165	36
25	258	106	9 696153	10 303847	35
26	512	043	470	530	34
27	767	9 951980	787	214	33
28	9 649020	917	9 697103	10 302897	32
29	274	854	420	580	31
30	527	791	736	264	30
	Co-fines	Sines	Co-tang	Tangents	M

63 Degrees

Sines and Tangents.

26 Degrees

M	Sines	Co-sines	Tangents	Co-tang.	
30	9 649527	9·951791	9·697736	10 302264	30
31	781	728	9·698053	10·301947	29
32	9·650034	665	369	631	28
33	287	602	685	315	27
34	540	539	9·699001	10 300999	26
35	792	476	316	684	25
36	9·651044	412	632	368	24
37	297	349	947	053	23
38	549	286	9·700263	10 299737	22
39	800	222	578	422	21
40	9·652052	159	893	107	20
41	304	096	9 701208	10 298792	19
42	555	032	523	477	18
43	806	9 950969	837	163	17
44	9 653057	905	9 702152	10 297848	16
45	308	841	466	534	15
46	558	778	781	220	14
47	808	714	9·703095	10 296905	13
48	9 654059	650	409	591	12
49	309	586	723	278	11
50	558	522	9·704036	10 295964	10
51	808	458	350	650	9
52	9·655058	394	663	337	8
53	307	330	977	024	7
54	556	266	9 705290	10·294710	6
55	805	202	603	397	5
56	9·656054	138	916	084	4
57	302	074	9·706228	10 293772	3
58	551	010	541	459	2
59	799	9 949945	854	147	1
60	9·657047	881	9 707166	10 292834	0
	Co-sines	Sines	Co-tang.	Tangents	M

63 Degrees.

A Table of

27 Degrees

M	Sines	Co-sines	Tangents	Co-tang	
0	9 657047	9 949881	9 707166	10·292834	60
1	295	817	478	522	59
2	542	752	790	210	58
3	790	688	9 708102	10·291898	57
4	9 658037	623	414	586	56
5	284	559	726	274	55
6	531	494	9 709037	10 290963	54
7	778	429	349	651	53
8	9·659025	365	660	340	52
9	271	300	971	029	51
10	517	235	9 710282	10 289718	50
11	763	170	593	407	49
12	9 660009	105	904	096	48
13	255	040	9 711215	10 288785	47
14	501	9 948975	525	475	46
15	746	910	836	164	45
16	991	845	9 712146	10 287854	44
17	9 661236	780	456	544	43
18	481	715	766	234	42
19	726	650	9 713076	10 286924	41
20	970	584	386	614	40
21	9 662215	519	696	304	39
22	459	454	9 714005	10 285995	38
23	703	388	315	686	37
24	946	323	624	376	36
25	9 663190	257	933	067	35
26	434	192	9 715242	10 284758	34
27	677	126	551	449	33
28	920	060	860	141	32
29	9 664163	9 947995	9 716168	10·283832	31
30	406	929	477	523	30
	Co-sines	Sines	Co-tang	Tangents	M

62 Degrees

Sines and Tangents

27 Degrees

M	Sines	Co-sines	Tangents	Co-tang	
30	9 664406	9 947929	9 716477	10 283523	30
31	648	863	785	215	29
32	891	797	9 717093	10 282907	28
33	9·665133	731	401	599	27
34	375	666	709	291	26
35	617	600	9 718017	10 281983	25
36	859	534	325	675	24
37	9 666100	467	633	367	23
38	342	401	940	060	22
39	583	335	9 719248	10 280752	21
40	824	269	555	445	20
41	9 667065	203	862	138	19
42	305	136	9 720169	10 279831	18
43	546	070	476	524	17
44	786	004	783	217	16
45	9 668027	9 946937	9 721089	10 278911	15
46	267	871	396	604	14
47	506	804	702	298	13
48	746	738	9 722009	10 277992	12
49	986	671	315	685	11
50	9 669225	604	621	379	10
51	464	538	927	073	9
52	703	471	9 723232	10 276768	8
53	942	404	538	462	7
54	9 670181	337	844	156	6
55	419	270	9 724119	10 275851	5
56	658	203	454	546	4
57	896	136	760	241	3
58	9 671134	069	9 725065	10 274935	2
59	372	002	370	631	1
60	609	9 945935	674	326	0
	Co-sines	Sines	Co-tang.	Tangents	M

62 Degrees.

A Table of

28 Degrees.

M	Sines	Co-sines	Tangents	Co-tang.	
0	9 671609	9 945935	9 725674	10 274326	60
1	847	868	979	021	59
2	9 672084	801	9 726284	9 273716	58
3	321	733	588	412	57
4	558	666	893	108	56
5	795	599	9 727197	9 272803	55
6	9 673032	531	501	499	54
7	268	464	805	195	53
8	505	396	9 728109	9 271891	52
9	741	329	412	588	51
10	977	261	716	284	50
11	9 674213	193	9 729020	9·270980	49
12	449	126	323	677	48
13	684	058	626	374	47
14	919	9·944990	930	071	46
15	9 675155	922	9 730233	9·269768	45
16	390	854	535	465	44
17	625	786	838	162	43
18	859	718	9·731141	9 268859	42
19	9·676094	650	444	556	41
20	328	582	746	254	40
21	562	514	9·732048	9 267952	39
22	796	446	351	649	38
23	9 677030	378	653	347	37
24	264	309	955	045	36
25	498	241	9 733257	9 266743	35
26	731	173	558	442	34
27	964	104	860	140	33
28	9 678197	036	9 734162	9 265838	32
29	430	9·943967	463	537	31
30	663	899	764	236	30
	Co-sines	Sines	Co-tang.	Tangents	M

61 Degrees.

SINES *and* TANGENTS.

28 Degrees

M	Sines	Co-sines	Tangents	Co-tang	
30	9 678663	9 943898	9 734763	10 265236	30
31	895	830	9 735066	10 264934	29
32	9 679128	761	367	633	28
33	360	693	668	332	27
34	592	624	968	032	26
35	824	555	9 736269	10 263731	25
36	9·680056	486	570	430	24
37	288	417	871	130	23
38	519	348	9 737171	10 262829	22
39	750	279	471	529	21
40	982	210	771	229	20
41	9 681213	141	9·738071	10 261929	19
42	443	072	371	629	18
43	674	003	671	329	17
44	905	9 942931	971	029	16
45	9 682135	864	9·739271	10 260729	15
46	365	795	570	430	14
47	595	726	870	130	13
48	825	656	9 740169	10 259831	12
49	9·683055	587	468	532	11
50	284	517	767	233	10
51	514	448	9 741066	10 258934	9
52	743	378	365	635	8
53	972	308	664	336	7
54	9 684201	239	962	038	6
55	430	169	9 742261	10 257739	5
56	658	099	559	441	4
57	887	029	858	142	3
58	9 685115	9·941959	9 743156	10 256844	2
59	343	889	454	546	1
60	571	819	752	248	0
	Co-fines	Sines	Co-t ng	Tangents	M

61 Degrees

29 Degrees

M	Sines	Co-fines	Tangents	Co-tang.	
0	9 685571	9 941819	9 743752	10 256248	60
1	799	749	9 744050	10 255950	59
2	9·686027	679	348	652	58
3	254	609	645	355	57
4	482	537	943	057	56
5	709	468	9·745240	10 254760	55
6	936	398	538	462	54
7	9 687163	328	835	165	53
8	389	258	9·746132	10·253868	52
9	616	187	429	571	51
10	843	117	726	274	50
11	9 688069	046	9 747023	10 252977	49
12	295	9 940975	319	681	48
13	521	905	616	384	47
14	747	834	912	088	46
15	972	763	9 748209	10 251791	45
16	9 689198	693	505	495	44
17	423	622	801	199	43
18	648	551	9 749097	10 250903	42
19	873	480	393	607	41
20	9 690098	409	689	311	40
21	323	338	985	015	39
22	548	267	9 750281	10 249719	38
23	772	196	576	424	37
24	996	125	872	128	36
25	9 691220	053	9 751167	10 248833	35
26	444	9·939982	462	538	34
27	668	911	757	243	33
28	892	840	9·752052	10 247948	32
29	9 692115	768	347	653	31
30	339	697	642	358	30
	Co-fines	Sines	Co-tang.	Tangents	M

60 Degrees.

SINES and TANGENTS.

29 Degrees.

M	Sines	Co-sines	Tangents	Co-tang	
30	9 692339	9 939697	9 752642	10 247358	30
31	562	625	937	063	29
32	785	554	9·753231	10 246769	28
33	9 693009	482	526	474	27
34	231	410	820	180	26
35	453	339	9·754115	10·245885	25
36	676	267	409	591	24
37	898	195	703	297	23
38	9 694120	123	997	003	22
39	342	051	9·755291	10 244709	21
40	564	9 938980	585	415	20
41	786	908	878	122	19
42	9 695007	836	9 756172	10·243828	18
43	229	763	465	535	17
44	450	691	759	241	16
45	671	619	9 757052	10·242948	15
46	892	547	345	655	14
47	9 696113	475	638	362	13
48	334	402	931	069	12
49	554	330	9 758224	10·241776	11
50	774	258	517	483	10
51	995	185	810	190	9
52	9 697215	113	9·759102	10·240898	8
53	435	040	395	605	7
54	654	9 937967	687	313	6
55	874	895	979	021	5
56	9 698094	822	9 760272	10·239728	4
57	313	749	564	436	3
58	532	676	856	1	2
59	751	603	9 761148	10 238852	1
60	970	531	439	561	0
	Co-sines	Sines	Co-tang.	Tangents	M

60 Degrees.

30 Degrees

M	Sines	Co-sines	Tangents	Co-tang	
0	9 698970	9 937531	9·761439	10 238561	60
1	699189	458	731	269	59
2	407	385	9 762023	10 237977	58
3	626	312	314	686	57
4	844	238	606	394	56
5	9 700062	165	897	103	55
6	280	092	9·763188	10·236812	54
7	498	019	479	521	53
8	716	9 936946	770	230	52
9	953	872	9 764061	10 235939	51
10	9 701151	799	352	648	50
11	368	725	643	357	49
12	585	652	933	067	48
13	802	578	9 765224	10 234776	47
14	9 702019	505	514	486	46
15	276	431	805	195	45
16	452	357	9 766095	10 233905	44
17	669	284	385	615	43
18	885	210	675	325	42
19	9 703101	136	965	035	41
20	317	062	9 767255	10 232745	40
21	533	9 935988	545	455	39
22	749	914	834	166	38
23	964	840	9·768124	10·231876	37
24	9 704179	766	413	587	36
25	395	692	703	297	35
26	610	618	992	008	34
27	825	543	9 769281	10 230719	33
28	9 705040	469	570	430	32
29	254	395	860	140	31
30	469	320	, 770148	10 229852	30
	Co sines	Sines	Co-tang	Tangents	M

59 Degrees

Sines and Tangents.

30 Degrees

M	Sines	Co-sines	Tangents	Co-tang	
30	9 705469	9 935320	9 770148	10 229852	30
31	683	246	437	563	29
32	897	171	726	274	28
33	9 706112	097	9 771015	10 228985	27
34	326	022	303	697	26
35	539	9 934948	592	408	25
36	753	873	880	120	24
37	967	798	9 772168	10 227832	23
38	9 707180	723	457	543	22
39	393	649	745	255	21
40	606	574	9 773033	10 226967	20
41	819	499	321	679	19
42	9 708032	424	608	392	18
43	245	349	896	104	17
44	457	274	9 774184	10·225816	16
45	670	199	471	529	15
46	882	123	759	241	14
47	9 709094	048	9 775046	10 224954	13
48	306	9·933973	333	667	12
49	518	898	621	379	11
50	730	822	908	092	10
51	942	747	9·776195	10 223805	9
52	9 710153	671	482	518	8
53	364	596	769	232	7
54	575	520	9 777055	10·222945	6
55	786	444	342	658	5
56	997	369	628	372	4
57	9 711208	293	915	085	3
58	419	217	9 778201	10·221799	2
59	629	142	487	513	1
60	839	066	774	226	0
	Co-sines	Sines	Co-tang.	Tangents	M

59 Degrees

31 Degrees

M	Sines	Co-sines	Tangents	Co-tang.	
0	9 711839	9 933066	9 778774	10·221226	60
1	9 712050	9 932990	9·779060	10 220940	59
2	260	914	346	654	58
3	469	838	632	368	57
4	679	762	918	082	56
5	889	685	9 780203	10·219797	55
6	9·713098	609	489	511	54
7	308	533	775	225	53
8	517	457	9 781060	10 218940	52
9	726	380	346	654	51
10	935	304	631	369	50
11	9 714144	228	916	084	49
12	352	151	9 782201	10 217799	48
13	561	075	486	514	47
14	769	9 931998	771	229	46
15	978	921	9 783056	10 216944	45
16	9 715186	845	341	659	44
17	394	768	626	374	43
18	601	691	910	090	42
19	809	614	9·784195	10·215805	41
20	9 716017	537	479	521	40
21	224	460	764	236	39
22	432	383	9·785048	10 214952	38
23	639	306	332	668	37
24	846	229	616	384	36
25	9 717053	152	900	100	35
26	259	075	9 786184	10 213816	34
27	466	9 930998	468	532	33
28	673	920	752	248	32
29	879	843	9 787036	10 212964	31
30	9 718085	766	319	681	30
	Co-sines	Sines	Co-tang	Tangents	M

58 Degrees

Sines and Tangents.

31 Degrees

M	Sines	Co-sines	Tangents	Co-tang	
30	9·718085	9·930766	9·787319	10·212681	30
31	291	688	603	397	29
32	497	611	886	114	28
33	703	533	9·788170	10·211830	27
34	909	456	453	547	26
35	9·719114	378	736	264	25
36	320	300	9·789019	10·210981	24
37	525	223	302	698	23
38	730	145	585	415	22
39	935	067	868	132	21
40	9·720140	9·929989	9·790151	10·209849	20
41	345	911	433	567	19
42	549	833	716	284	18
43	754	755	999	001	17
44	958	677	9·791281	10·208719	16
45	9·721162	599	563	437	15
46	366	521	846	154	14
47	570	442	9·792128	10·207872	13
48	774	364	410	590	12
49	978	286	692	308	11
50	9·722181	207	974	026	10
51	385	129	9·793256	10·206744	9
52	588	050	538	462	8
53	791	9·928972	819	181	7
54	994	893	9·794101	10·205899	6
55	9·723197	814	383	617	5
56	400	736	664	336	4
57	603	657	945	055	3
58	805	578	9·795227	10·204773	2
59	9·724007	499	508	492	1
60	210	420	789	211	0
	Co-sines	Sines	Co-tang	Tangents	M

58 Degrees.

A Table of
32 Degrees.

M	Sines	Co-fines	Tangents	Co-tang	
0	9 724210	9 928420	9 795789	10·204211	60
1	412	341	9 796070	10 203930	59
2	614	262	351	649	58
3	816	183	632	368	57
4	9 725017	104	913	087	56
5	219	025	9 797194	10 202806	55
6	420	9 927946	474	526	54
7	622	867	755	245	53
8	823	787	9 798036	10·201964	52
9	9 726024	708	316	684	51
10	225	628	596	404	50
11	426	549	877	123	49
12	626	470	9 799157	10 200843	48
13	827	390	437	563	47
14	9 727027	310	717	283	46
15	228	231	997	003	45
16	428	151	9 800277	10 199723	44
17	628	071	557	443	43
18	828	9·926991	836	164	42
19	9 728027	911	9 801116	10 198884	41
20	227	831	396	604	40
21	427	751	675	325	39
22	626	671	955	015	38
23	825	591	9 802234	10·197766	37
24	9·729024	511	513	487	36
25	223	431	793	208	35
26	422	351	9·803072	10 196928	34
27	621	270	351	649	33
28	816	190	630	370	32
29	9·730018	110	908	092	31
30	217	029	9·804187	10 195813	30
	Co-fines	Sines	Co-tang	Tangents	M

57 Degrees

SINES and TANGENTS.

32 Degrees

M	Sines	Co-sines	Tangents	Co-tang.	
30	9 730216	9·926029	9 804187	10 195813	30
31	415	9 925949	466	534	29
32	613	868	745	255	28
33	811	787	9·805023	10·194977	27
34	9·731009	707	302	698	26
35	206	626	580	420	25
36	404	545	859	141	24
37	601	465	9 806137	10·193863	23
38	799	384	415	585	22
39	996	303	693	307	21
40	9 732193	222	971	029	20
41	390	141	9 807249	10 192751	19
42	587	060	527	473	18
43	784	9 924979	805	195	17
44	980	897	9·808083	10 191917	16
45	9 733177	816	361	639	15
46	373	735	638	362	14
47	569	653	916	084	13
48	765	572	9·809193	10·190807	12
49	961	491	471	529	11
50	9·734157	409	748	252	10
51	353	328	9 810025	10·189975	9
52	548	246	302	698	8
53	744	164	580	420	7
54	939	083	857	143	6
55	9 735134	001	9 811134	10·188866	5
56	330	9 923919	410	590	4
57	525	837	687	313	3
58	729	755	964	036	2
59	914	673	9·812241	10·187759	1
60	9·736109	591	517	483	0
	Co-sines	Sines	Co-tang.	Tangents	M

57 Degrees.

A Table of
33 Degrees.

M	Sines	Co-fines	Tangents	Co-tang.	
0	9 736109	9 923591	9 812517	10·187483	60
1	303	509	794	206	59
2	498	427	9 813070	10 186930	58
3	692	345	347	653	57
4	886	263	623	377	56
5	9 737080	180	899	101	55
6	274	098	9 814175	10·185825	54
7	467	016	452	548	53
8	661	9·922933	728	272	52
9	855	851	9 815004	10·184996	51
10	9 738048	768	279	721	50
11	241	686	555	445	49
12	434	603	831	169	48
13	627	520	9·816107	10 183893	47
14	820	438	382	618	46
15	9 739013	355	658	342	45
16	205	272	934	067	44
17	398	189	9 817209	10·182791	43
18	590	106	484	516	42
19	783	023	759	241	41
20	975	9 921940	9 818035	10 181965	40
21	9·740167	857	310	690	39
22	359	774	585	415	38
23	550	691	860	140	37
24	742	607	9 819135	10 180865	36
25	934	524	410	590	35
26	9 741125	441	684	316	34
27	316	357	959	041	33
28	507	274	9 820234	10 179766	32
29	699	190	508	492	31
30	889	107	783	217	30
	Co-fines	Sines	Co-tang.	Tangents	M

56 Degrees.

SINES and TANGENTS

33 Degrees

M	Sines	Co-sines	Tangents	Co-tang	
30	9 714889	9 921107	9 820783	10 179217	30
31	9·742080	023	9 821057	10 178943	29
32	271	9·920939	332	668	28
33	462	855	606	394	27
34	652	772	880	120	26
35	842	688	9 822154	10 177846	25
36	9 743033	604	429	571	24
37	223	520	703	297	23
38	413	436	977	023	22
39	602	352	9 823251	10 176750	21
40	792	268	524	476	20
41	982	184	798	202	19
42	9 744171	099	9 824072	10 175928	18
43	361	015	345	655	17
44	550	9 919931	619	381	16
45	739	846	893	107	15
46	928	762	9 825166	10 174834	14
47	9 745117	677	439	561	13
48	306	593	713	287	12
49	494	508	986	014	11
50	683	424	9 826259	10·173741	10
51	871	339	532	468	9
52	9 746059	254	805	195	8
53	248	169	9 827078	10 172922	7
54	436	084	351	649	6
55	624	9·919000	624	376	5
56	811	915	897	103	4
57	999	830	9 828170	10 171830	3
58	9 747 87	744	442	558	2
59	374	659	715	285	1
60	562	574	987	013	0
	Co-sines	Sines	Co-tang	Tangents	M

56 Degrees

A Table of

34 Degrees

M	Sines	Co-sines	Tangents	Co-tang.	
0	9·747562	9·918574	9·828987	10·171013	60
1	749	489	9 829260	10 170740	59
2	936	404	532	468	58
3	9 748123	318	805	195	57
4	310	233	9·830077	10 169923	56
5	497	147	349	651	55
6	683	062	621	379	54
7	870	9 917976	893	107	53
8	9·749056	891	9·831165	10 168835	52
9	242	805	437	563	51
10	429	719	709	291	50
11	615	634	981	019	49
12	801	548	9 832253	10 167747	48
13	987	462	525	475	47
14	9·750172	376	796	204	46
15	358	290	9·833068	10·166932	45
16	543	204	339	661	44
17	729	118	611	389	43
18	914	032	882	118	42
19	9 751099	9 916945	9·834154	10·165846	41
20	284	859	425	575	40
21	469	773	696	304	39
22	654	687	967	033	38
23	838	600	9·835238	10·164762	37
24	9·752023	514	509	491	36
25	207	427	780	220	35
26	392	341	9 836051	10·163949	34
27	576	254	322	678	33
28	760	167	593	407	32
29	944	082	864	136	31
30	9·753128	9·915994	9·837134	10 162866	30
	Co-sines	Sines	Co-tang	Tangents	M

55 Degrees.

SINES and TANGENTS.

34 Degrees

M	Sines	Co-sines	Tangents	Co-tang	
30	9·753128	9 915994	9 837134	10·162866	30
31	312	907	405	595	29
32	495	820	675	325	28
33	679	733	946	054	27
34	862	646	9·838216	10 161784	26
35	9 754046	559	487	513	25
36	229	472	757	243	24
37	412	385	9 839027	10·160973	23
38	595	297	297	703	22
39	778	210	568	432	21
40	960	123	838	162	20
41	9 755143	035	9·840108	10 159892	19
42	326	9 914948	378	622	18
43	508	860	647	353	17
44	690	773	917	083	16
45	872	685	9·841187	10 158813	15
46	9 756054	598	457	543	14
47	236	510	726	274	13
48	418	422	996	004	12
49	600	334	9 842266	10·157734	11
50	782	246	535	465	10
51	963	158	805	195	9
52	9·757144	070	9 843074	10·156926	8
53	326	9·913982	343	657	7
54	507	894	612	388	6
55	688	806	882	118	5
56	869	718	9·844151	10·155849	4
57	9·758049	630	420	580	3
58	230	541	689	311	2
59	411	453	958	042	1
60	591	364	9·845227	10·154773	0
	Co-sines	Sines	Co-tang.	Tangents	M

55 Degrees.

A Table of

35 Degrees

M	Sines	Co-sines	Tangents	Co-tang.	
0	9 758591	9 913364	9 845227	10 154773	60
1	772	276	496	504	59
2	952	187	764	236	58
3	9·759132	099	9 846033	10·153967	57
4	312	010	302	698	56
5	492	9 912921	570	430	55
6	672	833	839	161	54
7	851	744	9·847107	10 152893	53
8	9·760031	655	376	624	52
9	211	566	644	356	51
10	390	477	913	087	50
11	569	388	9 848181	10·151819	49
12	748	299	449	551	48
13	927	210	717	283	47
14	9·761106	121	985	015	46
15	285	031	9 849254	10 150746	45
16	464	9·911942	522	478	44
17	642	853	790	210	43
18	821	763	9 850057	10 149943	42
19	999	674	325	675	41
20	9 762177	584	593	407	40
21	356	495	861	139	39
22	534	405	9 851128	10 148872	38
23	712	315	396	604	37
24	889	226	664	336	36
25	9 763067	136	931	069	35
26	245	046	9 852199	10·147801	34
27	422	9·910956	466	534	33
28	600	866	733	267	32
29	777	776	9·853001	10·146999	31
30	954	686	268	732	30
	Co-sines	Sines	Co-tang	Tangents	M

54 Degrees

Sines and Tangents.

35 Degrees

M	Sines	Co-sines	Tangents	Co-tang.	
30	9 763954	9 910686	9 853268	10 146732	30
31	9 764131	596	535	465	29
32	308	506	802	198	28
33	485	415	9 854069	10·145931	27
34	662	325	336	664	26
35	838	235	603	397	25
36	9·765015	144	870	130	24
37	191	054	9 855137	10 144863	23
38	367	9 909963	404	596	22
39	544	873	671	329	21
40	720	782	938	062	20
41	896	691	9 856204	10 143796	19
42	9·766071	601	471	529	18
43	247	510	737	263	17
44	423	419	9·857004	10 242996	16
45	598	328	270	730	15
46	774	237	537	463	14
47	949	146	803	197	13
48	9·767124	055	9·858069	10 141931	12
49	300	9 908964	336	664	11
50	475	873	602	398	10
51	649	781	868	132	9
52	824	690	9 859134	10 140866	8
53	999	599	400	600	7
54	9·768173	507	666	334	6
55	348	416	932	068	5
56	522	324	9·860198	10 139802	4
57	697	233	464	536	3
58	871	141	730	270	2
59	9 769045	049	995	005	1
60	219	9·907958	9·861261	10 138739	0
	Co-fines	Sines	Co-tang.	Tangents	M

54 Degrees.

A Table of

36 Degrees

M	Sines	Co-sines	Tangents	Co-tang.	
0	9 769219	9 907958	9 861261	10 138739	60
1	392	866	527	473	59
2	566	774	792	208	58
3	740	682	9·862058	10 137942	57
4	912	590	323	677	56
5	9 770087	498	589	411	55
6	260	406	854	146	54
7	433	314	9 863119	10 136881	53
8	606	222	385	615	52
9	779	129	650	350	51
10	952	037	915	085	50
11	9 771125	9 906945	9 864180	10 135820	49
12	298	852	445	555	48
13	470	760	711	289	47
14	643	667	975	025	46
15	815	574	9 865240	10 134760	45
16	987	482	505	495	44
17	9 772159	389	770	230	43
18	331	296	9 866035	10·133965	42
19	503	204	300	700	41
20	675	111	564	436	40
21	847	018	829	171	39
22	9 773018	9·905925	9 867094	10·132906	38
23	190	832	358	642	37
24	361	739	623	377	36
25	533	645	887	113	35
26	704	552	9 868152	10·131848	34
27	875	459	416	584	33
28	9·774046	366	680	320	32
29	217	272	945	055	31
30	388	179	9·869209	10 130791	30
	Co-sines	Sines	Co-tang.	Tangents	M

53 Degrees.

SINES and TANGENTS.

36 Degrees

M	Sines	Co-fines	Tangents	Co-tang	
30	9·774388	9·905179	9·869209	10·130791	30
31	558	085	473	527	29
32	729	9·904992	737	263	28
33	899	898	9·870001	10·129999	27
34	9·775070	804	265	735	26
35	240	711	529	471	25
36	410	617	793	207	24
37	580	523	9·871057	10·128943	23
38	750	429	321	679	22
39	920	335	585	415	21
40	9·776090	241	849	151	20
41	259	147	9·872112	10·127888	19
42	429	053	376	624	18
43	598	9·903959	640	360	17
44	768	864	903	097	16
45	937	770	9·873167	10·126833	15
46	9·777106	676	430	570	14
47	275	581	694	306	13
48	444	487	957	043	12
49	613	392	9·874220	10·125780	11
50	781	298	484	516	10
51	950	203	747	253	9
52	9·778119	108	9·875010	10·124990	8
53	287	014	273	727	7
54	455	9·902919	536	464	6
55	623	824	800	200	5
56	792	729	9·876063	10·123937	4
57	960	634	326	674	3
58	9·779128	539	589	411	2
59	295	444	851	149	1
60	463	349	9·877114	10·122886	0
	Co-fines	Sines	Co-tang	Tangents	M

53 Degree

4 D

37 Degrees

M	Sines	Co-sines	Tangents	Co-tang	
0	9·779463	9·902319	9·877114	10·122886	60
1	631	253	377	623	59
2	798	158	640	360	58
3	965	063	903	097	57
4	9·780133	9·901967	9·878165	10·121835	56
5	300	872	428	572	55
6	467	776	691	309	54
7	634	681	953	047	53
8	801	585	9·879216	10·120784	52
9	968	489	478	522	51
10	9·781134	394	741	259	50
11	301	298	9·880003	10·119997	49
12	467	202	265	735	48
13	634	106	528	472	47
14	800	010	790	210	46
15	966	9·900914	9·881052	10·118948	45
16	9·782132	818	314	686	44
17	298	722	576	424	43
18	464	626	839	161	42
19	630	529	9·882101	10·117899	41
20	796	433	363	637	40
21	961	337	625	375	39
22	9·783127	240	887	113	38
23	292	144	9·883148	10·116852	37
24	457	047	410	590	36
25	623	9·899951	672	328	35
26	788	854	934	066	34
27	953	757	9·884196	10·115804	33
28	9·784118	660	457	543	32
29	282	564	719	281	31
30	447	467	980	020	30
	Co-sines	Sines	Co-tang	Tangents	M

52 Degrees

SINES and TANGENTS

37 Degrees

M	Sines	Co-sines	Tangents	Co-tang	
30	9 784447	9 899467	9 884980	10 115020	30
31	612	370	9 885242	10 114758	29
32	776	273	503	497	28
33	941	176	765	235	27
34	9 785105	078	9 886026	10 113974	26
35	269	9 898981	288	712	25
36	433	884	549	451	24
37	597	787	810	190	23
38	761	689	9 887072	10 112928	22
39	925	592	333	667	21
40	9 786089	494	594	406	20
41	252	397	855	145	19
42	416	299	9 888116	10 111884	18
43	579	202	377	623	17
44	742	104	639	361	16
45	906	006	900	100	15
46	9 787069	9 897908	9 889160	10 110840	14
47	232	810	421	579	13
48	395	712	682	318	12
49	557	614	943	057	11
50	720	516	9 890204	10 109796	10
51	883	418	465	535	9
52	9 788045	320	725	275	8
53	208	222	986	014	7
54	370	123	9 891247	10 108752	6
55	532	025	507	493	5
56	694	9 896926	768	232	4
57	856	828	9 892028	10 107972	3
58	9 789018	729	289	711	2
59	180	631	549	451	1
60	342	532	810	190	0
	Co-sines	Sines	Co-tang	Tangents	M

52 Degrees.

4 D 2

38 Degrees

M	Sines	Co-sines	Tangents	Co-tang	
0	9·789342	9·896532	9·892810	10·107190	60
1	504	433	9·893070	10·106930	59
2	665	335	331	669	58
3	827	236	591	409	57
4	988	137	851	149	56
5	9 790149	038	9 894111	10·105889	55
6	310	9·895939	371	629	54
7	471	840	632	368	53
8	632	741	892	108	52
9	793	641	9 895152	10 104848	51
10	954	542	412	588	50
11	9 791115	443	672	328	49
12	275	343	932	068	48
13	436	244	9 896192	10 103808	47
14	596	144	452	548	46
15	757	045	712	288	45
16	917	9·894945	971	029	44
17	9 792077	846	9·897231	10 102769	43
18	237	746	491	509	42
19	397	646	751	249	41
20	557	546	9 898010	10 101990	40
21	716	446	270	730	39
22	876	346	530	470	38
23	9 793035	246	789	211	37
24	195	146	9·899049	10 100951	36
25	354	046	308	692	35
26	513	9·893946	568	432	34
27	673	846	827	173	33
28	832	745	9 900086	10 099914	32
29	991	645	346	654	31
30	9 794150	544	605	395	30
	Co-sines	Sines	Co-tang	Tangents	M

51 Degrees

SINES and TANGENTS.

38 Degrees

M	Sines	Co-sines	Tangents	Co tang	
30	9 794150	9 893544	9 900605	10 099395	30
31	308	444	864	136	29
32	467	343	9 901124	10 098876	28
33	626	243	383	617	27
34	784	142	642	358	26
35	942	041	901	099	25
36	9 795101	9 892940	9 902160	10 097840	24
37	259	839	419	581	23
38	417	738	679	321	22
39	575	637	938	062	21
40	733	536	9 903197	10 096803	20
41	891	435	455	545	19
42	9 796019	334	714	286	18
43	206	233	973	027	17
44	364	132	9 904232	10 095768	16
45	521	030	491	509	15
46	679	9 891929	750	250	14
47	836	827	9 905008	10 094992	13
48	993	726	267	733	12
49	9·797150	624	526	474	11
50	307	523	784	216	10
51	464	421	9 906043	10 093957	9
52	621	319	302	698	8
53	777	217	560	440	7
54	934	115	819	181	6
55	9 798091	013	9 907077	10 092923	5
56	247	9 890911	336	664	4
57	403	809	594	406	3
58	560	707	852	148	2
59	716	605	9 908111	10 091889	1
60	872	503	369	631	0
	Co-fines	Sines	Co-tang	Tangents	M

51 Degrees.

A Table of
39 Degrees.

M	Sines	Co-sines	Tangents	Co-tang.	
0	9 798872	9 890503	9 908369	10 091631	60
1	9 799028	400	627	373	59
2	184	298	886	114	58
3	339	195	9 909144	10 090856	57
4	495	093	402	598	56
5	651	9 889990	660	340	55
6	806	888	918	082	54
7	962	785	9 910177	10 089823	53
8	9 800117	682	435	565	52
9	272	579	693	307	51
10	427	476	951	049	50
11	582	374	9 911209	10 088791	49
12	737	271	467	533	48
13	892	167	724	276	47
14	9 801047	064	982	018	46
15	201	9 888961	9 912240	10 087760	45
16	356	858	498	502	44
17	511	755	756	244	43
18	665	651	9 913014	10 086986	42
19	819	548	271	729	41
20	973	444	529	471	40
21	9 802128	341	787	213	39
22	282	237	9 914044	10 085956	38
23	435	133	302	698	37
24	589	030	560	440	36
25	743	9 887926	817	183	35
26	897	822	9 915075	10 084925	34
27	9 803050	718	332	668	33
28	204	614	590	410	32
29	357	510	847	153	31
30	510	406	9 916104	10 083896	30
	Co-sines	Sines	Co-tang.	Tangents	M

50 Degrees.

Sines and Tangents.

39 Degrees.

M	Sines	Co-sines	Tangents	Co-tang	
30	9·803510	9·887406	9·916104	10·083896	30
31	664	302	362	638	29
32	817	198	619	381	28
33	970	093	876	124	27
34	9·804123	9·886989	9·917134	10·082866	26
35	276	885	391	609	25
36	428	780	648	352	24
37	581	676	905	095	23
38	734	571	9·918163	10·081837	22
39	886	466	420	580	21
40	9·805038	362	677	323	20
41	191	257	934	066	19
42	343	152	9·919191	10·080809	18
43	495	047	448	552	17
44	647	9·885942	705	295	16
45	799	837	962	038	15
46	951	732	9·920219	10·079781	14
47	9·806103	627	476	524	13
48	254	521	733	267	12
49	406	416	990	010	11
50	557	311	9·921247	10·078753	10
51	709	205	503	497	9
52	860	100	760	240	8
53	9·807011	9·884994	9·922017	10·077983	7
54	163	889	274	726	6
55	314	783	530	470	5
56	465	677	787	213	4
57	615	572	9·923044	10·076956	3
58	766	466	300	700	2
59	917	360	557	443	1
60	9·808067	254	813	187	0
	Co-fines	Sines	Co-tang	Tangents	M

50 Degrees.

A Table of

40 Degrees.

M	Sines	Co-sines	Tangents	Co-tang	
0	9.808068	9.884254	9.924813	10.076187	60
1	218	148	9.924070	10.075930	59
2	368	042	327	673	58
3	519	9.883936	583	417	57
4	669	829	840	160	56
5	819	723	9.925096	10.074904	55
6	969	617	352	648	54
7	9.809119	510	609	391	53
8	269	404	865	135	52
9	419	297	9.926121	10.073879	51
10	569	191	378	622	50
11	718	084	634	366	49
12	868	9.882977	890	110	48
13	9.810017	871	9.927147	10.072853	47
14	167	764	403	597	46
15	316	657	659	341	45
16	465	550	915	085	44
17	614	443	9.928171	10.071829	43
18	763	336	427	573	42
19	912	228	683	317	41
20	9.811061	121	940	060	40
21	210	014	9.929196	10.070804	39
22	358	9.881907	452	548	38
23	507	799	708	292	37
24	655	692	964	036	36
25	804	584	9.930219	10.069781	35
26	952	477	475	525	34
27	9.812100	369	731	269	33
28	248	261	987	013	32
29	397	153	9.931243	10.068757	31
30	544	045	499	501	30
	Co-sines	Sines	Co-tang	Tangents	M

49 Degrees.

SINES and TANGENTS.

40 Degrees

M	Sines	Co-sines	Tangents	Co-tang.	
30	9·812544	9 881045	9 931499	10 068501	30
31	692	[9·880938	755	245	29
32	840	830	9·932010	10·067990	28
33	988	721	266	734	27
34	9 813135	613	522	478	26
35	283	505	778	222	25
36	430	397	9 933033	10 066967	24
37	578	289	289	711	23
38	725	180	545	455	22
39	872	072	800	200	21
40	9 814019	9 879963	9·934056	10·065944	20
41	166	855	311	689	19
42	313	746	567	433	18
43	460	637	823	177	17
44	607	529	9·935078	10 064922	16
45	753	420	333	667	15
46	900	311	589	411	14
47	9 815046	202	844	156	13
48	193	093	9 936100	10·063900	12
49	339	9 878984	355	645	11
50	485	875	610	390	10
51	631	766	866	134	9
52	778	656	9 937121	10·062879	8
53	923	547	376	624	7
54	9 816069	438	632	368	6
55	215	328	887	113	5
56	361	219	9·938142	10·061858	4
57	507	109	397	603	3
58	652	9 877999	653	347	2
59	797	890	908	092	1
60	943	780	9·939163	10 060837	0
	Co-fines	Sines	Co-tang	Tangents	M

49 Degrees.

4 E

41 Degrees.

M	Sines	Co-sines	Tangents	Co-tang.	
0	9 816943	9 877780	9 939163	10 060837	60
1	9·817088	670	418	582	59
2	233	560	673	327	58
3	378	450	928	072	57
4	523	340	9 940183	10·059817	56
5	668	230	438	562	55
6	813	120	694	306	54
7	958	010	949	051	53
8	9·818103	9·876899	9·941204	10·058796	52
9	247	789	458	542	51
10	392	678	713	287	50
11	536	568	968	032	49
12	681	457	9 942223	10·057777	48
13	825	347	478	522	47
14	969	236	733	267	46
15	9 819113	125	988	012	45
16	257	014	9·943243	10·056757	44
17	401	9 875904	498	502	43
18	545	793	752	248	42
19	689	682	9·944007	10 055993	41
20	832	571	262	738	40
21	976	459	517	483	39
22	9 820120	348	771	229	38
23	263	237	9 945026	10 054974	37
24	406	126	281	719	36
25	550	014	535	465	35
26	693	9 874903	790	210	34
27	836	791	9 946045	10·053955	33
28	979	679	299	701	32
29	9·821122	568	554	446	31
30	265	456	808	192	30
	Co-sines	Sines	Co-tang	Tangents	M

48 Degrees.

Sines *and* Tangents.

41 Degrees

M	Sines	Co-sines	Tangents	Co-tang	
30	9·821265	9 874456	9·946808	10 053192	30
31	407	344	9·947063	10·052937	29
32	550	232	317	683	28
33	693	120	572	428	27
34	835	008	826	174	26
35	977	9 873896	9 948081	10 051919	25
36	9 822120	784	335	665	24
37	262	672	590	410	23
38	404	560	844	156	22
39	546	448	9 949099	10·050901	21
40	688	335	353	647	20
41	830	223	607	393	19
42	972	110	862	138	18
43	9 823114	9·872998	9·950116	10·049884	17
44	255	885	370	630	16
45	397	772	625	375	15
46	539	659	879	121	14
47	680	547	9·951133	10·048867	13
48	821	434	388	612	12
49	963	321	642	358	11
50	9·824104	208	896	104	10
51	245	094	9 952150	10·047850	9
52	386	9·871981	404	596	8
53	527	868	659	341	7
54	668	755	913	087	6
55	808	641	9 953167	10 046833	5
56	949	528	421	579	4
57	9 825090	414	675	325	3
58	230	301	929	071	2
59	370	187	9·954183	10·045817	1
60	511	073	437	563	0
	Co sines	Sines	Co-tang.	Tangents	M

48 Degrees.

A Table of
42 Degrees.

M	Sines	Co-sines	Tangents	Co-tang	
0	9·825511	9·871073	9·954437	10·045563	60
1	651	9·870960	691	309	59
2	791	846	945	055	58
3	931	732	9·955199	10·044801	57
4	9·826071	618	453	547	56
5	211	504	707	293	55
6	351	390	961	039	54
7	491	276	9·956215	10·043785	53
8	631	161	469	531	52
9	770	047	723	277	51
10	910	9·869933	977	023	50
11	9·827049	818	9·957231	10·042769	49
12	189	704	485	515	48
13	328	589	739	261	47
14	467	474	993	007	46
15	606	360	9·958246	10·041754	45
16	745	245	500	500	44
17	884	130	754	246	43
18	9·828023	015	9·959008	10·040992	42
19	162	9·868900	262	738	41
20	301	785	515	485	40
21	439	670	769	231	39
22	578	555	9·960023	10·039977	38
23	716	440	277	723	37
24	855	324	530	470	36
25	993	209	784	216	35
26	9·829131	093	9·961038	10·038962	34
27	269	9·867978	291	709	33
28	407	862	545	455	32
29	545	747	799	201	31
30	683	631	9·962052	10·037948	30
	Co-sines	Sines	Co-tang	Tangents	M

47 Degrees.

SINES and TANGENTS.

42 Degrees

M	Sines	Co-sines	Tangents	Co-tang.	
30	9 829683	9·867631	9 962052	10 037948	30
31	821	515	306	694	29
32	959	399	560	440	28
33	9 830097	283	813	187	27
34	234	167	9 963067	10·036933	26
35	372	051	320	680	25
36	509	9 866935	574	426	24
37	646	819	827	173	23
38	784	703	9 964081	10 035919	22
39	921	587	335	665	21
40	9 831058	470	588	412	20
41	195	353	842	158	19
42	332	237	9·965095	10 034905	18
43	469	120	349	651	17
44	606	004	602	398	16
45	742	9 865887	855	145	15
46	879	770	9 966109	10·033891	14
47	9 832015	653	362	638	13
48	152	536	616	384	12
49	288	419	869	131	11
50	425	302	9·967122	10 032878	10
51	561	185	376	624	9
52	697	068	630	370	8
53	833	9·864950	883	117	7
54	969	833	9·968136	10·031864	6
55	9·833105	716	389	611	5
56	241	598	643	357	4
57	377	481	896	104	3
58	512	363	9·969149	10 030851	2
59	648	245	403	597	1
60	783	127	656	344	0
	Co-fines	Sines	Co-tang.	Tangents	M

47 Degrees.

43 Degrees

M	Sines	Co-sines	Tangents	Co-tang	
0	9.833783	9.864127	9.969656	10.030344	60
1	919	010	909	091	59
2	9.834054	9.863892	9.970162	10.029838	58
3	189	774	416	584	57
4	325	656	669	331	56
5	460	538	922	078	55
6	595	419	9.971175	10.028825	54
7	730	301	429	571	53
8	865	183	682	318	52
9	999	064	935	065	51
10	9.835134	9.862946	9.972188	10.027812	50
11	269	827	441	559	49
12	403	709	695	305	48
13	538	590	948	052	47
14	672	471	9.973201	10.026799	46
15	807	353	454	546	45
16	941	234	707	293	44
17	9.836075	115	960	040	43
18	209	9.861996	9.974213	10.025787	42
19	343	877	466	534	41
20	477	758	719	281	40
21	611	638	973	027	39
22	745	519	9.975226	10.024774	38
23	878	400	479	521	37
24	9.837012	280	732	268	36
25	146	161	985	015	35
26	279	041	9.976238	10.023762	34
27	413	9.860921	491	509	33
28	546	802	744	256	32
29	679	682	997	003	31
30	812	562	9.977250	10.022750	30
	Co-sines	Sines	Co-tang	Tangents	M

46 Degrees

SINES and TANGENTS.

43 Degrees

M	Sines	Co-sines	Tangents	Co-tang.	
30	9·837812	9·860562	9 977250	10·022750	30
31	945	442	503	497	29
32	9 838078	322	756	244	28
33	211	202	9·978009	10 021991	27
34	344	082	262	738	26
35	477	9 859962	515	485	25
36	610	842	768	232	24
37	742	721	9·979021	10 020979	23
38	875	601	274	726	22
39	9·839007	480	527	473	21
40	140	360	780	220	20
41	272	239	9 980033	10·019967	19
42	404	119	286	714	18
43	536	9 858998	538	462	17
44	668	877	791	209	16
45	800	756	9 981044	10·018956	15
46	932	635	297	703	14
47	9 840064	514	550	450	13
48	196	393	803	197	12
49	328	272	9 982056	10·017944	11
50	459	151	309	691	10
51	591	029	562	438	9
52	722	9·857908	814	186	8
53	854	786	9·983067	10 016933	7
54	985	665	320	680	6
55	9·841116	543	573	427	5
56	247	421	826	174	4
57	378	300	9 984079	10 015921	3
58	509	178	331	669	2
59	640	056	584	416	1
60	771	9·856934	837	163	0
	Co-sines	Sines	Co-tang	Tangents	M

46 Degrees.

A Table of

44 Degrees

M	Sines	Co-sines	Tangents	Co-tang.	
0	9 841771	9 856934	9 984837	10 015163	60
1	902	812	9·985090	10 014910	59
2	9·842033	690	343	657	58
3	163	568	596	404	57
4	294	445	848	152	56
5	424	323	9 986101	10 013899	55
6	555	201	354	646	54
7	685	078	607	393	53
8	815	9·855956	860	140	52
9	946	833	9 987112	10 012888	51
10	9·843076	711	365	635	50
11	206	588	618	382	49
12	336	465	871	129	48
13	465	342	9 988123	10 011877	47
14	595	219	376	624	46
15	725	096	629	371	45
16	855	9 854973	882	118	44
17	984	850	9·989134	10 010866	43
18	9 844114	727	387	613	42
19	243	603	640	360	41
20	372	480	893	107	40
21	502	356	9 990145	10 009855	39
22	631	233	398	602	38
23	760	109	651	349	37
24	889	9 853986	903	097	36
25	9 845018	862	9 991156	10·008844	35
26	147	738	409	591	34
27	276	614	662	338	33
28	404	490	914	086	32
29	533	366	9 992167	10·007833	31
30	662	242	420	580	30
	Co-sines	Sines	Co-ting.	Tangents	M

45 Degrees.

SINES and TANGENTS.

44 Degrees

M	Sines	Co-sines	Tangents	Co-tang	
30	9·845662	9·853242	9·992420	10·007580	30
31	790	118	672	328	29
32	919	9·852994	925	075	28
33	9·846047	869	9·993178	10·006822	27
34	175	745	430	570	26
35	304	620	683	317	25
36	432	496	936	064	24
37	560	371	9·994189	10·005811	23
38	688	247	441	559	22
39	816	122	694	306	21
40	944	9·851997	947	053	20
41	9·847071	872	9·995199	10·004801	19
42	199	747	452	548	18
43	327	622	705	295	17
44	454	497	957	043	16
45	582	372	9·996210	10·003790	15
46	709	246	463	537	14
47	837	121	715	285	13
48	964	9·850996	968	032	12
49	9·848091	870	9·997221	10·002779	11
50	218	745	473	527	10
51	345	619	726	274	9
52	472	493	979	021	8
53	599	367	9·998231	10·001769	7
54	726	242	484	516	6
55	852	116	737	263	5
56	979	9·849990	989	011	4
57	9·849106	864	9·999242	10·000758	3
58	232	737	495	505	2
59	359	611	747	253	1
60	485	485	10·000000	10·000000	0
	Co-sines	Sines	Co-tang.	Tangents	M

45 Degrees.

4 F

STREET'S LOGISTICAL LOGARITHMS. 585

′	″	0	1	2	3	4	5	6	7	8	9	″
0.	0	00000	35563	32553	30792	29542	28573	27782	27112	26532	26021	0
	10	25563	5149	4771	4424	4102	3802	3522	3259	3010	2775	10
	20	2553	2341	2139	1940	1761	1584	1413	1249	1091	0939	20
	30	0792	0649	0512	0378	0248	0122	0000	9881	9765	9652	30
	40	19542	9435	9331	9229	9128	9031	8935	8842	8751	8661	40
	50	8575	8497	8303	8320	8239	8139	8081	8004	7929	7855	50
1	0	17782	710	639	570	501	434	368	302	238	175	60
	10	112	050	990	930	872	812	755	698	642	587	70
	20	16532	478	425	372	310	269	218	168	118	069	80
	30	021	973	925	878	832	786	740	695	651	607	90
	40	15563	520	477	435	393	351	310	269	229	189	100
	50	149	110	071	032	994	956	918	881	844	808	110
2	0	14771	735	699	664	629	594	559	525	491	457	120
	10	424	390	357	325	292	260	228	196	165	133	130
	20	102	071	040	010	979	949	919	890	860	831	140
	30	13802	773	745	716	688	660	632	604	576	549	150
	40	525	495	468	441	415	388	362	336	310	284	160
	50	259	233	208	183	158	133	108	083	059	034	170
3	0	010	986	962	936	915	891	868	845	821	798	180
	10	12775	753	730	707	685	663	640	618	596	574	190
	20	553	531	510	488	467	445	424	403	382	362	200
	30	341	320	300	279	259	239	218	198	178	159	210
	40	139	119	099	080	061	041	022	003	984	965	220
	50	11946	927	908	889	871	852	834	816	797	779	230
4.	0	761	743	725	707	689	671	654	636	619	601	240
	10	584	566	549	532	515	498	481	464	447	430	250
	20	414	397	380	363	347	331	314	298	282	266	260
	30	249	233	217	201	186	170	154	138	123	107	270
	40	09	076	061	045	030	015	999	984	969	954	280
	50	10939	924	909	894	880	865	850	835	821	806	290
5.	0	792	777	763	749	734	720	706	692	678	663	300
	10	649	635	621	608	594	580	566	552	539	525	310
	20	512	428	484	471	458	444	431	418	404	391	320
	30	378	365	352	339	326	313	300	287	274	261	330
	40	248	235	223	210	197	185	172	160	147	135	340
	50	122	110	098	085	073	061	049	036	024	012	350
6	0	000	988	976	964	952	940	928	916	905	893	360
	10	9881	869	858	846	834	823	811	800	788	777	370
	20	765	753	742	731	720	708	697	686	675	664	380
	30	652	641	630	619	608	597	586	575	564	553	390
	40	542	532	521	510	499	488	478	467	456	446	400
	50	435	425	414	404	393	383	372	362	351	341	410

′	″	0	1	2	3	4	5	6	7	8	9	″
7.	0	9·331	320	310	300	289	279	269	259	249	238	420
	10	228	218	208	198	188	178	168	158	148	138	430
	20	128	119	109	099	089	079	070	060	050	041	440
	30	031	021	012	002	992	983	973	964	954	945	450
	40	8·935	926	917	907	898	888	879	870	861	851	460
	50	842	833	824	814	805	796	787	778	769	760	470
8	0	751	742	733	724	715	706	697	688	679	670	480
	10	661	652	643	635	626	617	608	599	591	582	490
	20	573	565	556	547	539	530	522	513	504	496	500
	30	487	479	470	462	453	445	437	428	420	411	510
	40	403	395	386	378	370	361	353	345	337	328	520
	50	320	312	304	296	288	279	271	263	255	247	530
9.	0	82·39	31	23	15	07	99	91	83	75	67	540
	10	81 59	52	44	36	28	20	12	04	97	89	550
	20	80 81	73	66	58	50	43	35	27	20	12	560
	30	04	97	89	81	74	66	59	51	44	36	570
	40	79·29	21	14	06	99	91	84	77	69	62	580
	50	78 55	47	40	32	25	18	11	03	96	89	590
10.	0	77·82	74	67	60	53	45	38	31	24	17	600
	10	10	03	96	88	81	74	67	60	53	46	610
	20	76·39	32	25	18	11	04	97	90	83	77	620
	30	75·70	63	56	49	42	35	28	22	15	08	630
	40	01	94	88	81	74	67	61	54	47	41	640
	50	74·34	27	21	14	07	01	94	87	81	74	650
11.	0	73·68	61	54	48	41	35	28	22	15	09	660
	10	02	96	89	83	76	70	64	57	51	44	670
	20	72·38	32	25	19	12	06	00	93	87	81	680
	30	71·75	68	62	56	49	43	37	31	24	18	690
	40	12	06	00	93	87	81	75	69	63	57	700
	50	70·50	44	38	32	26	20	14	08	02	96	710
12.	0	69 90	84	78	72	66	60	54	48	42	36	720
	10	30	24	18	12	06	00	94	88	82	77	730
	20	68·71	65	59	53	47	41	36	30	24	18	740
	30	12	07	01	95	89	84	78	72	66	61	750
	40	67 55	49	43	38	32	26	21	15	09	04	760
	50	66 96	92	87	81	76	70	64	59	53	48	770
13.	0	42	37	31	25	20	14	09	03	98	92	780
	10	65 87	81	76	70	65	59	54	48	43	38	790
	20	32	27	21	16	10	05	00	94	89	84	800
	30	64·78	73	67	62	57	51	46	41	35	30	810
	40	25	20	14	09	04	98	93	88	83	77	820
	50	63·72	67	62	57	51	46	41	36	31	25	830

Street's Logicacal Logarithms.

′	″	0	1	2	3	4	5	6	7	8	9	″
14.	0	20	15	10	05	00	94	89	84	79	74	840
	10	62·69	64	59	54	48	43	38	33	28	23	850
	20	·18	13	08	03	98	93	88	83	78	73	860
	30	61·68	63	58	53	48	43	38	33	28	23	870
	40	18	13	08	03	99	94	89	84	79	74	880
	50	60 69	64	59	55	50	45	40	35	30	25	890
15	0	21	16	11	06	01	97	92	87	82	77	900
	10	59·73	68	63	58	54	49	44	39	35	30	910
	20	25	20	16	11	06	02	97	92	88	83	920
	30	58·78	74	69	64	60	55	50	46	41	36	930
	40	32	27	23	18	13	09	04	00	95	90	940
	50	57 86	81	77	72	68	63	58	54	49	45	950
16.	0	57·40	36	31	27	22	18	13	09	04	00	960
	10	56·95	91	86	82	77	73	69	64	60	55	970
	20	51	46	42	37	33	29	24	20	15	11	980
	30	07	02	98	94	89	85	80	76	72	67	990
	40	55·63	59	54	50	46	41	37	33	28	24	1000
	50	20	16	11	07	03	98	94	90	86	81	1010
17.	0	54 77	73	69	64	60	56	52	47	43	39	1020
	10	35	30	26	22	18	14	09	05	01	97	1030
	20	53 93	89	84	80	76	72	68	64	59	55	1040
	30	51	47	43	39	35	31	26	22	18	14	1050
	40	10	06	02	98	94	90	85	81	77	73	1060
	50	52·69	65	61	57	53	49	45	41	37	33	1070
18.	0	29	25	21	17	13	09	05	01	97	93	1080
	10	51·89	85	81	77	73	69	65	61	57	53	1090
	20	49	45	41	37	33	29	25	22	18	14	1100
	30	10	06	02	98	94	90	86	82	79	75	1110
	40	50 71	67	63	59	55	51	48	44	40	36	1120
	50	32	28	25	21	17	13	09	05	02	98	1130
19.	0	49·94	90	86	83	79	75	71	67	64	60	1140
	10	56	52	49	45	41	37	33	30	26	22	1150
	20	18	15	11	07	03	00	96	92	89	85	1160
	30	48 81	77	74	70	66	63	59	55	52	48	1170
	40	44	41	37	33	30	26	22	19	15	11	1180
	50	08	04	00	97	93	89	86	82	78	75	1190
20.	0	47 71	68	64	60	57	53	50	46	42	39	1200
	10	35	32	28	24	21	17	14	10	07	03	1210
	20	46 99	96	93	89	85	82	78	75	71	68	1220
	30	64	60	57	53	50	46	43	39	36	32	1230
	40	29	25	22	18	15	11	08	04	01	97	1240
	50	45·94	90	87	84	80	77	73	70	66	63	1250

588 Street's Logistical Logarithms.

"	'	0	1	2	3	4	5	6	7	8	9	"
21	0	59	56	52	49	46	42	39	35	32	28	1260
	10	25	22	18	15	11	08	05	01	98	94	1270
	20	44 91	88	84	81	77	74	71	67	64	60	1280
	30	57	54	50	47	44	40	37	34	30	27	1290
	40	24	20	17	14	10	07	04	00	97	94	1300
	50	43 90	87	84	80	77	74	70	67	64	60	1310
22.	0	57	54	51	47	44	41	38	34	31	28	1320
	10	25	21	18	15	11	08	05	02	98	95	1330
	20	42 92	89	85	82	79	76	73	69	66	63	1340
	30	60	56	53	50	47	44	40	37	34	31	1350
	40	28	24	21	18	15	12	09	05	02	99	1360
	50	41 96	93	89	86	83	80	77	74	71	67	1370
23	0	64	61	58	55	52	49	45	42	39	36	1380
	10	33	30	27	24	20	17	14	11	08	05	1390
	20	02	99	96	92	89	86	83	80	77	74	1400
	30	40 71	68	65	62	59	55	52	49	46	43	1410
	40	40	37	34	31	28	25	22	19	16	13	1420
	50	10	07	04	01	98	95	91	88	85	82	1430
24	0	39 79	76	73	70	67	64	61	58	55	52	1440
	10	49	46	43	40	37	34	31	28	25	22	1450
	20	19	17	14	11	08	05	02	69	96	93	1460
	30	38 90	87	84	81	78	75	72	69	66	63	1470
	40	60	57	55	52	49	46	43	40	37	34	1480
	50	31	28	25	22	20	17	14	11	08	05	1490
25.	0	02	99	96	93	91	88	85	82	79	76	1500
	10	37 73	70	68	65	62	59	56	53	50	47	1510
	20	45	42	39	36	33	30	27	25	22	19	1520
	30	16	13	10	08	05	02	99	96	93	91	1530
	40	36 88	85	82	79	77	74	71	68	65	63	1540
	50	60	57	54	51	49	46	43	40	37	35	1550
26	0	32	29	26	23	21	18	15	12	10	07	1560
	10	04	01	98	96	93	90	87	85	82	79	1570
	20	35 76	74	71	68	65	63	60	57	55	52	1580
	30	49	46	44	41	38	35	33	30	27	25	1590
	40	22	19	16	14	11	08	06	03	00	97	1600
	50	34 95	92	89	87	84	81	79	76	73	71	1610
27.	0	68	65	63	60	57	54	52	49	46	44	1620
	10	41	38	36	33	31	28	25	23	20	17	1630
	20	15	12	09	07	04	01	99	96	93	91	1640
	30	33 98	86	83	80	78	75	72	70	67	65	1650
	40	62	59	56	53	51	49	46	44	41	38	1660
	50	36	33	31	28	25	23	20	18	15	13	1670

Street's Logistical Logarithms.

′ ″	0	1	2	3	4	5	6	7	8	9	″
28. 0	10	07	05	02	00	97	94	92	89	87	1680
10	32·84	82	79	76	74	71	69	66	64	61	1690
20	59	56	53	51	48	46	43	41	38	36	1700
30	33	31	28	25	23	20	18	15	13	10	1710
40	08	05	03	00	98	95	93	90	88	85	1720
50	31·83	80	78	75	73	70	68	65	63	60	1730
29. 0	58	55	53	50	48	45	43	40	38	35	1740
10	33	30	28	25	23	20	18	15	13	10	1750
20	08	05	03	01	98	96	93	91	88	86	1760
30	30·83	81	78	76	73	71	69	66	64	61	1770
40	59	56	54	52	49	47	44	42	39	37	1780
50	34	32	30	27	25	22	20	18	15	13	1790
30. 0	10	08	05	03	01	98	96	93	91	89	1800
10	29·86	84	81	79	77	74	72	69	67	65	1810
20	62	60	58	55	53	50	48	46	43	41	1820
30	39	36	34	31	29	27	24	22	20	17	1830
40	15	12	10	08	05	03	01	98	96	94	1840
50	28 91	89	87	84	82	80	77	75	73	70	1850
31. 0	68	66	63	61	59	56	54	52	49	47	1860
10	45	42	40	38	35	33	31	28	26	24	1870
20	21	19	17	15	12	10	08	05	03	01	1880
30	27·98	96	94	92	89	87	85	82	80	78	1890
40	75	73	71	69	66	64	62	60	67	55	1900
50	53	50	48	46	44	41	39	37	35	32	1910
32. 0	27·30	28	25	23	21	19	16	14	12	10	1920
10	07	05	03	01	98	96	94	92	89	87	1930
20	26 85	83	81	78	76	74	72	69	67	65	1940
30	63	60	58	56	54	52	49	47	45	43	1950
40	40	38	36	34	32	39	27	25	23	21	1960
50	18	16	14	17	10	07	05	03	01	99	1970
33. 0	25·96	94	92	90	88	85	83	81	79	77	1980
10	74	72	70	68	66	64	61	59	57	55	1990
20	53	51	48	46	44	42	40	38	35	33	2000
30	31	29	27	25	22	20	18	16	14	12	2010
40	10	07	05	03	01	99	97	94	92	90	2020
50	24·88	86	84	82	80	77	75	73	71	69	2030
34. 0	67	65	62	60	58	56	54	52	50	48	2040
10	45	43	41	39	37	35	33	31	29	26	2050
20	24	22	20	18	16	14	12	10	08	05	2060
30	03	01	99	97	95	93	91	89	87	84	2070
40	23·82	80	78	76	74	72	70	68	66	64	2080
50	61	59	57	55	53	51	49	47	45	43	2090

STREET's LOGISTICAL LOGARITHMS.

′	″	0	1	2	3	4	5	6	7	8	9	″
35.	0	41	39	37	35	33	31	28	26	24	22	2100
	10	20	18	16	14	12	10	08	06	04	02	2110
	20	00	98	96	94	91	89	87	85	83	81	2120
	30	22 79	77	75	73	70	69	67	65	63	61	2130
	40	59	57	55	53	51	49	47	45	43	41	2140
	50	39	37	35	33	31	29	27	25	23	20	2150
36.	0	18	16	14	12	10	08	06	04	02	00	2160
	10	21 98	96	94	92	90	88	86	84	82	80	2170
	20	78	76	74	72	70	69	67	65	63	61	2180
	30	59	57	55	53	61	49	47	45	43	41	2190
	40	39	37	35	33	31	39	27	25	23	21	2200
	50	19	17	15	13	11	09	07	05	03	01	2210
37.	0	20 99	98	96	94	92	90	88	86	84	82	2220
	10	80	78	76	74	72	70	68	66	64	62	2230
	20	60	59	57	55	53	51	49	47	45	43	2240
	30	41	39	37	35	33	32	30	28	26	24	2250
	40	22	20	18	16	14	12	10	09	07	05	2260
	50	03	01	99	97	95	93	91	89	87	86	2270
38.	0	19 84	82	80	78	76	74	72	70	68	67	2280
	10	65	63	61	59	57	55	53	51	50	48	2290
	20	46	44	42	40	38	36	34	33	31	29	2300
	30	27	25	23	21	19	18	16	14	12	10	2310
	40	08	06	04	03	01	99	97	95	93	91	2320
	50	18 89	88	86	84	82	80	78	76	75	73	2330
39.	0	71	69	67	65	63	62	60	58	56	54	2340
	10	52	50	49	47	45	43	41	39	38	36	2350
	20	34	32	30	28	27	25	23	21	19	17	2360
	30	16	14	12	10	08	06	05	03	01	99	2370
	40	17 97	95	94	92	90	88	86	85	83	81	2380
	50	79	77	75	74	72	70	68	66	65	63	3390
40.	0	17 61	59	57	55	54	52	50	48	46	45	2400
	10	43	41	39	37	36	34	32	30	28	27	2410
	20	25	23	21	19	18	16	14	12	11	09	2420
	30	07	05	03	02	00	98	96	94	92	91	2430
	40	16 89	87	86	84	82	80	78	77	75	73	2440
	50	71	70	68	66	64	62	61	59	57	55	2450
41.	0	54	52	50	48	47	45	43	41	40	38	2460
	10	36	34	33	31	29	27	26	24	22	20	2470
	20	19	17	15	13	12	10	08	06	05	03	2480
	30	01	99	98	96	94	92	91	89	87	85	2490
	40	15 84	82	80	78	77	75	73	71	70	68	2500
	50	66	65	63	61	59	58	56	54	52	51	2510

′	″	0	1	2	3	4	5	6	7	8	9	″
42	0	49	47	46	44	42	40	39	37	35	34	2520
	10	32	30	28	27	25	23	22	20	18	16	2530
	20	15	13	11	10	08	06	04	03	01	99	2540
	30	14 98	96	94	93	91	89	87	86	84	82	2550
	40	81	89	77	76	74	72	70	69	67	65	2560
	50	64	62	60	59	57	55	54	52	50	49	2570
43	0	47	45	43	42	40	38	37	35	33	32	2580
	10	30	28	27	25	23	22	20	18	17	15	2590
	20	13	11	10	08	07	05	03	02	00	98	2600
	30	13·97	95	93	92	90	88	87	85	83	82	2610
	40	80	78	77	75	73	72	70	68	67	65	2620
	50	63	62	60	59	57	55	54	52	50	49	2630
44.	0	47	45	44	42	40	39	37	35	34	32	2640
	10	31	29	27	26	24	22	21	19	17	16	2650
	20	14	13	11	09	08	06	04	03	01	00	2660
	30	12 98	96	95	94	91	90	88	87	85	83	2670
	40	82	80	78	77	75	74	72	70	69	68	2680
	50	66	64	62	61	59	57	56	54	53	51	2690
45.	0	49	48	46	45	43	41	40	38	37	35	2700
	10	33	32	30	29	27	25	24	22	21	19	2710
	20	17	16	14	13	11	09	08	06	05	03	2720
	30	01	00	98	97	95	94	92	90	89	87	2730
	40	11·86	84	82	81	79	78	76	74	73	71	2740
	50	70	68	67	65	63	62	60	59	57	56	2750
46.	0	54	52	51	49	48	46	45	43	41	40	2760
	10	38	37	35	34	32	30	29	27	26	24	2770
	20	23	21	19	18	16	15	13	12	10	09	2780
	30	07	05	04	02	01	99	98	96	95	93	2790
	40	10·91	90	88	87	85	84	82	81	79	78	2800
	50	76	74	73	71	70	68	67	65	64	62	2810
47.	0	61	59	57	56	54	53	51	50	48	47	2820
	10	45	44	42	41	39	37	36	34	33	31	2830
	20	30	28	27	25	24	22	21	19	18	16	2840
	30	15	13	12	10	08	07	05	04	02	01	2850
	40	9 99	98	96	95	93	92	90	89	87	86	2860
	50	84	83	81	80	78	77	75	74	72	71	2870
48.	0	9·69	68	66	65	63	62	60	59	57	56	2880
	10	54	53	51	50	48	47	45	44	42	41	2890
	20	39	38	36	35	33	32	30	29	27	26	2900
	30	24	23	21	20	18	17	15	14	12	11	2910
	40	09	08	06	05	03	02	00	99	97	96	2920
	50	8·94	93	91	90	88	87	85	84	83	82	2930

4 G

Street's Logistical Logarithms.

′	″	0	1	2	3	4	5	6	7	8	9	″
49	0	80	78	77	75	74	72	71	69	68	66	2940
	10	65	63	62	60	59	57	56	55	54	53	2950
	20	50	49	47	46	44	43	41	40	38	37	2960
	30	35	34	33	31	30	28	27	25	24	22	2970
	40	21	19	18	16	15	14	12	11	09	08	2980
	50	06	05	03	02	01	99	98	96	95	93	2990
50	0	7 92	90	89	87	86	85	83	82	80	79	3000
	10	77	76	74	73	72	70	69	67	66	64	3010
	20	63	62	60	59	57	56	54	53	51	50	3020
	30	49	47	46	44	43	41	40	39	37	36	3030
	40	34	33	32	30	29	27	26	24	23	21	3040
	50	20	19	17	16	14	13	11	10	09	07	3050
51	0	06	04	03	02	00	99	97	96	94	93	3060
	10	6 92	90	89	87	86	85	83	82	80	79	3070
	20	78	76	75	73	72	70	69	68	66	65	3080
	30	63	62	61	59	58	56	55	54	52	51	3090
	40	49	48	47	45	44	42	41	40	38	37	3100
	50	35	34	33	31	30	28	27	26	24	23	3110
52	0	21	20	19	17	16	15	13	12	10	09	3120
	10	08	06	05	03	02	01	99	98	96	95	3130
	20	5 94	92	91	90	88	87	85	84	83	81	3140
	30	80	79	77	76	74	73	72	70	69	68	3150
	40	66	65	63	62	61	59	58	57	55	54	3160
	50	52	51	50	48	47	46	44	43	41	40	3170
53	0	39	37	36	35	33	32	31	29	28	26	3180
	10	25	24	22	21	20	18	17	16	14	13	3190
	20	12	10	09	07	06	05	03	02	01	99	3200
	30	4 98	96	95	94	93	91	90	89	87	86	3210
	40	84	83	82	80	79	78	76	75	74	72	3220
	50	71	70	68	67	66	64	63	62	60	59	3230
54	0	58	56	55	54	52	51	50	48	47	46	3240
	10	44	43	42	40	39	38	36	35	34	32	3250
	20	31	30	28	26	24	23	22	21	20	19	3260
	30	18	16	15	14	12	11	10	08	07	06	3270
	40	04	03	02	00	99	98	96	95	94	92	3280
	50	3 91	90	88	87	86	84	83	82	81	79	3290
55	0	78	77	75	74	73	71	70	69	67	66	3300
	10	65	63	62	61	59	58	57	56	54	53	3310
	20	52	50	49	48	46	45	44	42	41	40	3320
	30	39	37	36	35	33	32	31	29	28	27	3330
	40	26	24	23	22	20	19	18	16	15	14	3340
	50	13	11	10	09	07	06	05	04	02	01	3350

STREET's LOGISTICAL LOGARITHMS.

′	″	0	1	2	3	4	5	6	7	8	9	″
56.	0	3 00	98	97	96	94	93	92	91	89	88	3360
	10	2 87	85	84	83	82	80	79	78	76	75	3370
	20	74	73	71	70	69	67	66	65	64	62	3380
	30	61	60	58	57	56	55	53	52	51	50	3390
	40	48	47	46	44	43	42	41	39	38	37	3400
	50	35	34	33	32	30	29	28	27	25	24	3410
57.	0	23	21	20	19	18	16	15	14	13	11	3420
	10	10	09	08	06	05	04	02	01	00	99	3430
	20	1·97	96	95	94	92	91	90	89	87	86	3440
	30	85	84	82	81	80	79	77	76	75	74	3450
	40	72	71	70	69	67	66	65	63	62	61	3460
	50	60	58	57	56	55	53	52	51	50	48	3470
58	0	47	46	45	43	42	41	40	39	37	36	3480
	10	35	34	32	31	30	29	27	26	25	24	3490
	20	22	21	20	19	17	16	15	14	12	11	3500
	30	10	09	07	06	05	04	03	01	00	99	3510
	40	0·98	96	95	94	93	91	90	89	88	87	3520
	50	85	84	83	82	80	79	78	77	75	74	3530
59	0	73	72	71	69	68	67	86	64	63	62	3540
	10	61	60	58	57	56	55	53	52	51	50	3550
	20	49	47	46	45	44	42	41	40	39	38	3560
	30	36	35	34	33	31	30	29	28	27	25	3570
	40	24	23	22	21	19	18	17	16	15	13	3580
	50	12	11	10	8	7	6	5	4	2	1	3590
60	0	0										3600

F I N I S.

E R R A T A.

Page 78, line 19, dele 7″ —p. 167, l 15, for *one fourth*, read *the Square of one fourth*.—p. 167, l. 7, dele *or the Sine of the Arch* BE —p 173, l 8, for $\frac{AB}{2} \frac{AE}{2}$ read $\frac{AB}{2} - \frac{AL}{2}$.——p 243, .24, for *intended*, read *included*.

CPSIA information can be obtained
at www.ICGtesting.com
Printed in the USA
LVHW080232130519
617599LV00005B/58/P